Evidence-Based Leadership, Innovation, and Entrepreneurship in Nursing and Healthcare

Bernadette Mazurek Melnyk, PhD, APRN-CNP, FAANP, FNAP, FAAN is the Vice President for Health Promotion, University Chief Wellness Officer, and Professor and Dean of the College of Nursing at The Ohio State University. She also is a Professor of Pediatrics and Psychiatry at Ohio State's College of Medicine. In addition, she is the Executive Director of the Helene Fuld Health Trust National Institute for Evidence-based Practice in Nursing and Healthcare. Dr. Melnyk earned her bachelor of science in nursing degree from West Virginia University, her master of science degree with a specialization in nursing care of children and pediatric nurse practitioner from the University of Pittsburgh, and her PhD in clinical research from the University of Rochester, where she also completed her post-master's certificate as a psychiatric mental health nurse practitioner. She is a nationally/internationally recognized expert in evidence-based practice, intervention research, child and adolescent mental health, and health and wellness, and is a frequent keynote speaker at national and international conferences on these topics. Dr. Melnyk has consulted with hundreds of healthcare systems and colleges throughout the nation and globe on how to improve quality of care and patient outcomes through implementing and sustaining evidence-based practice. Her record includes over $33 million of sponsored funding from federal agencies and foundations as principal investigator and over 400 publications. Dr. Melnyk is coeditor of six other books, including *Implementing the Evidence-Based Practice (EBP) Competencies in Healthcare: A Practical Guide for Improving Quality, Safety, and Outcomes*; *Evidence-Based Practice in Nursing & Healthcare: A Guide to Best Practice* (Fourth Edition), an *American Journal of Nursing* Research Book of the Year Award winner; *Implementing EBP: Real World Success Stories; A Practical Guide to Child and Adolescent Mental Health Screening, Early Intervention and Health Promotion* (Second Edition); *Intervention Research and Evidence-Based Quality Improvement: Designing, Conducting, Analyzing and Funding* (Second Edition), also an *American Journal of Nursing* Research Book of the Year Award winner, and *Evidence-Based Health and Well-Being Assessment. A Guide to Best Practice.* Dr. Melnyk is an elected fellow of the National Academy of Medicine, the American Academy of Nursing, the National Academies of Practice, and the American Association of Nurse Practitioners. She served a 4-year term on the 16-member United States Preventive Services Task Force and the National Institutes of Health's National Advisory Council for Nursing Research and was a board member of the National Guideline Clearinghouse and the National Quality Measures Clearinghouse (NGC/NQMC). She currently serves as a member of the National Quality Forum's (NQF) Behavioral Health Standing Committee. Dr. Melnyk also serves as editor of the journal *Worldviews on Evidence-Based Nursing* and is a member of the National Academy of Medicine's Action Collaborative on Clinician Well-Being and Resilience as well as an elected board member for the National Forum for Heart Disease & Stroke Prevention.

Dr. Melnyk has received numerous national and international awards, including the Audrey Hepburn Award; Mary Tolle Wright Excellence in Leadership Award; and the International Nursing Research Hall of Fame Award from Sigma Theta Tau International; the Jessie Scott Award from the American Nurses Association for the improvement of healthcare quality through the integration of research, education and practice; the 2012 Midwest Nursing Research Society Senior Scientist award; the NIH/National Institute of Nursing Research's inaugural director's lectureship award; the American Association of Nurse Practitioners (AANP) Sharp Cutting Edge Award, and the National Organization of Nurse Practitioner Faculties Lifetime Achievement Award. She has been recognized as an *Edge Runner* three times by the American Academy of Nursing for founding and directing the National Association of Pediatric Nurse Practitioners' KySS child and adolescent mental health program, her Creating Opportunities for Personal Empowerment (COPE) program for parents of critically ill children and preterm infants, and her COPE cognitive behavioral skills-building program for depressed and anxious children, teens, and college students, which is being implemented in 44 states throughout the United States and five countries. She is also the founder of two companies that disseminate her evidence-based intervention programs.

Dr. Melnyk founded the National Interprofessional Education and Practice Collaborative to advance the Department of Health and Human Services' Million Hearts® initiative to prevent 1 million heart attacks and strokes, which is a collaboration of over 150 organizations and academic institutions across the United States. She also created and chaired the first three National Summits on Building Healthy Academic Communities and is the founder and the current President of the National Consortium for Building Healthy Academic Communities, a collaborative organization to improve population health in the nation's institutions of higher learning, and also served as its first president.

Tim Raderstorf, DNP, RN, is the Chief Innovation Officer at The Ohio State University College of Nursing. As the first nurse to hold this academic title in the United States, he takes great pride in educating the nation on the role of the nurse as an innovator and entrepreneur. In 2017, he founded The Innovation Studio, a makerspace/incubator that provides interprofessional healthcare teams with the tools and mentorship needed to turn ideas into actions. This work at the Innovation Studio led to Tim being named the 2018 Early Career Innovator of the Year at The Ohio State University. Outside of Ohio State, Tim is the founder of Quality Health Communications, a digital Clinical Decision Support System that communicates real-time patient quality and safety metrics to the healthcare team.

Evidence-Based Leadership, Innovation, and Entrepreneurship in Nursing and Healthcare

A Practical Guide to Success

Bernadette Mazurek Melnyk, PhD, APRN-CNP, FAANP, FNAP, FAAN

Tim Raderstorf, DNP, RN

Editors

SPRINGER PUBLISHING COMPANY

Springer Publishing Company, LLC
11 West 42nd Street
New York, NY 10036
www.springerpub.com
http://connect.springerpub.com

Acquisitions Editor: Joseph Morita
Compositor: S4Carlisle Publishing Services

ISBN: 978-0-8261-9618-7
e-book ISBN: 978-0-8261-9625-5
Instructor's Manual: 978-0-8261-8621-8
Instructor's PowerPoints: 978-0-8261-8613-3
DOI: 10.1891/9780826196255

Instructor's Materials: Qualified instructors may request supplements by emailing textbook@springerpub.com

*Visit https://connect.springerpub.com/content/book/978-0-8261-9625-5/front-matter/fmatter6
to access accompanying podcasts.*

22 23 24 / 5 4 3

The author and the publisher of this Work have made every effort to use sources believed to be reliable to provide information that is accurate and compatible with the standards generally accepted at the time of publication. The author and publisher shall not be liable for any special, consequential, or exemplary damages resulting, in whole or in part, from the readers' use of, or reliance on, the information contained in this book. The publisher has no responsibility for the persistence or accuracy of URLs for external or third-party Internet websites referred to in this publication and does not guarantee that any content on such websites is, or will remain, accurate or appropriate.

Library of Congress Cataloging-in-Publication Data

Names: Melnyk, Bernadette Mazurek, editor. | Raderstorf, Tim, editor.
Title: Evidence-based leadership, innovation, and entrepreneurship in
  nursing and healthcare : a practical guide to success / [edited by]
  Bernadette Mazurek Melnyk, Tim Raderstorf.
Description: New York : Springer Publishing Company, [2021] |
Identifiers: LCCN 2019032688 (print) | ISBN 9780826196187 (paperback) |
  ISBN 9780826196255 (epub) | ISBN 9780826186218 (instructors manual) |
  ISBN 9780826186133 (instructors powerpoints)
Subjects: MESH: Evidence-Based Nursing | Nursing–organization &
  administration | Leadership | Organizational Innovation |
  Entrepreneurship | United States
Classification: LCC RT86.7 (print) | LCC RT86.7 (ebook) | NLM WY 100.7 |
  DDC 610.73068–dc23
LC record available at https://lccn.loc.gov/2019032688
LC ebook record available at https://lccn.loc.gov/2019032689

Contact us to receive discount rates on bulk purchases.
We can also customize our books to meet your needs.
For more information please contact: sales@springerpub.com

Printed in the United States of America by Hatteras, Inc.

I dedicate this book to my loving husband, John; my three wonderful daughters, Kaylin, Angela, and Megan; and my awesome grandsons, Alexander and Bradley, who support me to achieve my dreams and who are all the light of my life! I also dedicate it to my terrific executive team at The Ohio State University College of Nursing, including Drs. Margaret Graham, Cindy Anderson, Mary Beth Happ, Wendy Bowles, Kristy Browning, and Laurel Van Dromme; my innovative university-wide wellness team, Drs. Megan Amaya, Brenda Buffington, Dave Hrabe, Sharon Tucker, Lauren Battista, Josh Winn, Nicole Johnson, Brian Keller, and Abby Ewert; and my outstanding executive assistants, Kathy York, Jackie Hollins, and Rebecca Momany, who are all the wind beneath my wings and a major reason that I can still pursue many of my own passions, including the writing of books that equip people with the knowledge and skills to make a positive impact in the real world.

—Bernadette Mazurek Melnyk

This book is dedicated to my wonderful wife, Jill, and our three curious children, who continually remind me that asking "why" is always an appropriate question. I also dedicate this book to Jackie Hoying, Jason Walsh, and Bern Melnyk, who all provided me with opportunities that have changed my life; to my parents, Rex and Sherri, who made me realize what it means to set others up for success; and to the nursing staff at The Hole in the Wall Gang Camp for being such an amazing testament of what it means to be a nurse that I had to join the profession just to try to be like them. This book is also dedicated to Josh Wooten, Liz McClurg, Laurel Van Dromme, Scott Osborne, Mary Beth Happ, our amazing student team at the Innovation Studio, and the clinicians whom we have the privilege of working with every day to turn their ideas into actions.

—Tim Raderstorf

Contents

UNIT I. LEADERSHIP

UNIT II. INNOVATION

UNIT III. ENTREPRENEURSHIP

Contributors

Nancy Albert, PhD, CCNS, CHFN, CCRN, NE-BC, FAHA, FCCM, FAAN   Associate Chief Nursing Officer, Research and Innovation, Cleveland Clinic, Cleveland, Ohio

Adrienne Boissy, MD, MA   Chief Experience Officer, Cleveland Clinic, Cleveland, Ohio

Courtney Campbell-Saxton, MBA   VP Patient Services Finance, Cincinnati Children's Hospital Medical Center, Lebanon, Ohio

Bonnie Clipper, DNP, RN, MA, MBA, CENP, FACHE   Vice President, Practice & Innovation, American Nurses Association, Silver Spring, Maryland

Caroline Crisafulli, BS, PMP   Director of Innovation, Ohio State ADVANCE, The Ohio State University, Columbus, Ohio

Suratha Elango, MD, MSHP   Assistant Professor, Department of Pediatrics, Baylor College of Medicine and Texas Children's Hospital, Houston, Texas

Lynn Gallagher-Ford, PhD, RN, NE-BC, DPFNAP, FAAN   Senior Director, The Helene Fuld Institute for Evidence-based Practice in Nursing and Healthcare, The Ohio State College of Nursing, Columbus, Ohio

T. Scott Graham, PhD   Director, Ohio State University Leadership Academy, Clinical Professor of Leadership, The Ohio State University, The Ohio State College of Nursing, Columbus, Ohio

Linsey Grove, DrPH, CPH, CHES   eunoia Media Lab, LLC, St. Petersburg, Florida

Mary Beth Happ, PhD, RN, FAAN, FGSA   Associate Dean for Research and Innovation, The Ohio State University College of Nursing, Columbus, Ohio

Alma Helping, BBA, CPA   Vice President and Chief Financial Officer, The Christ Hospital, Cincinnati, Ohio

Cheryl L. Hoying, PhD, RN, NEA-BC, FAAN, FACHE, FAONL   Chief Nursing Executive and Patient Care Services Officer, The Ohio State University, Columbus, Ohio

Stefanie Lyn Kaufman, AB   Founder/Executive Director, Project LETS, Westbury, New York

Sidney Kushner, BS Executive Director and Founder, Connecting Champions, Pittsburgh, Pennsylvania

Eli MacLaren, MS Former Chief Market Maker, Business Innovation Factory, Providence, Rhode Island

Kathy Malloch, PhD, MBA, RN, FAAN President, KMLS, LLC, Lepisic, Ohio; Clinical Professor, The Ohio State University College of Nursing, Columbus, Ohio

John J. McNamara, AuD Owner and Audiologist, Ontario Hearing Centers, Rochester, New York

Christine W. Meehan, BSN, MA Entrepreneur in Residence, Adjunct Professor, University of Connecticut, Storrs, Connecticut

Bernadette Mazurek Melnyk, PhD, APRN-CNP, FAANP, FNAP, FAAN Vice President for Health Promotion; University Chief Wellness Officer; Dean and Professor, College of Nursing; Professor of Pediatrics & Psychiatry, College of Medicine; Executive Director, the Helene Fuld Health Trust National Institute for EBP, The Ohio State University, Columbus, Ohio

Deborah Mills-Scofield CEO, Mills-Scofield, LLC, Visiting Scholar, Cognitive Science Department, Brown University, Oberlin, Ohio

Dianne Morrison-Beedy, PhD, RN, WHNP, FNAP, FAANP, FAAN Chief Talent and Global Strategy Officer, Centennial Professor of Nursing, The Ohio State University College of Nursing, Columbus, Ohio

Susan Neale, MFA Senior Writer/Editor, The Ohio State University, Columbus, Ohio

Joseph Novello IV, BSN, BA Entrepreneur, NurseGrid, Portland, Oregon

Michelle Podlesni, RN President, National Nurses in Business Association, CEO, Bloom Service Group, Inc., Henderson, Nevada

Tim Porter-O'Grady, DM, EdD, APRN, FAAN Clinical Professor, Emory University, Atlanta, Georgia

David Putrino, PT, PhD Director of Rehabilitation Innovation, Icahn School of Medicine at Mt Sinai, New York, New York

Tim Raderstorf, DNP, RN Chief Innovation Officer and Assistant Professor of Nursing Practice, The Ohio State University College of Nursing, Columbus, Ohio

Candy Rinehart, DNP, CRNP, FAANP CEO/Director, Ohio State University Total Health and Wellness, The Ohio State University College of Nursing, Columbus, Ohio

Jess Roberts, MARCH   Founder and Lead, Culture of Health by Design, Minnesota Design Center, University of Minnesota, Minneapolis, Minnesota

Betsy Sewell, BS   Head of Marketing, Aware, Columbus, Ohio

Gary L. Sharpe, MBA, BA, DH (hon)   Chairman and CEO, Health Care Logistics, Inc., Circleville, Ohio

Robert Smith   College Football Analyst, Fox, Arlington, Texas

Sharon Tucker, PhD, RN, APRN-CNS, FNAP, FAAN   Grayce Sills Endowed Professor in Psychiatric Mental Health Nursing, Translational/Implementation Research Core Director, Helene Fuld Health Trust National Institute for Evidence-based Practice, Nurse Scientist, Wexner Medical Center, The Ohio State University College of Nursing, Columbus, Ohio

Jonathon Vinocur, JD   Partner, Thompson Hine, LLP, Cleveland, Ohio

Dan Weberg, PhD, MHI, BSN, RN   Head of Clinical Innovation, Trusted Health, San Francisco, California; Clinical Assistant Professor, The Ohio State University College of Nursing, Columbus, Ohio

Vibeke Westh, RN   Former President, Danish Nurse Organization Capital Region, Copenhagen, Denmark

Pamala Wilson, DNAP, CRNA, MA, BSN, RN   CEO, Freelance Anesthesia, Owasso, Oklahoma

Tami H. Wyatt, PhD, RN, CNE, CHSE, ANEF, FAAN   Associate Dean of Research, University of Tennessee–Knoxville, Knoxville, Tennessee

Preface

Evidence from numerous studies supports that leadership and innovation are critical factors for organizational success and improved outcomes. Further, no change takes place and sustains without strong leadership. Although the United States spends more money on healthcare than any other country in the Western world, our health outcomes are poor. For example, the United States is the worst such country in which to give birth. Sick care continues to be the predominant paradigm and this needs to shifted to well care as 80% of chronic conditions can be prevented with healthy lifestyle behaviors. We are also living during a period when over 50% of clinicians are suffering from burnout, which affects the quality and safety of care. Solutions, including employing strong leaders and innovators, are urgently needed.

As leaders, innovators, entrepreneurs, and educators, we are painfully aware that the unknowns in healthcare are growing more rapidly and more broadly than what is known. With that in mind, we have developed this book on leadership, innovation, and entrepreneurship to provide you with an evidence-based approach to maximize your leadership and innovation potential. Our practical guide will prepare you to lead your organization into the uncertainty of the future so as to make a positive impact on the world.

This book is organized into three distinct sections: leadership, innovation, and entrepreneurship. The first two sections may be named for terms that are very familiar to you, but as health professionals, principles of entrepreneurship are not typically integrated into our daily practice. However, it is important to note that entrepreneurship and its principles can be applied to leadership and innovation in almost any industry. Some of the greatest minds were entrepreneurial leaders, including Einstein, Gates, and Buffet. Who says your name can't be added to the list? By studying and applying the evidence-based principles of leadership, innovation, and entrepreneurship offered in this book, you will emerge as a more confident and prepared leader to advance your team and organization to its optimal potential, no matter what lies ahead.

PURPOSE

The purpose of this book is to stimulate you to think and act differently by strengthening your leadership, innovation, and entrepreneurial skills. As you will see time and time again throughout this book, our system is broken. We know it will take a new generation of leaders and innovators to solve healthcare's complex problems. That next generation of leaders consists of individuals who consistently base their practices on the best available evidence and, when no evidence exists, creates it.

FEATURES

We believe this book is unlike any other text you have ever read. Many of the chapters are written in the first person using storytelling as a common thread. You are going to study multiple real-world examples with direct applicability to your practice as a leader, innovator, and entrepreneur. You will not find heavy theoretical content in our book as we wanted to create content that would be relatable and help you to put key content into real-world practice. Here are just a few examples of how this book is different than what you have been probably exposed to in the past.

Quotes—Each chapter is filled with motivational quotes related to the content that will inspire and challenge you to put the lessons into practice.

Calls to Action—Embedded within each chapter, our multiple *calls to action* are practical exercises to help you develop specific skills related to the content in each chapter. We promised this book would provide a practical guide to leadership success. These *calls to action* are an exceptional way to position you, the reader, for success. However, you have to do your part and be diligent about putting the *calls to action* into practice.

Podcasts—Each section of the book contains a podcast recorded by one of the world's most engaging leaders on the topic under discussion. This is a unique opportunity to hear how these leaders have put our book's content into practice and how they learned from their experiences.

Key Takeaway Points—You are not going to find long-winded summaries in this book. Instead, each chapter contains four to seven key takeaway points. These represent the essential content that each chapter's authors found to be most valuable and practical when developing their leadership, innovation, and entrepreneurship skills.

A FINAL WORD FROM THE AUTHORS

What would you do in the next 5 to 10 years if you knew you could fail? It is critical to write your dreams down, put a date on them, and place this list where you see it every day. Then, believe you can achieve your list and persist through the "character-builders" until those dreams come to fruition. Evidence supports that these ingredients are key to achieving your dreams.

It is past time for change; this is not meant to be an alarming statement. It is not meant to make current leaders feel inadequate or that their work has not had a positive impact. Leaders are doing the best job they can with what they have learned in their academic programs and the tools that have been available. However, our book offers a new approach as well as novel ways of thinking and acting in order to develop a new set of leaders, innovators, and entrepreneurs who will positively disrupt healthcare and substantially improve health and well-being. The leadership principles of innovation and entrepreneurship offered in this book are evidence-based methods that provide you with the most effective tools to improve healthcare and health outcomes well into the future.

As you work to achieve your own dreams, do not forget the importance of disconnecting to connect with the special important people in your life and to take good self-care. If you do not, you will have to take time for illness in the future. Now, let us dream, discover, and deliver a healthier world!

Bernadette (Bern) Mazurek Melnyk and Tim Raderstorf

Qualified instructors may obtain access to the supplementary material (Instructor's Manual and PowerPoints) by emailing textbook@springerpub.com

Acknowledgments

We acknowledge the many healthcare leaders who have come before us, blazed a solid foundation, and laid a trail to be followed. We are very appreciative of their work and the advancements they made to improving healthcare and enhancing the lives of others. A special acknowledgment goes to David Bergeron for contributing his photography to this text. Thank you also to Kathy York, Liz McClurg, and Brian Keller for their assistance in helping to make this book a reality. Thank you to our spouses, children, grandchildren, friends, and family who have supported and inspired us as this book came to life.

List of Podcasts

PODCAST 1: BE CURIOUS!

In this first episode, we meet Tim (Dr. Tim Raderstorf) and Bern (Dr. Bernadette Melnyk) as they offer an introductory breakdown of the subjects covered throughout the text and why this book is unlike anything else on the market for those looking to be successful leaders in today's healthcare environment. They talk about their personal journeys and express why learning from the successes and failures of other leaders, innovators, and entrepreneurs could save you a few missteps on your own journey to leadership.

PODCAST 2: UNLEARNING AND DOING THINGS DIFFERENT

Tim and Bern talk with chapter contributor Cheryl Hoying about the importance of healthcare finance and what leaders should be teaching their team about organizational budgets. She discusses the different ways healthcare leaders can shift the financial paradigm, from using fewer supplies to changing "sick care" into well care, to keep people out of the hospital.

PODCAST 3: WHAT EVERY LEADER SHOULD KNOW ABOUT COMPLEX SYSTEMS

Tim talks to chapter contributor Dan Weberg about the *innovation* portion of this text—specifically, understanding complex systems and how to effectively navigate them as a leader. Dr. Weberg has committed his life's work to healthcare innovation, and he was the first PhD graduate of the Healthcare Innovation Leadership program at Arizona State University. He went on to found the Master's in Healthcare Innovation program at The Ohio State University College of Nursing.

PODCAST 4: DO WHAT YOU SAY YOU WOULD DO

Tim talks to chapter contributor Gary Sharpe, the chairman and CEO of Healthcare Logistics, Inc. After Gary graduated from college, he took a job that no one wanted, in the human pharmaceutical branch at Philips Electronics, reporting directly to the CEO. When his boss refused to listen to the requests of customers wanting new products, Gary decided to quit and go out on his own. This inspiring conversation between Tim and Gary will motivate any aspiring entrepreneur.

Visit https://connect.springerpub.com/content/book/978-0-8261-9625-5/front-matter/fmatter6 to access the podcasts.

Evidence-Based Leadership, Innovation, and Entrepreneurship in Nursing and Healthcare

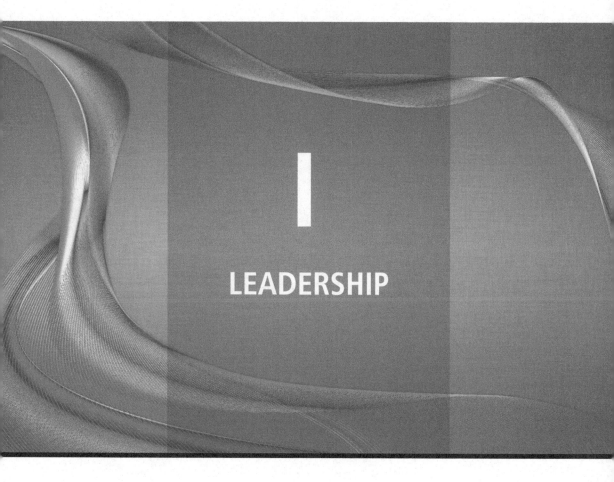

I

LEADERSHIP

Making the Case for Evidence-Based Leadership and Innovation

Bernadette Mazurek Melnyk and Tim Raderstorf

"Innovation distinguishes between a leader and a follower."
—Steve Jobs, Apple Co-founder

LEARNING OBJECTIVES

- Define *evidence-based decision-making, evidence-based practice*, and *evidence-based leadership*.

- Discuss outcomes that result when leaders implement evidence-based decision-making and create a culture that supports evidence-based practice.

- Discuss innovation, the evidence on its impact, and how to create innovation cultures in healthcare systems.

- Describe various leadership styles and the evidence on their association with organizational outcomes.

- Identify the steps that leaders need to take when having crucial conversations.

INTRODUCTION

As optimists, it is really hard to say this; after all, every contributor in this book believes that healthcare leaders are doing the best they can. However, the evidence is just too overwhelming; we cannot ignore it any more. *It is time to sound the alarm. Our healthcare system is broken.* Here is the good news: **with every broken system comes boundless opportunities**—those that will be capitalized on by the most creative leaders, which include those with the ability to understand the complexity of healthcare; those who empathize with patients, providers, and payers; and those who innovate solutions to the most pressing health and healthcare problems. This book presents evidence-based approaches to becoming that type of leader. Through the principles of innovation and entrepreneurship, you will gain insights into how you can become a leader who can help your organization to understand the task at hand, develop a comprehensive strategic approach to tackling the mountain of issues that impact your system, and address those issues head-on in order to facilitate the best outcomes.

UNDERSTANDING THE PROBLEM

Before diving deeply into the content of this text, you must first develop an understanding of our dire (not an exaggeration) need for improved evidence-based innovative leadership, more rapid innovation, and the need for healthcare professionals to become more involved in companies that are designing the future of healthcare. Some statistics and key points will be frequently repeated throughout this book. Although this may seem redundant, the frequency and repetition is meant to drive important points home. Our healthcare system is broken, and, by reading this book, you are being asked to commit yourself to helping this cause by developing solutions to resolve the inherent problems that are threatening healthcare quality, safety, and patient outcomes as well as driving an increase in costs.

Preventable Medical Errors: The Third Leading Cause of Death in America

Estimates indicate that between 250,000 and 400,000 people die each year in the United States owing to preventable healthcare errors (James, 2013; Makary & Daniel, 2016). On the high end of these estimates, this would be the same number of lives lost if eight (yes, eight) fully loaded 737 jet airliners crashed and killed *every passenger on board every day*, in the United States alone. This makes preventable medical errors the third leading cause of death in this country (Makary & Daniel, 2016). Would you ever get on an airplane if even one 737 crashed just once a month or if airplane accidents led to the 10th largest cause of death in the United States? This statistic is easy to dismiss or ignore, but healthcare leaders must keep this information as ammunition for implementing evidence-based practice, driving innovation, and encouraging clinicians to engage in solving this massive problem.

Clinician Burnout, Depression, and Compassion Fatigue

Over 50% of clinicians in the United States are currently affected by burnout, depression, and compassion fatigue (Dzau, Kirch & Nasca, 2018; McHugh, Kutney-Lee, Cimiotti, Sloane & Aiken, 2011; Melnyk et al., 2018; Shanafelt et al., 2015); as a result, the quality and safety of healthcare are being compromised as health professionals who are experiencing poor mental and physical health are at greater risk of making medical errors. In a recent national study, depression was the leading cause of medical errors in nurses (Melnyk et al., 2018). Clinicians typically invest in taking great care of their patients, but do not tend to prioritize their own self-care. Burnout also is very costly to the American healthcare system as turnover rates soar. Nursing turnover costs an organization nearly $90,000 per vacancy (Kurnat-Thoma, Ganger, Peterson, & Channell, 2017), and estimates of the cost of replacing a physician are as high as $1,000,000 (Shanafelt, Goh, & Sinsky, 2017). As a result of this alarming public health epidemic, the National Academy of Medicine launched the Action Collaborative on Clinician Well-Being and Resilience (see nam.edu/initiatives/clinician-resilience-and-well-being), a national initiative to raise awareness of the problem and generate evidence-based solutions to combat it. In order to improve this situation, healthcare leaders must invest in a system that prioritizes clinician well-being and provides a culture and resources that support it.

Gross Domestic Product Versus Outcomes

Gross domestic product (GDP) is an economics term that represents the total value of the goods and services of a country produced over a specific time (Kramer, 2018). It is commonly viewed as one of the most important indicators of the health of a nation's economy. In the United States, health spending accounted for 17.9% of the GDP in 2017. To provide some perspective, in 1940, health spending accounted for 4.5% of the nation's GDP. In 1990, health spending reached 12.2% of the GDP (Centers for Medicare & Medicaid Services [CMS], 2018). Is spending a large portion of GDP on healthcare such a bad thing? Isn't health, as is said, our greatest wealth? The issue lies in the fact that Americans are not seeing a comparable return on investment for this astronomically high level of health spending. The United States ranks highest in healthcare spending (Organisation for Economic Co-operation and Development [OECD], 2018) but falls to an abysmal ranking of 34 in life expectancy outcomes (World Health Organization [WHO], 2018). Leaders need to create more value (i.e., innovate) for care and challenge the status quo to develop new methods that improve outcomes while simultaneously reducing cost.

The Opioid and Mental Health Crises

Almost as alarming as the number of deaths per day related to preventable medical errors is the fact that over 115 people die every day in the United States owing to an opioid overdose (Centers for Disease Control and Prevention/National Center for Health Statistics, 2017). More alarming is the rate at which opioid overdoses are increasing; the Midwest region has seen a 70% increase in opioid overdoses from July 2016 through September 2017 (Vivolo-Kantor et al., 2017). Multiple innovations are being piloted across the country, and healthcare leaders are reminded on a daily basis just how challenging it can be to change human behaviors and the mental health of the population.

Mental health problems are a contributing factor to the addiction epidemic and are in urgent need of solutions. Currently, one in four to five children, adolescents, and adults has a mental health problem, such as depression and anxiety (as common as broken bones), yet the majority do not receive treatment (see www.nimh.nih.gov/health/statistics/mental-illness.shtml for current data; Wainberg et al., 2017). Untreated depression is now the second leading cause of death among 10- to 34-year-olds (www.nimh.nih.gov/health/statistics/suicide.shtml). Although the United States Preventive Services Task Force recommends depression screening in primary care for both adolescents and adults (www.uspreventiveservicestaskforce.org/Page/Document/UpdateSummaryFinal/depression-in-children-and-adolescents-screening), it is often not performed because of lack of reimbursement for screening or because there are inadequate systems in place to deal with mental health problems once diagnosed. Further, even though there is a strong body of evidence to support cognitive behavioral therapy (CBT) as the gold standard evidence-based treatment for depression and anxiety (Weershing et al., 2017), few individuals receive it because of inadequate numbers of mental health providers, especially in rural and underserved areas. More innovative solutions, such as the evidence-based Creating Opportunities for Personal Empower-ment (COPE) program, a manualized seven-session CBT-based program that can be delivered by nonmental health practitioners in primary care settings and schools, are needed. Multiple stud-ies have found that COPE is effective in decreasing depression, anxiety, behavior problems, and overweight/obesity and in improving self-esteem and academic performance in children, teens, and young adults (Hoying & Melnyk, 2016; Hoying, Melnyk, & Arcoleo, 2016; Kozlowski, Lusk, & Melnyk, 2015; Lusk & Melnyk, 2018; Melnyk et al., 2013, 2015; Melnyk, Kelly, & Lusk, 2014). Healthcare providers in 44 states who are using this program with depressed and anxious children and teens are receiving reimbursement for it in primary care settings. More information about the research-based COPE program is described in Chapter 24, Key Strategies for Moving From Research to Commercialization With Real-World Success Stories.

The Chronic Disease Epidemic

Although cardiovascular disease remains the leading killer of Americans, considering all causes of death and disease in the United States, behaviors are truly the number one killer owing to physical inactivity, unhealthy eating, smoking, and alcohol/drug abuse. One out of two Americans has a chronic condition, such as high blood pressure, diabetes, and heart disease. Yet, 80% of chronic disease is totally preventable with the adoption of healthy lifestyle behaviors, such as engaging in 30 minutes of physical activity 5 days a week, eating at least five fruits and vegetables per day, not smoking, and limiting alcohol intake (Ford, Zhao, Tsai, & Li, 2011). In addition, 7 hours of sleep per night and the practice of regular stress reduction (e.g., mindful-ness, cognitive behavioral skills-building) could nearly obliterate chronic disease.

However, behavior change is not easy. Most people do not change their behaviors unless a crisis occurs or their emotions are raised. Obesity, which is largely preventable with the adop-tion of healthy lifestyle behaviors, will soon surpass smoking as the leading cause of prevent-able death and disease in the United States. Although people should be counseled in regard to healthy lifestyle behaviors at every healthcare visit, we still live in a sick care healthcare system. We desperately need to turn sick care into well care, even for those patients at the end of life; every person should be helped to achieve his or her optimal state of well-being.

Need for Emphasis on "So What" Outcomes

"So what" outcomes are factors that are highly significant to the current healthcare system, including rehospitalizations and complications that are currently not reimbursed (e.g., falls, pressure ulcers), as well as costs (Melnyk & Morrison-Beedy, 2019). Researchers do not often include these types of "so what" outcomes in their studies. As a result, they often have much difficulty scaling their evidence-based interventions into real-world clinical settings. When de-signing studies, it is critical that "so what" outcomes are incorporated into the evaluation plan so that if an intervention is found to positively impact outcomes through research, healthcare systems will be more likely to adopt that intervention and implement it in practice.

The Social Determinants of Health

Integrating the **social determinants of health** into the care of all people has become a major global priority. According to the WHO, the social determinants of health are the conditions in which people are born, grow, live, work, and age (e.g., housing, schools, employment, food); in other words, they are factors aside from healthcare (Braveman & Gottlieb, 2014). The social determinants of health are largely responsible for health inequities, which are the unfair and avoidable differences in health status seen within and between countries. However, the manner in which health systems are designed, operate, and financed also act as a powerful determinant of health. Changes in healthcare, including value-based reimbursement, increased health system and provider accountability, and the addition of millions of Americans to health insurance rosters, have created incentives and demand social determinants of health are addressed (Robert Wood Johnson Foundation, 2016).

Small Percentage of Healthcare Start-Ups Being Founded by Clinicians

As healthcare tends to move at a much less rapid pace than other industries, it can be very challenging to keep up with new technologies that could be applied in healthcare settings. Health professionals tend to maintain their focus on the challenges they face on a daily basis, placing little emphasis on strategizing about the future. If healthcare leaders are not involved in the creation of the new technologies, products, processes, and services that are being developed, then these leaders are essentially allowing nonhealthcare professions to determine the future of healthcare. Conversely, if companies looking to develop a new technology or service for healthcare do not involve healthcare professionals in the creation of the new technology or service, then they are less likely to develop something that can be readily adopted in practice. This proverbial double-edged sword showcases the need for clinicians and healthcare professionals to become more involved with start-ups and for companies implementing new healthcare technologies and services to ensure that clinicians provide meaningful input into the future of healthcare.

EVIDENCE-BASED DECISION-MAKING AND PRACTICE: A MUST FOR LEADERS

With so many problems to address, it can be intimidating and challenging to know where to begin. The innovative leader knows it's always best to start with the evidence. Findings from a strong body of research indicate that healthcare quality, population health outcomes, costs, and clinician engagement and satisfaction, otherwise known as the *Quadruple Aim* in healthcare (Bodenheimer & Sinsky, 2014), are improved when decisions and care are based on solid evidence versus care that is steeped in tradition (e.g., "that is the way we do it here; that is the way the outdated policy says it needs to be done"). Further, clinicians are empowered and more satisfied when they engage in evidence-based practice (EBP) and work in a culture that supports it, ultimately leading to higher job satisfaction and less turnover (Kim et al., 2016, 2017; Melnyk, Fineout-Overholt, Giggleman, & Choy, 2017). Despite all of its positive impactful outcomes, **EBP**, which was initially defined in medicine as the conscientious use of current best evidence to make decisions about patient care (i.e., **evidence-based decision- making**; Sackett, Straus, Richardson, Rosenberg, & Haynes, 2000), is not consistently implemented by clinicians and leaders in healthcare systems across the nation and globe. Since the earlier definition appeared, EBP has been broadened to include a lifelong problem-solving approach to the way that healthcare is delivered, one that integrates the best evidence from high-quality studies with a clinician's expertise and a patient's preferences and values (Melnyk & Fineout-Overholt, 2019). Within the scope of a clinician's expertise are (a) clinical judgment; (b) internal evidence from the patient's history and physical exam, and data gathered from EBP, evidence-based quality improvement, or outcomes management projects; and (c) an evaluation of available resources required to deliver the best practices (Melnyk & Fineout-Overholt, 2019). **Evidence-based leadership** is a problem-solving approach to leading and influencing organizations or groups to achieve a common goal that integrates the conscientious use of best evidence with leadership expertise and stakeholders' preferences and values (Gallagher-Ford, Buck, & Melnyk, 2019).

It typically takes a number of years or even decades to translate findings from research into real-world clinical practice settings to improve outcomes. A recent national study of 276 chief nurses from across the United States found that their implementation of EBP was low, even though their beliefs about the value of EBP were high (Melnyk et al., 2016). Although these chief nurses named healthcare quality and safety as their first and second priorities, respectively, EBP fell to the bottom of their priority list. The majority of the chief nurses also invested a very small percentage of their budgets in ensuring their clinicians were skilled in EBP, indicating that they did not recognize evidence-based care as a potent direct pathway to quality and safety. As a result, a large number of their hospitals did not meet benchmark data on the CMS's Core Measures (e.g., falls, pressure ulcers) and the National Database of Nursing Quality (NDNQI) Indicators.

Innovation typically involves the creation of a solution to something when a solution or evidence does not exist (Ackerman, Porter-O'Grady, Malloch, & Melnyk, 2018). In this book, *innovation* is defined as the process of implementing new products, services, and/or solutions that *create new value*. However, for an innovation to "stick" or sustain, evidence must be generated that supports its value or outcomes. Studies have found that clinicians who are involved in innovations that generate solutions to healthcare problems are more satisfied in their roles (Warmelink et al., 2015).

Unfortunately, EBP is not the standard of care in healthcare systems throughout the United States and globally because of several barriers that have persisted over recent decades, including (a) inadequate knowledge of and skills in EBP by clinicians; (b) lack of cultures and environments that support EBP; (c) misperceptions that EBP takes too much time; (d) organizational politics and policies that are outdated; (e) limited resources and tools available for point of care providers, including budgetary investment in EBP by chief nurse executives; (f) resistance from colleagues, nurse managers, and leaders; (g) inadequate numbers of EBP mentors in healthcare systems; and (h) academic programs that continue to teach baccalaureate and master's students the rigorous process of how to conduct research instead of taking an evidence-based approach to care (Melnyk & Fineout-Overholt, 2019; Melnyk, Fineout-Overholt, Gallagher-Ford, & Kaplan, 2012; Melnyk et al., 2016; Titler, 2009).

Given that evidence-based clinical decision-making leads to the highest quality of safe and cost-effective care, leaders must implement evidence-based clinical decisions, role model EBP, and provide the resources/support for the seven-step EBP process if evidence-based care is to be delivered consistently in their healthcare system.

The seven steps of EBP, as outlined by Melnyk and Fineout-Overholt (2019), adapted to a leader's role in implementing and supporting them, are outlined in the following text.

Step #0. Cultivate a Spirit of Inquiry Within an EBP Culture and Environment

Leaders must have an ongoing spirit of inquiry, continually asking questions about the current practices followed in their hospital or healthcare system, such as: Does using an evidence-based fall-prevention protocol reduce fall rates in older adults? Is mindfulness or cognitive behavioral skills-building better at reducing burnout and turnover rates in clinicians? Does early ambulation in the ICU lead to reduced episodes of ventilator-associated pneumonia? A continual spirit of inquiry will lead to a search for the best evidence to answer questions that will improve healthcare quality, safety, and outcomes.

Leaders must also cultivate this spirit of inquiry in clinicians and build an EBP culture and environment where they have easy access to EBP resources (computers, databases, librarians), opportunities for EBP education and skills-building, space for reading and reflective thinking, opportunities for interprofessional collaboration, consistent access to EBP mentors, time to read and critically appraise the literature, and autonomy to change practice based on best evidence when indicated (Melnyk et al., 2017; Pryse, McDaniel, & Schafer, 2016; Spiva et al., 2017). EBP should be included in the organization's vision, mission, and goals, staff performance evaluations, and clinical ladders to set the expectation that all clinicians will meet the EBP competencies (see Chapter 8, Achieving the Quadruple Aim in Healthcare With Evidence-Based Practice: A Necessary Leadership Strategy for Improving Quality, Safety, Patient Outcomes, and Cost Reductions). When evidence-based clinical decision-making is the standard approach or norm for all decision-making, an EBP environment and culture are actualized (Gallagher-Ford et al., 2019).

Step #1. Ask the Burning Clinical Question in PICO(T) Format (Patient/population, Intervention/area of interest, Comparison, Outcome(s), Time)

To conduct a successful search of the literature in a time-efficient way, leaders must place their questions in the PICO(T) format to avoid countless hours or weeks of searching for best evidence. For example, reformatting the preceding clinical questions according to the following PICO(T) format will yield the quickest search for the best evidence.

1. In hospitalized older adults (P), how does using an evidence-based fall-prevention protocol (I) versus not using an evidence-based fall-prevention protocol (C) affect fall rates (O)?

2. In clinicians (P), how does mindfulness training (I) versus cognitive behavioral skills-building (C) affect burnout and turnover rates (O) 6 months after training (T)?

3. In adults in intensive care (P), how does early ambulation (I) versus delayed ambulation (C) affect rates of ventilator-associated pneumonia (O)?

Leaders can stimulate clinicians to ask PICO(T) questions through a variety of mechanisms, including the placement of PICO(T) boxes on units throughout a healthcare system and unit–unit contests that recognize clinicians for their spirit of inquiry. Meetings can also be started by asking clinicians for their latest burning PICO(T) questions.

CALL TO ACTION

Formulate three PICO(T) questions from issues that you see in your healthcare system.

Step #2. Search for and Collect the Most Rlevant Best Evidence

Once a leader's clinical question is posed in the PICO(T) format, each of the key words in the PICO(T) question should be used to systematically search for the best evidence; this strategy is referred to as *key word searching*. For example, to gather the evidence needed to answer the intervention PICO(T) questions noted earlier, you would first search databases, such as the Cochrane Database of Systematic Reviews, MEDLINE, and the Cumulative Index of Nursing and Allied Health Literature (CINAHL), for systematic reviews and randomized controlled trials as they provide the strongest levels of evidence to guide practice decisions. However, the search should extend to include all evidence that answers the clinical question. Each key word or phrase from the second PICO(T) question noted earlier (e.g., clinicians, mindfulness-based training, cognitive behavioral skills-building, burnout, turnover) should be entered individually and searched. Searching controlled vocabulary that matches the key words is the next step in a systematic approach to searching. In the final step, each key word and the controlled vocabulary that was previously searched is combined, typically yielding a few studies that should answer the PICO(T) question. This systematic approach to searching for evidence usually yields a few studies to answer the PICO(T) question versus a less systematic approach that typically produces a large number of irrelevant studies.

A leader needs to ensure that his or her clinicians have the knowledge and infrastructure support to search for best evidence to answer their PICO(T) questions. Having access to a librarian, or better yet one on staff specifically assigned to assist with evidence searches, as well as having designated EBP mentors with expertise in evidence-based care, is key to assisting clinicians with the steps in the process (Melnyk & Fineout-Overholt, 2019).

Step #3. Critically Appraise the Evidence

Leaders need critical appraisal skills to evaluate the evidence once the search is completed. As a first step, conduct a rapid critical appraisal (RCA) of each of the studies from the search to determine whether or not it is one of your "keeper studies" (i.e., those that indeed answer the clinical question; Melnyk, Gallagher-Ford, & Fineout-Overholt, 2017). This process includes answering the following questions:

1. Are the results of the study valid (i.e., did the researchers use the best methods to conduct the study (**study validity**)? For example, assessment of a study's validity determines whether the methods used to conduct the study were rigorous.

2. What are the results (i.e., do the results matter, and can I get similar results in my practice; **study reliability**)?

3. Will the results help me in caring for my patients (e.g., is the treatment feasible to use with my patients; **study applicability**; Melnyk & Fineout-Overholt, 2019)?

RCA checklists can help evaluate the validity, reliability, and applicability of a study in a time-efficient way (see Melnyk and Fineout-Overholt [2019] for a variety of rapid critical appraisal checklists). After an RCA is completed on each study and it is found to be a keeper, it is included in the evaluation and synthesis of the body evidence to determine whether a practice change should be made.

Leaders must provide their clinicians with time and skills-building to learn the art of critical appraisal, evaluation, and synthesis. This step is often the most difficult for clinicians, and practice is absolutely necessary to learn these skills. Again, EBP mentors have this expertise and should be available to work with clinicians on this critical step in EBP.

Step #4. Integrate the Best Evidence With One's Clinical Expertise and Patient/Family Preferences

Once the body of evidence from the search is critically appraised, evaluated, and synthesized, it is integrated with a leader or clinician's expertise and the patient's preferences and values to decide whether a practice change should be made. Providing the patient with existing evidence and involving the patient in the decision regarding whether a certain intervention or treatment is performed is an important step in EBP. Patient decision support tools that provide evidence-based information in an understandable format should be used when they are available (Elwyn et al., 2015).

Leaders must provide a culture that empowers and supports clinicians through the process of making EBP changes. Clinicians should all be oriented to the process through which practice changes can be made. Bureaucratic systems that make it cumbersome to effect change based on best evidence will diminish enthusiasm for EBP and be disempowering for clinicians. Therefore, leaders must ensure that the process is workable in a timely fashion for clinicians and population health outcomes.

Step #5. Evaluate Outcomes of the Practice Decision or Change Based on Evidence

An *outcome* is the consequence of an intervention or treatment. For example, an outcome of providing evidence-based CBT is a decrease in depressive symptoms. Outcomes evaluation is absolutely critical to assess the impact of an EBP change on healthcare quality and patient outcomes. Consider and include "so what" hard outcomes that the current healthcare system considers important, such as complication rates, length of stay, rehospitalization rates, and costs, because hospitals are currently being reimbursed on the basis of their performance on these outcomes (Melnyk & Morrison-Beedy, 2019).

In their national study of chief nursing executives, Melnyk et al. (2016) reported that over 50% of the executives reported that they were not sure how to measure outcomes of the care that was being delivered in their hospitals and healthcare systems. Outcomes management is a critical skill for leaders to use to garner the evidence needed to demonstrate the positive impact and cost savings of their initiatives.

Step #6. Disseminate the Outcomes of the EBP Decision or Change

The outcomes of an EBP change should be disseminated so that findings can be scaled or spread to benefit other units or healthcare systems. Various mechanisms for disseminating evidence-based change projects—including institutional EBP rounds; poster and podium presentations at local, regional, and national conferences; and publications—can overcome barriers to spreading the results, such as silos even within the same healthcare organization. Leaders should allocate a percentage of their budgets for such dissemination efforts. Not only will staff feel appreciated for being supported in the effort to disseminate their terrific work, but also the organization will gain considerable visibility.

TABLE 1.1 Similarities and Differences in the Seven Steps of Evidence-Based Practice and Innovation-Based Practice

Evidence-Based Practice	Innovation-Based Practice
Step #0. Cultivate a spirit of inquiry within an EBP culture and environment.	Step #0. Cultivate a spirit of inquiry within an EBP culture and environment.
Step #1. Ask the burning clinical question in PICO(T) format.	Step #1. Ask the burning clinical question in PICO(T) format.
Step #2. Search for and collect the most relevant best evidence.	Step #2: Search for and collect the most relevant best evidence.
Step #3. Critically appraise the evidence.	Step #3. Critically appraise the evidence.
Step #4. Integrate the best evidence with one's clinical expertise and patient or family preferences in making a practice decision or change.	Step #4. Innovate a solution, which could be an intervention, product, technology, or process, when high-quality evidence is lacking.
Step #5. Evaluate outcomes of the practice decision or change based on evidence.	Step #5. Conduct research to generate the efficacy or impact of the innovation on "so what" outcomes in order to increase its potential to scale and sustainability.
Step #6. Disseminate the outcomes of the EBP decision or change.	Step #6. Disseminate the findings of the study.
EBP, evidence-based practice.	
Source: Copyright 2019, Bernadette Mazurek Melnyk.	

 CALL TO ACTION

Name two issues within your healthcare system for which innovation is necessary because evidence does not currently exist to guide the current practices.
What innovative solutions might you suggest to address these issues?

INNOVATION-BASED PRACTICE

When evidence does not exist to support a change in care, a leader must generate innovative solutions to address problems in healthcare systems with a view to ultimately improving healthcare quality and patient outcomes. Innovation-based practice occurs at the intersection of what is known on the basis of evidence and what is needed or desired (Ackerman et al., 2018). In practice, evidence should guide clinical decisions about what is best or works best for patient outcomes.

When there is a lack of evidence to support a certain practice, clinicians are uncertain about what is best practice, which stimulates a spirit of inquiry (step #0 in EBP). The clinician must decide on the best approach to patient care, and this becomes difficult when faced with no or poor-quality evidence, conflicting evidence, or only opinion to guide practice. These types of uncertainties that lack quality evidence encourage clinicians to innovate or implement "work-arounds," which are a source of potential struggle because, although innovation arises in response to a need, there exists a lag in evidence to support the innovation. Without evidence, the innovation is often discarded. The degree of disruption that the innovation presents has an impact on the rate of adoption, giving the highest chance of adoption to those innovations that cause minimal disruption (Ackerman et al., 2018). Whenever possible, evidence should be generated of the innovation's impact through research as it is typically critical for the innovation to be sustained.

HEALTHCARE IMPROVEMENT THROUGH INTERPROFESSIONAL INNOVATION AND AN EBP MODEL

When a problem becomes evident in healthcare (e.g., an increase in the number of patient falls or rehospitalizations), leaders must make a decision about how to solve that problem. That decision must be based on the best evidence available and, therefore, both leaders and clinicians throughout an organization must be proficient in evidence-based decision-making and practice, possessing skills in the critical appraisal of evidence. After a decision is made and a change is implemented on the basis of best evidence, an evaluation must be conducted to determine the impact of the EBP change. When high-quality evidence is not available to guide strategic decisions, leaders and their interprofessional team members must innovate new solutions. **Innovation** is more than having good ideas; **it adds measurable value to a system.**

The Healthcare Improvement Through Interprofessional Innovation and Evidence-based practice (HITI^{2}E) Model is a framework that can be used to improve clinician and healthcare outcomes. The first step in this model is assessing organizational culture and readiness for interprofessional EBP and innovation. Once this assessment is conducted, an infrastructure should be created or the current structure strengthened to support both EBP and innovation. A critical mass of interprofessional innovation and EBP facilitators should then be developed to work with point-of-care clinicians at the grassroots level on how to implement EBP to improve healthcare quality and patient outcomes.

Without quality evidence to drive positive practice change, these facilitators must work with point-of-care clinicians to spark innovation to solve important practice challenges. Having this critical mass of innovation and EBP facilitators throughout the grassroots of the organization

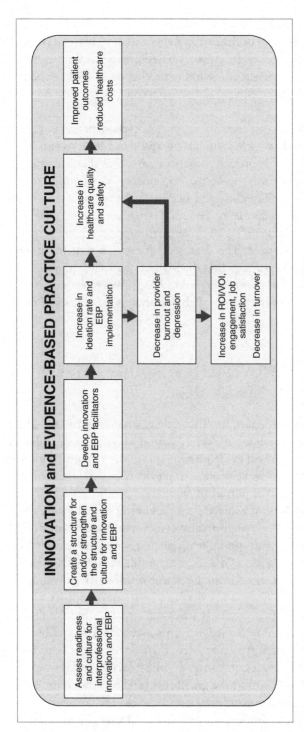

Figure 1.1 The Healthcare Improvement Through Interprofessional Innovation and Evidence-based practice Model.
EBP, evidence-based practice; ROI, return on investment; VOI, value of investment.

Source: Copyright 2019, Bernadette Melnyk and Tim Raderstorf.

should result in an increase in ideation rate and EBP implementation, eventually bringing about a decrease in clinician burnout/depression and an increase in return on investment/value of investment, including improved clinician engagement and job satisfaction as well as decreased turnover rate. In addition, an increase in EBP implementation and ideation rate should result in improved healthcare quality and safety. The final outcomes should be improved patient outcomes and decreased healthcare costs (Figure 1.1).

Interprofessional teams at the grassroots of the organization should be skilled in EBP and encouraged to innovate solutions to the healthcare problems that they are encountering in their daily practice. In fact, innovation and EBP should be inherent in the values of an organization and set as an expectation for all interprofessional clinicians. Leaders must understand that for innovations to sustain, evidence must be generated to support them and their positive outcomes. Both innovation and EBP take investment from leaders, but the return on investment and value of investment will be well worth it.

BUILDING A STRUCTURE AND CULTURE TO ADVANCE INNOVATION

Although a structure and a culture of innovation are often used interchangeably, they are, in fact, two dichotomous elements that are heavily dependent on each other. It is not a chicken-or-egg scenario, it is the chicken *and* the egg. Regardless of the culture of an organization, innovation cannot flourish without a solid structure to advance innovation. The inverse of that statement also is true. You can build the most beautiful innovation center in the world, but if the end users do not experience a positive culture where innovation is the norm, organizational innovation will wither and die on the vine.

You can see the structure of innovation through organizational policies on intellectual property (IP) creation, the designation of physical space for employees to use to collaborate on new ideas, and the appointment of a chief innovation officer whose role is to advance innovations within the organization. These elements (and surely many others) provide the structure for innovation to occur. The structure for innovation is not as fragile as the culture for innovation. The people who fill chief innovation officer positions will come and go, but the role continues to exist. The structure to make innovation possible remains.

Building a culture of innovation is much more challenging, and the concept will be explored in depth. Perceived barriers of innovation (such as *it costs too much money, it takes too much time, that is not part of my job description*) should be eliminated to build a culture of innovation. Three simple steps set the foundation:

1. **Provide the permission to innovate.** "We do not just want you to innovate in our organization; we expect it to be a foundational component of your work."

2. **Provide validation that all ideas are worth perusing.** "We hired you because you are an intelligent problem solver. We rely on your problem-solving skills to be successful."

3. **Showcase your structure to innovate.** "Let's reach out to the innovation team to find out how we can set you up for success."

Clearly, this is an oversimplification of a complex process, but you will hear from top-tier organizations that have used the core model of eliminating the barriers to innovation to find success. Innovation can take years to complete and gobble up a budget, but with the proper innovation structure and culture in place, innovation is often timely, rewarding, and financially beneficial (see medtechboston.medstro.com/blog/2018/11/09/300-days-240-20-2-empowered -nurses-1-makerspace-and-endless-impact).

COMMON LEADERSHIP STYLES

All leadership styles have positive attributes. Leaders typically have one predominant leadership style, but many individuals display attributes of two or more styles. Leadership style and organizational culture should match, as "dis-"synchrony can result in adverse outcomes for both the leader and the organization.

Innovation Leadership

Innovation leaders create an infrastructure that integrates innovation into the DNA of their organization (Gallagher-Ford et al., 2019). Within a culture of innovation, employees are both empowered and encouraged to develop innovative solutions to solve healthcare issues for systems to operate smoothly and to produce positive patient outcomes. Today, leaders are constantly faced with the need to improve healthcare quality and safety while reducing costs. Innovation leaders support innovation and oversee change effectively (Porter-O'Grady & Malloch, 2017).

Innovation leaders create the context for innovation to occur, developing both (infra)structure and culture. They provide the roles, decision-making structures, physical space, partnerships, and networks that support innovative thinking and testing (Malloch & Porter-O'Grady, 2009). Malloch (2010) contends that the following competencies are necessary for innovation leaders:

- Assessment for innovation: Personal knowledge of one's propensity, ability, and skill with innovation work
- Future focused: Actively plans for a better future and understands the value of change
- Value-driven: Believes new ideas will advance performance and value

Transformational Leadership

Transformational leadership is defined as a state in which leaders and followers "find meaning and purpose in their work, and grow and develop as a result of their relationship" (Barker, Sullivan, & Emery, 2006, p. 16). Because of this special relationship, leaders and followers become partners in pursuing common goals. Transformational leaders are enthusiastic, energetic, and compassionate. They generate an exciting vision and inspire others to engage in a journey to achieve that vision. They support and encourage people within the organization and regularly recognize and appreciate them for their efforts. Followers typically respect, admire, and trust a transformational leader. The culture created by transformational leaders is innovative and change oriented, supportive of new ideas, and open (Klainberg & Dirschel, 2010). Transformational leaders create cultures in which staff are creative, innovative, and open to change (Guerrero, Padwa, Fenwick, Harris, & Aarons, 2016).

Servant Leadership

Robert K. Greenleaf first described the concept of a servant leader in 1970. Servant leadership is based on a focus on others along with trust, empathy, and caring (Greenleaf Center for Servant Leadership, 2013). Greenleaf asserted that great leadership grows from service and that great leaders are servants first (Gersh, 2006). A servant leader practices shared power and focuses on enhancing the growth and optimal well-being of his or her followers. What counts is not power, but whether those being served become more autonomous, healthier, independent, wiser, and likely to become servant leaders themselves (Greenleaf for Servant Leadership, 2013). Spears (2010) describes 10 foundational characteristics central to servant leadership: listening, empathy, healing, awareness, persuasion, conceptualization, foresight, stewardship, commitment to growth of people, and building community.

Authentic Leadership

Authentic leaders are transparent, confident, hopeful, optimistic, resilient, and of high moral character. These leaders are keenly aware of how they think and behave and have firm convictions of who they are and where they stand on issues, values, and beliefs (Wong & Cummings, 2009). They are role models, focusing on ethics and working to develop others. Followers perceive them as being transparent and valuing others' perspectives and strengths (Avolio, Gardner, Walumbwa, Luthans, & May, 2004). Authentic leaders create and sustain high-quality relationships with their followers. They build trust and healthy work environments. Authentic leaders conduct thorough self-assessments and objectively analyze data for the purpose of informing their decisions. They hold high moral and ethical standards for themselves and their people and are transparent in their communication. Authentic leaders listen to others and take their opinions into consideration when making decisions. This leads to open and trusting cultures where people feel free to share innovative ideas (Avolio et al., 2004; Walumbwa, Peterson, Avolio, & Hartnell, 2010; Wong & Cummings, 2009).

Autocratic Leadership

Also known as *authoritarian leadership*, *autocratic leadership* is characterized by high control over decisions with little input from others. Autocratic leaders typically make decisions based on their ideas, knowledge, and judgment. They typically do not accept feedback or constructive criticism well and move forward with their ideas and decisions without much regard for others' opinions. Although this style of leadership is usually not favored by people in an organization, it is common. At the extreme, autocratic leadership is stifling and can damage the morale of an organization. Autocratic leaders are often perceived as micromanagers who have no consideration for people's feelings and emotions. On a positive note, this style of leadership is helpful when decisions need to be made quickly to turn a poor-performing organization around. People with low and unstable self-esteem tend to prefer autocratic leaders whose powerful abilities they believe in and in whom they can place their trust and hope (Schoel, Bluemke, Mueller, & Stahlberg, 2011).

> **CALL TO ACTION**
> Which of these styles capture your type of leadership?
> Are you satisfied with your leadership style?
> If not, what specific steps will you take in the next 90 days to come more in alignment with the leadership style you most desire?

 ## EVIDENCE ON THE VARIOUS LEADERSHIP STYLES AND ORGANIZATIONAL OUTCOMES

A growing body of studies indicates the many positive outcomes associated with a transformational leadership style. To be specific, transformational leadership has been found to be significantly related to increased satisfaction and well-being in nurses as well as decreased burnout, stress, and incivility among them (Kaiser, 2017; Weberg, 2010). Another study of emergency room nurse leadership style and its impact on nurse turnover indicated that a transformational leadership style was related to less nurse turnover, although there was no association between transformational leadership and patient satisfaction (Raup, 2008). Another study with primary care clinicians also found that the transformational leadership style is linked to high job satisfaction (Jodar, Badia, Hito, Osaba, & Del Val Garcia, 2016). Transformational leadership by surgeons also has been associated with better team performance in the operating room (Hu et al., 2016).

Marmo and Berkman (2018), in a study of 203 hospice social workers, found that the perception of servant leadership was related to higher job satisfaction. Other variables linked to job satisfaction were interdisciplinary collaboration and feeling valued by the hospice physician.

A recent systematic review by McCay, Lyles, and Larkey (2018) found that relational leadership traits, similar to authentic leadership traits, contribute to greater nurse satisfaction, whereas task-oriented styles decrease nurse satisfaction. The high-quality relationships that authentic leaders create and sustain result in increased engagement, increased motivation, commitment, and job satisfaction (Avolio et al., 2004; Wong & Laschinger, 2013).

In a systematic review of 20 studies (Wong, Cummings, & Ducharme, 2013), findings indicated that there are associations among positive relational leadership styles and higher patient satisfaction and lower patient mortality, medication errors, restraint use, and hospital-acquired infections. However, more rigorous studies are needed to generate additional evidence regarding specific leadership characteristics, including the innovation leadership style, and patient as well as clinician outcomes.

CRUCIAL CONVERSATIONS: A NECESSARY LEADERSHIP SKILL

Regardless of the type of leadership style an individual has, he or she must be effective at having **crucial conversations**, that is, a discussion between two people in which the stakes are high, opposing positions, and emotions are strong (Patterson et al., 2012). Leaders must possess the ability to speak up even when it is not comfortable to do so and to engage in conversations when there is disagreement in order to achieve a positive outcome.

The book *Crucial Conversations* (Patterson et al., 2012) teaches a seven-step process for managing difficult conversations, including:

1. Start with the heart, which includes asking yourself what you really want and what's at stake.

2. Learn to look. Observe carefully when safety may be at risk.

3. Make it safe. … learn how to step out of the content, create a mutual purpose, resolve conflict, and return to a healthy dialogue.

4. Master your story. … what we tell ourselves is the cause of all emotions. Learn how to retell your story and create emotions that make you want to resume a healthy dialogue; separate facts from stories.

5. State your path. … learn to say things in ways that decrease the other person's defensiveness; the best way to start is to share facts (e.g., "I was expecting to receive this at 3 p.m. and now it's 4 p.m.; this lateness leads me to conclude that meeting a deadline isn't a goal"; avoid "you" statements that appear to fix blame).

6. Explore others' paths … ask the other person to share his or her story so you can understand his or her point of view (e.g., "Can you help me to better understand where you are coming from?").

7. Move to action (who does what by when; the follow-up).

In conclusion, leaders must act as role models in evidence-based decision-making and innovation if they expect their employees to also engage in these practices. Leaders must also create cultures and environments that allow their staff to consistently engage in evidence-based practice and innovation. In addition, they must be aware of their own leadership style and understand its impact on clinician and organizational outcomes as well as having the necessary skills to engage in crucial conversations.

🔑 KEY TAKEAWAY POINTS

- Evidence-based decision-making and practice are key to achieving the Quadruple Am in healthcare.

- When evidence does not exist or is of weak quality, it is critical to innovate new solutions.

- When an innovation is created, it is important to generate evidence through research on its efficacy or impact so that it will be likely to be sustainable.

- Building cultures that promote EBP and innovation is necessary to make them the norm in a healthcare system.

- It is essential that leaders learn the skills of having crucial conversations.

REFERENCES

Ackerman, M. H., Porter-O'Grady, T., Malloch, K., & Melnyk, B. M. (2018). Innovation-based practice (IBP) versus evidence-based practice (EBP): A new perspective that assesses and differentiates evidence and innovation (Editorial). *Worldviews on Evidence-based Nursing, 15*(3), 159–169.

Avolio, B., Gardner, W., Walumbwa, F., Luthans, F., & May, D. (2004). Unlocking the mask: A look at the process by which authentic leaders impact follower attitudes and behaviors. *Leadership Quarterly, 15*, 801–823.

Barker, A. M., Sullivan, D. T., Emery, M. J. (2006). *Leadership competencies for clinical managers: The renaissance of transformational leadership.* Sudbury, MA: Jones and Bartlett.

Bodenheimer, T., & Sinsky, C. (2014). From Triple to Quadruple Aim: Care of the patient requires care of the provider. *Annals of Family Medicine, 12*, 573–576.

Braveman, P., & Gottlieb, L. (2014). The social determinants of health. It's time to consider the causes of the causes. *Public Health Reports, 129* (Suppl. 2), 19–31.

Centers for Disease Control and Prevention/National Center for Health Statistics. (2017). Mortality. Retrieved from https://wonder.cdc.gov

Centers for Medicare & Medicaid Services. (2018). *National health expenditure data.* Retrieved from https://www.cms.gov/Research-Statistics-Data-and-Systems/Statistics-Trends-and-Reports/NationalHealthExpendData/index.html

Dzau, V. J., Kirch, D. G., Nasca, T. J. (2018). To care is human—Collectively confronting the clinician-burnout crisis. *New England Journal of Medicine, 378*(4), 312–314. doi: 10.1056/NEJMp1715127

Elwyn, G., Quinlan, C., Mulley, A., Agoritsas, T., Vandik, P. O., & Guyatt, G. (2015). Trustworthy guidelines-excellent; customized care tools-even better. *BioMed Central Medicine, 13*(1), 199.

Ford, E. S., Zhao, G., Tsai, J., & Li, C. (2011). Low-risk lifestyle behaviors and all-cause mortality: Findings from the national health and nutrition examination survey III mortality study. *American Journal of Public Health, 101*, 1922–1929. doi:10.2105/AJPH.2011.300167

Gallagher-Ford, L., Buck, J. S., & Melnyk, B. M. (2019). Leadership strategies for creating and sustaining evidence-based practice organizations. In B. M. Melnyk & E. Fineout-Overholt (Eds.), *Evidence-based practice in nursing and healthcare. A guide to best practice* (4th ed., pp. 328–347). Philadelphia, PA: Wolters Kluwer.

Gersh, M. R. (2006). Servant-leadership: A philosophical foundation for professionalism in physical therapy. *Journal of Physical Therapy Education, 20*(2), 12.

Greenleaf Center for Servant Leadership. (2013). Retrieved from http://www.greenleaf.org

Guerrero, E., Padwa, H., Fenwick, K., Harris, L., & Aarons, G. (2016). Identifying and ranking implicit leadership strategies to promote evidence-based practice implementation in addiction health services. *Implementation Science, 11*(69), 1–13.

Hoying, J., & Melnyk, B. M. (2016). COPE: A pilot study with urban-dwelling minority sixth grade youth to improve physical activity and mental health outcomes. *Journal of School Nursing, 32*(5), 347–356. doi:10.1177/1059840516635713

Hoying, J., Melnyk, B. M., & Arcoleo, K. (2016). Effects of the COPE Cognitive Behavioral Skills Building TEEN Program on the healthy lifestyle behaviors and mental health of Appalachian early adolescents. *Journal of Pediatric Health Care, 30*(1), 65–72.

Hu, Y. Y., Parker, S. H., Lipsitz, S. R., Arriaga, A. F., Peyre, S. E., Corso, K. A., … Greenberg, C. C. (2016). Surgeons' leadership styles and team behavior in the operating room. *Journal of the American College of Surgeons, 222*(1), 41–51. doi:10.1016/j.jamcollsurg.2015.09.013

James, J. T. (2013). A new, evidence-based estimate of patient harms associated with hospital care. *Journal of Patient Safety, 9*(3), 122–128. doi:10.1097/PTS.0b013e3182948a69

Jodar, I. S. G., Badia, G. I., Hito, P. D., Osaba, M. A., & Del Val Garcia, J. L. (2016). Self-perception of leadership styles and behaviour in primary health care. *BMC Health Services Research, 16*(1), 572.

Kaiser, J. A. (2017). The relationship between leadership style and nurse-to-nurse incivility: Turning the lens inward. *Journal of Nursing Management, 25*(2), 110–118. doi:10.1111/jonm.12447

Kim, S. C., Ecoff, L., Brown, C. E., Gallo, A. M., Stichler, J. F., & Davidson, J. E. (2017). Benefits of a regional evidence-based practice fellowship program: A test of the ARCC model. *Worldviews on Evidence-Based Nursing, 14*(2), 90–98. doi:10.1111/wvn.12199

Kim, S. C., Stichler, J. F., Ecoff, L., Brown, C. E., Gallo, A. M., & Davidson, J. E. (2016). Predictors of evidence-based practice implementation, job satisfaction, and group cohesion among regional fellowship program participants. *Worldviews on Evidence-Based Nursing, 13*(5), 340–348. doi:10.1111/wvn.12171

Klainberg, M., & Dirschel, K. (Eds.). (2010). *Today's nursing leader: Managing, succeeding, excelling.* Sudbury, MA: Jones & Bartlett Learning.

Kozlowski, J., Lusk, P., & Melnyk, B. M. (2015). Pediatric nurse practitioner management of child anxiety in the rural primary care clinic with the evidence-based COPE. *Journal of Pediatric Health Care, 29*(3), 274–282.

Kramer, L. (2018). *What is GDP and Why is it so important to economists and investors?* Retrieved from https://www.investopedia.com/ask/answers/what-is-gdp-why-its-important-to-economists-investors/

Kurnat-Thoma, E., Ganger, M., Peterson, K., & Channell, L. (2017). Reducing annual hospital and registered nurse staff Turnover—A 10-element onboarding program intervention. *SAGE Open.* doi:10.1177/2377960817697712

Lusk, P., & Melnyk, B. M. (2018). Decreasing depression and anxiety in college youth using the Creating Opportunities for Personal Empowerment program (COPE). *Journal of the American Psychiatric Nurses Association, 25*, 89–98. doi:10.1177/1078390318779205

Makary, M. A. & Daniel, M. (2016). Medical error—the third leading cause of death in the U.S. *BMJ, 353.* doi: https://doi.org/10.1136/bmj.i2139

Malloch, K. (2010). Innovation Leadership: New perspectives for new work. *Nursing Clinics of North America, 45*, 1–9.

Malloch, K., & Porter-O'Grady, T. (2009). *Introduction to evidence-based practice in nursing and healthcare*. Sudbury, MA: Jones & Bartlett.

Marmo, S., & Berkman, C. (2018). Social workers' perceptions of job satisfaction, interdisciplinary collaboration, and organizational leadership. *Journal of Social Work in End of Life and Palliative Care, 14*(1), 8–27.

McCay, R., Lyles, A. A., & Larkey, L. (2018). Nurse leadership style, nurse satisfaction, and patient satisfaction: A systematic review. *Journal of Nursing Care Quality, 33*(4), 361–367. doi:10.1097/NCQ.0000000000000317

Melnyk, B. M., & Fineout-Overholt, E. (2019). *Evidence-based practice in nursing & healthcare. A guide to best practice* (4th ed.). Philadelphia, PA: Wolters Kluwer.

Melnyk, B. M., Fineout-Overholt, E., Gallagher-Ford, L., & Kaplan, L. (2012). The state of evidence-based practice in US nurses: Critical implications for nurse leaders and educators. *Journal of Nursing Administration, 42*(9), 410–417.

Melnyk, B. M., Fineout-Overholt, E., Giggleman, M., & Choy, K. (2017). A test of the ARCC© model improves implementation of evidence-based practice, healthcare culture, and patient outcomes. *Worldviews on Evidence-Based Nursing, 14*(1), 5–9.

Melnyk, B. M., Gallagher-Ford, L., & Fineout-Overholt, E. (2017). *Implementing the EBP competencies in healthcare: A practical guide for improving quality, safety and outcomes.* Indianapolis, IN: Sigma Theta Tau International.

Melnyk, B. M., Gallagher-Ford, L., Koshy, B., Troseth, M., Wyngarden, K., & Szalacha, L. (2016). A study of chief nurse executives indicates low prioritization of evidence-based practice and shortcomings in hospital performance metrics across the United States. *Worldviews on Evidence-based Nursing, 13*(1), 6–14. doi:10.1111/wvn.12133

Melnyk, B. M., Jacobson, D., Kelly, S., Belyea, M., Shaibi, G., Small, L., … Marsiglia, F. F. (2013). Promoting healthy lifestyles in high school adolescents: A randomized controlled trial. *American Journal of Preventive Medicine, 45*(4), 407–415. doi:10.1016/j.amepre.2013.05.013

Melnyk, B. M., Jacobson, D., Kelly, S. A., Belyea, M. J., Shaibi, G. Q., Small, L., … Marsiglia, F. F. (2015). Twelve-month effects of the COPE Healthy Lifestyles TEEN Program on overweight and depression in high school adolescents. *Journal of School Health, 85*(12), 861–870.

Melnyk, B. M., Kelly, S., & Lusk, P. (2014). Outcomes and feasibility of a manualized cognitive-behavioral skills building intervention: Group COPE for depressed and anxious adolescents in school settings. *Journal of Child and Adolescent Psychiatric Nursing, 27*(1), 3–13. doi:10.1111/jcap.12058

Melnyk, B. M., & Morrison-Beedy, D. (2019). *Intervention research and evidence-based quality improvement* (2nd ed.). New York, NY: Springer Publishing Company.

Melnyk, B. M., Orsolini, L., Tan, A., Arslanian-Engoren, C., Melkus, G. D., Dunbar-Jacob, J., … Lewis, L. M. (2018). A national study links nurses' physical and mental health to medical errors and perceived worksite wellness. *Journal of Occupational & Environmental Medicine, 60*(2), 126–131.

Organisation for Economic Co-operation and Development. (2018). *Health expenditure.* Retrieved from https://www.oecd.org/els/health-systems/health-expenditure.htm

Patterson, K., Grenny, J., McMillan, R., & Switzier, A. (2012). *Crucial conversations. Tools for talking when stakes are high.* New York, NY: McGraw-Hill Education.

Porter-O'Grady, T., & Malloch, K. (2017). *Quantum leadership. Creating sustainable value in healthcare* (5th ed.). Sudbury, MA: Jones & Bartlett.

Pryse, Y., McDaniel, A., & Schafer, J. (2016). Psychometric analysis of two new scales: The evidence-based practice nursing leadership and work environment scales. *Worldviews on Evidence-based Nursing, 11*(4), 240–247.

Raup, G. H. (2008). The impact of ED nurse manager leadership style on staff nurse turnover and patient satisfaction in academic health center hospitals. *Journal of Emergency Nursing, 34*(5), 403–409.

Robert Wood Johnson Foundation. (2016). *Using social determinants of health data to improve health care and health: A learning report.* Princeton, NJ: Author.

Sackett, D. L., Straus, S. E., Richardson, W. S., Rosenberg, W., & Haynes, R. B. (2000). *Evidence-based medicine: How to practice and teach EBM.* London, England: Churchill Livingstone.

Schoel, C., Bluemke, M., Mueller, P., & Stahlberg, D. (2011). When autocratic leaders become an option. *Journal of Personality and Social Psychology, 101*(3), 521–540. doi:10.1037/a0023393

Shanafelt, T., Goh, J., & Sinsky C. (2017). The business case for investing in physician well-being. *JAMA Internal Medicine, 177*(12):1826–1832.

Shanafelt, T. D., Hasan, O., Dyrbye, L. N., Sinsky, C., Satele, D., Sloan, J. & West, C. P. (2015). Changes in burnout and satisfaction with work-life balance in physicians and the general U.S. working population between 2011 and 2014. *Mayo Clinic Proceedings, 90*(12), 1600–1613. doi: 10.1016/j.mayocp.2015.08.023.

Spears, L. C. (2010). Character and servant leadership: Ten Characteristics of effective, caring leaders. *The Journal of Virtues & Leadership, 1*(1), 25–30.

Spiva, L., Hart, P. L., Patrick, S., Waggoner, J., Jackson, C., & Threatt, J. L. (2017). Effectiveness of an evidence-based practice nurse mentor training program. *Worldviews on Evidence-Based Nursing, 14*(3), 183–191.

Titler, M. G. (2009). Developing an evidence-based practice. In G. LoBiondo-Wood & J. Haber (Eds.), *Nursing research: Methods and critical appraisal for evidence-based practice* (7th ed., pp. 385–437). St Louis, MO: Mosby.

Vivolo-Kantor, A. M., Seth, P., Gladden, R. M., Mattson, C. L., Baldwin, G. T., Kite-Powell, A., & Coletta, M. A. (2017). Vital signs: Trends in emergency department visits for suspected opioid overdoses—United States, July 2016–September 2017. *Centers for Disease Control and Prevention, 67*(9), 279–285.

Wainberg, M. L., Scorza, P., Schultz, J. M., Helpman, L., Mootz, J. J., Johnson, K. A., … Arbuckle, M. R. (2017). Challenges and opportunities in global mental health: A research-to-practice perspective. *Current Psychiatry Reports, 19*(5), 28. doi:10.1007/s11920-017-0780-z

Walumbwa, F. O., Peterson, S. J., Avolio, B. J., & Hartnell, C. A. (2010). An investigation of the relationships among leader and follower psychological capital, service climate, and job performance. *Personnel Psychology, 63*(4), 937–963.

Warmelink, J. C., Hoijtink, K., Noppers, M., Wiegers, T. A., de Cock, T. P., Klomp, T., & Hutton, E. K. (2015). An explorative study of factors contributing to the job satisfaction of primary care midwives. *Midwifery, 31*(4), 482–488. doi:10.1016/j.midw.2014.12.003

Weberg, D. (2010). Transformational leadership and staff retention: An evidence review with implications for healthcare systems. *Nursing Administration Quarterly, 34*(3), 246–258.

Weersing, V. R., Jeffreys, M., Minh-Chau, T., Do, M. S., Schwarts, K. T. G., & Bolano, C. (2017). Evidence-base update of psychosocial treatments for child and adolescent depression. *Journal of Clinical Child and Adolescent Psychology, 46*(1), 11–43. doi:10.1080/153 74416.2016.1220310

Wong, C., & Cummings, G. (2009). Authentic leadership: A new theory for nursing or back to basics? *Journal of Health Organization and Management, 23*(5), 522–538.

Wong, C., & Laschinger, H. (2013). Authentic leadership, performance, and job satisfaction: The mediating role of empowerment. *Journal of Advanced Nursing, 69*(4), 947–959. doi:10.1111/j.1365-2648.2012.06089

Wong, C. A., Cummings, G. G., & Ducharme, L. (2013). The relationship between nursing leadership and patient outcomes: A systematic review update. *Journal of Nursing Management, 21*(5), 709–724. doi:10.1111/jonm.12116

World Health Organization (2018). *Life expectancy*. Retrieved from https://www.who.int/gho/mortality_burden_disease/life_tables/situation_trends/en/

Important Lessons Learned From a Personal Leadership, Innovation, and Entrepreneurial Journey

Bernadette Mazurek Melnyk

"Tough times never last, but tough people do." —Robert H. Schuller

LEARNING OBJECTIVES

- Describe the three "Ds" and how they lead to success.
- Discuss key characteristics that result in great leadership.
- Reflect on the strengths and limitations of leaders whom you have had the opportunity to observe.
- Identify leadership characteristics that you will work to develop over the next 2 to 5 years.
- Recognize important lessons that you have learned throughout your life and how they will influence your future behaviors.
- Identify what you will accomplish in the next 5 to 10 years if you cannot fail.

INTRODUCTION

This chapter offers content that is not typically found in an academic book on leadership. It includes excerpts from my personal and career stories, one that is packed with what I believe are several "pearls of wisdom." Sometimes, hindsight is better than foresight. It is my hope that the lessons I have learned in looking back at my journey and the calls to action presented throughout this chapter help you to avoid common pitfalls typically made and propel you forward to flourish in your own leadership, innovation, and/or entrepreneurial journey. To get the most value out of this chapter so as to enhance your own journey, it will be important for you to stop and spend some good reflection time responding to the "calls to action." I am going to start this chapter by providing what I believe are some of the most important pieces of advice that I have learned as a leader, innovator, and entrepreneur. Then I weave in several other key lessons that I have learned throughout my life by sharing my own personal story. Many of these and similar lessons reemerge again throughout future chapters of this book—as they are key to success.

Remember the Three Ds: Dream, Discover, and Deliver!

DREAM BIG AND DON'T LET ANYONE STEAL YOUR DREAMS!

"*Nothing happens unless first we dream.*"—Carl Sandburg

There is truly magic in thinking big. If you do not tend to dream big, the book *The Magic of Thinking Big* is a great classic that can help you to stretch your thinking (Schwartz, 1987). However, you will achieve your dreams faster if you write them down, put a date on your list, and place it where you can see it every day. If people look at you skeptically when you share a big dream, say to yourself, "I'm on the right track!" Don't let people discourage you from pursuing your dreams. If you take on roles that align with your dreams and passions, you will have great energy that sustains you throughout the day and never feel like you work a day in your life.

Discover. Always have a questioning spirit—constantly think about better and new innovative ways to do things and gaps that need to be filled. Part of discovery is risk-taking. The most successful people are the biggest dreamers and risk-takers. Learn to question and risk more.

Deliver. Any big dream is worth the persistent effort it takes to achieve it. Remain persistent through your challenges or what I call "character-builders." With every rejection, think "I'm one step closer to a yes." Stay focused on your dream.

Remember, how you think impacts how you feel and how you behave. Practice daily positive thinking and talking. Putting positive thoughts into your brain will result in positive emotions and behaviors. For nearly 30 years, I have woken up every morning and have read a positive-thinking book for 5 to 10 minutes. Starting the day with positive thoughts arms you against the negativity that tends to zap daily energy. Some of my favorite books include the *How Successful People Think* (Maxwell, 2009), *The Power of Positive Thinking* (Peale, 1956), and *The Present* (Johnson, 2010).

Count your blessings daily. Make it a habit to count at least three blessings every morning as an attitude of gratitude paves the way for a happy, fulfilled life.

Take great self-care. You can't take great care of others and be your most productive if you are not taking the time to take good care of yourself. You will learn more about optimizing your own health and well-being in Chapter 4, Key Strategies for Optimizing Personal Health and Well-being: A Necessity for Effective Leadership.

Stay humble and relatable. So many individuals develop big egos as they become successful. The most successful leaders are humble and empower others to accomplish their dreams. They serve others. Don't let leadership harden you because you will see the good, bad, and the sometimes ugly come out in people.

Don't feel guilty about saying no. Overcommitting can result in stress and burnout as you work to uphold all of your commitments. Learn to prioritize and invest your time in those activities that are most important in achieving your and your team's dreams.

Build teams that work well together. TEAM = together everyone accomplishes more. Construct teams very thoughtfully and deliberately as a team that has a cohesive vision and commitment to working together will accomplish its dreams and goals. Hire people with great attitudes; you can always build their skills. Empower your team and provide them with the necessary guidance and resources to succeed.

Be clear with expectations. So often, people don't perform to expectations because they are not aware of what exactly is expected. Upon hiring, inform people of what you expect in their roles and review those periodically.

Do not micromanage. Micromanagement will squash innovation. Allow your team to innovate and learn to solve problems.

Throw up, not down. Every leader will experience frustration from time to time. However, throwing negativity down on your team will have adverse effects on them. Find a trusted person who outranks you or an outside friend to share frustrations and talk through solutions.

Learn to have crucial conversations and to provide constructive comments. You will not do people any favors if you do not learn to provide helpful constructive feedback to them. I practice giving feedback using the "Oreo cookie" approach—always give positive first, then constructive feedback next, then finish with a positive. You also will not do your organization good if you do not call people out on less-than-desired or unacceptable behaviors.

Be open, transparent, caring, and appreciative. People do not know how much you know until they know how much you care. It is important to be open, transparent, and caring. Transparency builds trust in an organization, so never underestimate its value. Also, remember to show regular appreciation and recognize your people when they perform well.

Focus on the important, not urgent. Many leaders feel they have to respond to issues immediately without letting the team handle them. If the captain of a ship needs to keep going down to the bowels to fix problems, the ship will lose its direction. Similarly, if a leader has to focus on urgent daily problems, the vision and the direction of the organization will be lost.

MY PERSONAL STORY WITH LESSONS LEARNED

Now, I will use my own personal story to relate other key lessons that I have learned along the course of my own leadership, innovation, and entrepreneurship journey. I grew up in Republic, a small coal-mining town in southwestern Pennsylvania, which was near the West Virginia border and approximately an hour's drive from Pittsburgh. Republic was a relatively close-knit town with a population just under 1,000 people. My dad was a coal miner and my mom worked off and on as a cook and a baker. I have one brother, Fred, who is 14 years older than me and a cousin, Chris, who my mom and dad raised from infancy. Chris is 13 years older than me and I have always viewed her as my sister. My family lived in half of a small house, which was approximately 950 square feet. My mom and dad believed it was important to instill a strong foundation of faith in me, so we attended church every Sunday. They also sent me to Catholic school for 8 years at a time when guilt was heavily instilled in students.

Throughout this book, you are going to read about perseverance and resiliency as common traits of leaders, innovators, and entrepreneurs. **Resiliency** is an ability to adapt or cope with and recover quickly from adversity or challenges. These traits were woven into the fabric of my family from the days when both sets of my grandparents migrated to the United States from Poland. Since then, my family's ability to persevere and demonstrate resiliency were necessary in response to multiple tragedies. When my dad was only 3 years of age, his mom and baby sister died a few days apart from each another during the horrendous 1918 flu epidemic. From then on, the hits kept coming, but we found ways to successfully cope with adversity and multiple challenges.

My brother, Fred, was a gifted football player. He received scholarship offers from top university football programs across the country. During his junior year in high school, Fred sustained a severe head injury and coded on the football field. After a few days in a coma at a local rural hospital, he was transferred to a Pittsburgh medical center to undergo brain surgery for a subdural hematoma. People found it hard to believe he came back to play football again after that severe traumatic head injury. Call it that Mazurek (my maiden name) perseverance, but Fred was given a full college scholarship to the University of Pittsburgh and ended up being their starting quarterback from 1961 to 1965. He then went on to play for the Washington Redskins for a few years before having to leave football because of a back injury. My mom found it difficult to attend football games after that awful day when my brother was badly injured, so it was often my dad and me who traveled around the country to watch Fred play ball. My dad taught me every college fight song on those football trips and I grew up to love the game. In fact, to this day, I still have football in my DNA and am an avid fan at all of The Ohio State University's home football games.

Another leadership and entrepreneurial trait you will read about in this book is **optimism**. I was born seeing through rose-colored glasses, am an eternal optimist, and am as resilient as the day is long. These traits have come in handy throughout the numerous "character-building" times in my life, especially on a cold snowy winter day in January of 1973 when I was 15 years old and a sophomore in high school. My best friend had stayed overnight at my home and my mom made us a delicious breakfast and joined us in lively conversation with lots of laughter after my dad went to work that morning. Shortly after breakfast, my best friend went home and my mom sat down on our living room couch to pay bills. I started walking up the stairs to gather my clothes to take a shower when my mom sneezed. I said "Bless you, Mom" for the second time as I continued walking up the stairs because my mom did not respond to me the first time. Alarmed when there was no response from her, I walked back down the stairs to check on her. My mom's head was laying back on the couch and she was unconscious. I shook her and tried to get her to respond to me with no success. In complete terror and helplessness, I saw my mom die from a stroke right in front of me. Sadly, my mom had a history of headaches. She finally went to her doctor the week before she died, was diagnosed with high blood pressure and given a prescription for a blood pressure medication. My dad found the unfilled script in her purse after she died at the age of 52. Just maybe if my mom would have taken that medication and lowered her blood pressure that week, the sneeze may not have resulted in her death on that cold winter day.

Leadership Lesson Learned

Although cardiovascular disease is still technically the leading cause of death in the United States today, behaviors are truly the number one killer due to physical inactivity, unhealthy eating, smoking, drug overdoses, and nonadherence to medication or treatment regimens. As leaders, we must take care of our own health as well as the health and well-being of the people in our organization.

CALL TO ACTION

What lifestyle behaviors are you currently engaging in that are preventing you from achieving optimal health and full engagement as a leader?

Commit to one healthy lifestyle behavior change today!

I suffered from terrible posttraumatic stress disorder for many months after my mom's death. I would wake up with nightmares and cold sweats regularly as well as startle every time someone sneezed. I had difficulty with my schoolwork and lost my appetite. My anxiety was almost unbearable as I worried constantly about my dad dying, too; he was now the most significant person in my life. I also felt intense guilt about my mom's death, thinking that if I had been a better daughter, she may not have been taken from my family. After a few months of these distressing symptoms, my cousin, Chris, took me to my family physician and asked him to help me. He did what so many healthcare providers still do today and wrote a prescription for Valium, advising me to take one every night. He said I would sleep and be just fine. There was no counseling available for me in my little hometown of Republic, Pennsylvania. I remember taking one of those pills that evening; I slept for the first time in months, but woke up the next morning groggy. It was that day that I decided I had to lean on my faith, focus on my strengths, and count my blessings for a wonderful dad and good close friends whom I could count on for support. This experience also lit a spark within me that would eventually lead to my success as a nurse, leader, innovator, and entrepreneur.

Leadership Lessons Learned

The two most wasted emotions are worry about the future and guilt about the past as most of what we worry about never happens and guilt does not help to improve things.

We must learn to live in the present moment and be thankful for every day.

What doesn't break us only makes us stronger.

Our personal life struggles often instill in us a dream and passion to go on and accomplish meaningful and impactful things in life.

CALL TO ACTION

Reflect back on the times in your life that were difficult, or what I call "character-building."

How did those times help you to grow stronger and develop the strengths that you currently have today?

Today, one out of four to five children and teens suffer from a mental health disorder, yet less than 25% get any treatment (Merikangas et al., 2010). If they do get treatment, it often is not evidence based. The gold standard first-line evidence-based treatment for mild to moderate depression and anxiety is **cognitive behavioral therapy (CBT)**, yet so few children, teens, and adults receive it due to a severe shortage of mental health providers (Lusk & Melnyk, 2013; Weersing et al., 2017). CBT is a type of psychotherapy in which individuals learn how to turn negative thoughts into positive ones so that they feel better emotionally and behave in healthy ways. Findings from a recent study supported brief CBT in primary care as a cost-effective treatment option that generates cost savings over 2 years (Dickerson et al., 2018). Another meta-analysis supported that CBT may be even more effective at reducing symptoms and at resolving anxiety disorders than medications (Wang et al., 2017). My own mental health struggles as a teenager following my mom's death instilled in me a dream and passion to become a nurse so that I could help youth who also were suffering from mental or physical health challenges. That dream and passion gave me such purpose in life and fueled in me the drive to become a pediatric nurse practitioner (PNP), then a psychiatric mental health nurse practitioner, and a PhD scientist so that I could acquire the skills needed to innovate and test programs to improve mental health outcomes and foster healthy lifestyle behaviors in children, teens, and their parents. If not for the traumatic life event of losing my mom at a young age, I may not have gone on to develop and conduct multiple studies to generate the evidence to support my COPE (Creating Opportunity for Personal Empowerment) cognitive behavioral skills-building programs as an effective intervention in reducing depression/anxiety and improving healthy lifestyle behaviors in children and adolescents (Hoying, Melnyk, & Arcoleo, 2016; Kozlowski, Lusk, & Melnyk, 2015; Lusk & Melnyk, 2013; Melnyk, Amaya, et al., 2015; Melnyk et al., 2013; Melnyk, Jacobson, et al., 2015). Early on, I had to start thinking about ways that I could disseminate these evidence-based COPE programs to help children, teens, and college students who were suffering from depression and anxiety if my studies showed they produced great outcomes. After multiple studies showed the positive benefits of these programs, I started a company called *COPE2Thrive, LLC*, which is now bringing these evidence-based programs to children and youth in over 40 states across the United States and in five countries who might not otherwise get any help for their mental health problems.

Leadership and Entrepreneurial Lessons Learned

Dreams and purpose help sustain the energy to accomplish important life goals, especially during difficult times.

It is important to start thinking about entrepreneurial venues to disseminate your innovations early in the invention stage.

INNOVATION CALL TO ACTION

What would you do in the next 5 to 10 years if you knew that you could not fail?

Write those dreams down now, put a date on them, and place them where they can be seen every day—research supports these actions will increase your chances of success.

After my mom died, it was just my dad and me. I had to learn how to cook and clean our home. No matter how awful a meal was that I cooked, my dad would always tell me how grateful he was for me and my cooking; he never complained as he drank three to four glasses of milk with his meals, which I am sure were often needed to wash down many unpalatable dishes. In fact, I don't think I ever heard my dad complain. He was always appreciative for what he had and always let me know it. I learned a deep sense of appreciation from him. Even today, under stressful circumstances, I count my blessings daily.

Leadership Lesson Learned

An attitude of gratitude makes for a joyful and content heart.
   It is important to tell your loved ones and your team that you appreciate them often.

CALL TO ACTION

Every morning, name three people or things for which you are grateful.
   Tell at least two people a day that you appreciate them or something they did.
   When feeling anxious this week, say to yourself, "I'm too blessed to be stressed!"

In order to cope with my mom's sudden death, my dad turned to bowling five nights a week. I would often go to the bowling alley with him to avoid being alone in the home where my mom died. I became quite a bowler on the women's league by the time I was 17; I had a 172 bowling average and learned to love the game. Bowling was therapeutic for both my dad and me. It provided me with an outlet for my stress and kept me from being alone at night in the home where I experienced such a traumatic event.

During my junior and senior years in high school, I volunteered as a candy striper at our local small-town hospital. I so loved caring for people and knew that becoming a nurse was my true calling. At the hospital, I saw healthcare providers who knew a lot, but often came across as "business like" with their patients and provided information to them that was far above their level of understanding. During that time, I resolved to be like the clinicians who took time to listen to their patients and have a caring bedside manner.

Leadership Lesson Learned

People don't know how much you know unless they first know how much you care.
   As a leader, your people also must know that you care about and appreciate them.
   Tell them often.

CALL TO ACTION

Think about the best and poorest leaders you have seen in your life.
What were their best qualities? What were their worst qualities?
Which of those qualities will you adopt?

I dreamed of going to West Virginia University with several of my good friends, but knew my dad could not afford for me to attend an out-of-state academic institution. One of my family members advised me to go to a hospital school of nursing instead of a university, which at the time was more affordable. My dad, who only had a high school education, said that if he had to work double shifts 7 days a week, he would do so in order for me to have a 4-year college degree as he, himself, did not have one and knew how important it was for my future. At West Virginia University, students were admitted to pre-nursing, not directly into nursing. If you were an out-of-state student, the odds of getting into the nursing program were slim as they gave preference to in-state students. I knew that in order to stand a chance at getting into the program, I would have to earn at least a 3.9 or 4.0 grade point average (GPA). When all of my friends were socializing, I was studying and often was the last student to leave the library at night when it was closing. My friends often teased me, saying I was such a "bookworm." However, I stayed focused on my dream of getting into the nursing program and did not let my friends steer me off course. Throughout this book, you will continue to hear about the importance of focusing on your dreams.

Those who dream, innovate; and those who innovate, dream.

Although I had a nearly 3.9 GPA in my first semester in college, my admittance to the nursing program became a little tentative when I received a C in handball and tennis after suffering a severe ankle sprain during the first month of the academic semester. However, my perseverance, focus, and resiliency paid off as I was only one of six out-of-state students to get accepted into the nursing program that spring. My dad had a heart attack when I was a sophomore in college, but thankfully he lived another 9 years before passing. After his heart attack and advice from his physician to walk regularly, my dad built up to and walked an average of 3 miles a day—he had such a strong belief that he could beat his heart disease and had a tremendous will to live. He ended up getting remarried to a terrific woman during my college years; I was ecstatic that the two of them found each other.

I worked as a nurse's aide on the night shift during most of my college years to help out with living expenses. Three years later, I graduated with my bachelor of science degree and took my first job as a nurse in the pediatric intensive care unit at Children's Hospital in Pittsburgh.

Leadership Lessons Learned

If you keep your dream in front of you and work at it consistently and persistently, you are likely to achieve it.

Anything the mind can conceive and believe, it can achieve!

Dreams + belief + execution = outcomes.

CALL TO ACTION

Reflect on one or two successes you have had so far in your career.
What factors contributed to your success?

A few months before my mom died, I started dating a guy who was a year ahead of me in high school. Because of the sudden loss of my mom, I formed an anxious attachment to this person. We dated off and on for 9 years before marrying; it was a turbulent relationship. The night before my wedding, a close friend of mine called and asked whether I was sure I was making the right decision. Although I knew it was not a healthy relationship and my instincts told me not to follow through with the wedding that night, I walked down the aisle and got married the next morning. Seventeen months later, I had my daughter, Angela, after starting my master's degree program at the University of Pittsburgh to become a PNP. My husband took a job in upstate New York when I had two semesters left to finish my program; he urged me not to complete the degree, but I was driven by my dream to become a PNP, so I moved back to my dad's home in Republic with my baby daughter and finished my master's degree. My dad would often stroll Angela around our neighborhood for hours on Saturdays and Sundays so that I could write my master's thesis. It was fortunate that I completed that degree because my husband and I divorced approximately 3 years later.

Leadership Lesson learned

Listen to and follow your dreams and instincts!

CALL TO ACTION

Reflect back on times in your life when you did not follow your dream(s) and listen to your instincts.
What outcomes resulted? What lessons did **you** learn?

After the divorce, Angela and I moved from a beautiful home to a small apartment in Ithaca, New York. At that time, I was teaching in a baccalaureate nursing program at Keuka College, a small liberal arts college in Upstate New York. I also practiced as a PNP with three pediatricians in a private pediatric practice in Ithaca while consulting for a child and adolescent inpatient psychiatric unit in Elmira, New York. Those extra jobs helped me to pay the bills. It was tough being a single mom who was working full time and beyond, but I was thankful I had finished my master's degree and had the ability to support the two of us. I lost my dad shortly after my husband and I separated, which left a huge void in my life. However, I was comforted by the fact that he knew how much I loved and appreciated him.

During my time at Keuka College, I became good friends with a biology professor who also went through a challenging marriage and divorce. John had an adopted 5-year-old daughter, Megan. Megan and Angela quickly became friends and our families enjoyed outings together.

I had dreamed of teaching at a research-intensive university and knew that I would need a PhD for that dream to come to fruition. I explored and interviewed for two PhD programs: Boston College and the University of Rochester. When I interviewed at the University of Rochester, I was told by one of the professors who interviewed me that it was their most competitive year with 36 applicants and that they never had a PhD student who was a single mother. The faculty who interviewed me asked how I thought I could possibly undertake the program as a single mom. I remember thinking how odd of and discouraging a question that was because I always believed that I could do anything that I made up my mind to do. A quote I often referred to was:

"Anything the mind can believe and conceive, it can achieve!"—Napoleon Hill

I left my interviews at the University of Rochester thinking that it was probably a long shot for me to get selected for the program as admission would only be offered to six individuals. To my surprise the following week, I was not only offered admission to the PhD program, but it came with a full-tuition scholarship. Some of my relatives and close friends told me that it was very risky to move to Rochester where I knew no one to pursue my PhD. They questioned my judgment. However, I knew deep down that I had to pursue my dream and felt I had to take that risk.

"You can never discover new oceans unless you lose sight of the shore."—André Gide

That August, I moved into graduate housing on campus with Angela and began the PhD program at Rochester in 1988. John also took a big risk and left Keuka College to pursue his dream of becoming an optometrist by attending the accelerated optometry program at the New England College of Optometry in Boston. He took out enormous school loans to pursue his dream and could not work to earn income as the full-time program was so demanding. Our decisions led to "character-building" journeys for both of us. Shortly after John moved to Boston and I moved to Rochester, we realized we cared deeply about each other, but we both needed to finish what we started and earn those degrees to fulfill our dreams.

The coursework in my PhD program was the toughest I had ever encountered. I remember walking around in a daze on campus the first couple of months questioning my decision. Throughout my PhD program, I continued a side job consulting as a nurse practitioner at the Elmira Psychiatric Center, which entailed a drive of nearly 2 hours from Rochester. The job there was not just a job to me—it was a life's calling: to work with vulnerable children and youth who had mental health problems, many who just needed to hear that someone really cared about them as several never knew what it was like to be cared about or loved. It was at this psychiatric center that I started thinking innovatively about programming to help these children and teens. I began to develop my Creating Opportunities for Personal Empowerment (COPE) cognitive behavioral skills-building healthy lifestyle program to help the children and teens develop badly needed skills to deal with all of the adversity that they were experiencing in their lives and to engage in healthy behaviors. I am so grateful that I had the opportunity to care for so many psychologically distressed children and teens at that center; they taught me so much about their emotional pain and I learned how best to help them.

Leadership Lessons Learned

Anything worth having is worth risking.
People do not often regret what they did; they regret what they do not do.
If there is will, there is a way.

CALL TO ACTION

Think about a time in your life when you wanted to accomplish something, but were afraid to risk it? Do you regret not pursuing it?
What do you want to accomplish in the next year or 2?
What are you willing to risk to achieve it?

My life during the 4 years of my PhD program at Rochester was not easy for me. There were months I had to charge groceries as I did not have enough cash to pay for them. It was my dream of making a huge impact on improving outcomes in vulnerable children, teens, and parents that kept me going. When things got rough or my fears caused me stress, I learned to stay focused on my dreams, which gave me renewed energy and helped me through those "character-building" times.

Leadership Lesson Learned

Staying focused on your dreams, not your fears and uncertainties, gives you the strength and energy to persist through the "character-builders" during your journey.

CALL TO ACTION

Reflect on times in your life when your fears and uncertainties caused you to slow down in the pursuit of your dream. What is slowing down your success now?
Put your dream back in front of you again; stay focused on it and not your fears, and watch the progress that happens.

John and I continued our relationship during our academic programs and were married after he finished his optometry program; I was then a year away from completing my PhD. I conducted a complex randomized clinical trial to test the intervention I developed to enhance mental health outcomes in young hospitalized children and their parents for my dissertation study. I spent 7 days a week at the hospital for a whole year collecting data for that trial, including holidays. I was focused and driven to finish the program and would not let myself get distracted by life's daily small stressors. After 4 years of intense effort, I was the first in my cohort of six people to finish the PhD.

Leadership Lesson Learned

Stay focused on your dream and do not let distractions or unimportant things slow you down!

CALL TO ACTION

Think about the times in your life when your progress slowed toward goals you were aiming to achieve.

What slowed you down? What will you do from now on to ensure success in accomplishing your goals?

After I completed my PhD, I interviewed at and was offered a tenure-track faculty position at five top schools throughout the country. A **tenured appointment** at a university is a long-term appointment that can usually only be terminated for cause or extraordinary circumstances (American Association of University Professors, 2017). Tenure is important to people because it provides position stability over time. Some of the schools told me exactly what I would do if I joined them, never asking me what my dreams were and what it was that I was passionate about and wanted to do. I immediately ruled out those places. I knew I wanted an opportunity where I could be a leader and explore innovative pathways to improve mental health outcomes in children, teens, and their families. Rochester was not going to offer me a tenure-track faculty position at first as they had a rule about not offering these types of positions to their own graduates. I told the dean that I was not willing to stay on board with the school if I could not enter a tenure-track faculty position. She broke the rule and I decided to stay in Rochester as I had built a great team and had colleagues whom I valued there. John and I also believed it was best to stay in Rochester to provide Angela and Megan with stability as they also were adjusted there.

Leadership Lessons Learned

Don't settle for something less than what you really want or you will regret it.

When in a leadership position, ask people about their dreams and passions; help them to achieve them. Doing so will result in people being fully engaged and productive.

Don't fit round pegs into square holes; match people to their strengths and watch them soar.

CALL TO ACTION

Reflect on a time in your life when you "settled" for something.
What was the outcome? Would you do it again? Why or why not?

As an assistant professor on the tenure track, I was teaching in and directing the PNP program, publishing papers, writing grants like wildfire, and still practicing part time at the children and youth inpatient unit at Elmira Psychiatric Center. Criteria for success and promotion at a research-intensive university include excellent teaching, scholarly publishing, and funded research, preferably from the **National Institutes of Health** (**NIH**). The NIH, a part of the U.S. Department of Health and Human Services, is the nation's medical research agency, which makes important discoveries that improve health and save lives. I received several small grants from foundations and national organizations for pilot work to adapt my COPE program for parents of critically ill and preterm infants. I also applied to the NIH to conduct a randomized controlled trial at two study sites to test my COPE program for parents of critically ill children. To my and my research team's delight, we received a good score on our very first NIH grant application, so we worked hard to address the reviewers' critique and resubmitted the grant. The outcome of that second submission was not good: in fact, we only improved our score by 2 points. I took the reviewers' critique of that grant resubmission to five senior NIH-funded researchers to ask them for their advice. All five of those researchers told me that I should give up on the grant because coping research was not fundable. I was initially devastated to hear their advice. This area of research was my passion. There were so few evidence-based interventions for parents of young critically ill children to help them and their children cope with the stressful experience. I so wanted to develop an evidence-based intervention that could be used to help these vulnerable children and parents all throughout the world. That Mazurek perseverance kicked in as my gut told me to keep trying. I just could not let myself and my team give up on our dream. In the 1990s, the NIH allowed investigators to resubmit a grant twice. So I pulled my team together, gave them a big pep talk, and said we were going to try one last time. That third submission of our grant resulted in a terrific score, which was funded by the National Institute for Nursing Research 1 month before my tenure materials were due. Without that NIH-funded grant, I am convinced that I would have never received tenure and would be on a different path than the one I am on today. In looking back, if I did not have the willingness to take risks, manage uncertainty, and persevere with my NIH grant applications, I would have not gone on to make the impact that I have throughout the globe as so many hospitals and healthcare systems are now using my evidence-based programs to improve outcomes of critically ill children, preterm infants, and their parents.

Leadership Lesson Learned

If you never swing, you will never hit, so keep swinging!
   If you know something is right in your gut, don't let others talk you out of it.
   Persistence pays off!

CALL TO ACTION

Think about the times in your life when people tried to talk you out of a dream or pursuing your passion.

Did you persist? If not, do you regret it?

How will you respond the next time when people try and talk you out of pursuing one of your dreams, innovations, or passions?

Be prepared as there are many "negatoids" in the world who will tell you what you can't do instead of encourage you to do it.

Stay away from those negative people and do not allow them to steal your dreams!

Shortly after I received my first large NIH grant and was tenured, I was offered the opportunity to take on a leadership role in the school as associate dean for research. Our school had been slipping terribly in NIH-research rankings for about a decade, so I knew this role would be a big challenge. I also knew it would be character-building as several professors who had taught me throughout my PhD program would now be directly reporting to me. However, it was an exceptional opportunity for me to determine who I was as a leader and to test my leadership skills.

I was glad that I was familiar with Tony Robbins's **DISC (Dominant, Inspiring, Supportive, Cautious) personality types** and knew my areas of strength along with my limitations, which would require organizing a team that could round out those limitations. Reflecting on my strengths and a personality that is a high D (Dreamer, Discoverer/risk-taker, and fast Deliverer or persistent in accomplishing one's dreams) and high I (Interactive, Inspirational), I felt confident that I could get people excited about a common dream and encourage them to persist through the challenges that come with grant writing, but I also knew I had to build a team that complemented my personality style, one that was composed of people whose personalities were high S (Supportive, Steady) and moderately high C (Conscientious, detail oriented, and great at process implementation) but not so rule bound that it would slow down our progress. I also needed a team composed of people with positive "can do" attitudes who were willing to work hard to accomplish the dream. It meant putting the right people in key positions on my team and surrounding myself with "can-do" individuals.

Leadership Lessons Learned

Know your personality strengths and limitations. Surround yourself with positive people who complement your limitations.

When you put the right people on the bus, magic happens and dreams are accomplished!

CALL TO ACTION

Complete the DISC personality inventory at www.tonyrobbins.com/disc

What are your predominant personality styles?

How can you best work with others who have different personality styles?

The first 90 days in a leadership position are critical, they offer a terrific window of opportunity to build a team vision and begin executing it. I pulled our school's researchers together in the first month after my appointment to craft an exciting dream (i.e., a top NIH-funding ranking with research that would improve outcomes of people in the real world) and outline a bold strategic plan to accomplish it. As part of the plan, we needed to decide on a few areas of focus to invest in and become known for as being spread too thin zaps resources and does not afford the opportunity to build a strong, sustainable foundation. The plan entailed working harder and submitting many more grants as well as recognizing people regularly for their efforts. I always believed in valuing colleagues and team members, showing them how much they are appreciated. I made a frequent habit of writing notes of appreciation and often gave out well-deserved awards. In 5 years, we raised our NIH-ranking for colleges/schools of nursing in the United States from the 70s to #13 in the country. Never forget the power of a dream, a focused team effort, and persistence.

Leadership Lesson Learned

When people become weary, one of the best things you can do is recognize them for their efforts and let them know you appreciate them.

Priority setting, belief, focus, and execution are necessary to accomplish dreams.

CALL TO ACTION

Think back on a time when you were successful at accomplishing a dream or certain goals,

What helped you when you became tired or weary?

What contributed to your success?

During my time as associate dean for research, I had a big vision for accelerating evidence-based practice (EBP). Medicine was at least 20 years ahead of nursing in what was called *evidence-based medicine* and there was a huge need to develop solutions to more rapidly accelerate the translation of research into practice to improve nursing care and population health outcomes. As part of this vision, I created a Center for Research and Evidence-based Practice in 1999 and dreamed of launching a national/international conference that would attract thousands of participants from around the country and the world. I ended up hiring one of my PhD classmates who had just graduated, Dr. Ellen Fineout-Overholt, as associate director of this Center, who was charged with assisting me in leading EBP. Ellen shared my dream and we eventually built a booming EBP enterprise, both in academia and healthcare systems.

For the very first national/international EBP conference we held in 1999, only 40 people attended. So many of our "well-meaning" colleagues said it was embarrassing that so few people came to the conference. My response was "40 people came; isn't that great!" We had the belief, fortitude, and perseverance to keep on pursing the EBP dream. In 2002, I also envisioned an

EBP book that would help nurses and other clinicians learn the EBP process and implement best practices to ultimately improve patient outcomes. I approached an acquisitions editor from Lippincott about producing this book; it would be the first book written on EBP by nurses in the United States. That book, *Evidence-based Practice in Nursing and Healthcare. A Guide to Best Practice*, was published in 2004 with my co-editor, Ellen Fineout-Overholt. It is now in its fourth edition and is a heavily used book by clinicians, healthcare systems, and faculty in academic programs throughout the world.

Since our book was published, EBP has made great strides throughout the United States and the world. However, much opportunity still lies in front of us to reach the Institute of Medicine's (IOM) recommendation that 90% of all healthcare decisions be evidence based by 2020. I have always been an entrepreneur at heart, so after we established a national reputation in EBP, Ellen and I launched a successful consulting company called *ARCC, LLC*, which focused specifically on assisting hospitals and healthcare systems in implementing and sustaining EBP with our Advancing Research and Clinical practice with close Collaboration (ARCC) Model (Melnyk, Fineout-Overholt, Giggleman, & Choy, 2017). My passion for EBP led to an entrepreneurial enterprise for me so that I could broadly disseminate my expertise and passion. Most healthcare professionals are uncomfortable with putting a price on their expertise as most of us didn't pursue our passion for the money. However, in truth, entrepreneurship and commercialization is a key path for disseminating your work so it has lasting impact.

Entrepreneurship Lesson Learned

You will be more successful in launching a consulting company when you have a known reputation in your field. If that is your desire, become credible by speaking and publishing on the topic.

Due to escalating mental health issues in children and teens, I also had a vision for a national mental health promotion campaign that would not only raise awareness on youth mental health disorders but would also teach providers how to better screen for, identify, and provide evidence-based treatment to those affected. I was a member of the National Association of Pediatric Nurse Practitioners (NAPNAP) and felt that this would be the best place to position and lead this national initiative. After several evidence-based pitches to the NAPNAP board, the board voted to approve the launch of this campaign, which I entitled KySS (Keep your children/yourself Safe and Secure). Some of the board members thought the vision I had was too big and were skeptical, but I persevered by pitching the need for this initiative with convincing evidence and stories with emotional appeal. Shortly thereafter, I wrote a Health Resources & Services Administration (HRSA) grant that was awarded to fund a National KySS Summit that brought together leaders from over 20 major national organizations to provide recommendations and collaborate on next steps for action. These organizations included the American Academy of Pediatrics, the American School Health Association, and the Society for Adolescent Medicine.

Findings from the highly successful KySS Summit, including a keynote by the 16th U.S. Surgeon General, Dr. David Satcher, were published in the *Journal of Pediatric Health Care*. This summit led to many positive outcomes, including research that informed clinical practice, a KySS online continuing-education program that provided mental health education and skills-building to hundreds of healthcare providers across America, and a KySS walkathon to raise awareness on children and teen's mental health issues that involved NAPNAP chapters throughout the United States. This national KySS initiative was operative for 10 years and achieved its aims. The KySS online education mental health program is still in existence today at The Ohio State University College of Nursing (see www.nursing.osu.edu), continuing to educate thousands of healthcare providers across the United States on how to promote mental health and provide evidence-based management for child and adolescent mental health disorders.

Leadership Lessons Learned

When you share a big dream and people look at you like you have two heads, say to yourself "I'm on the right track" and keep on working toward that dream.

Great pitches include best evidence and stories that appeal to people's emotions.
If there is will, there is a way.
Anything is possible with a big dream, belief, and persistence.
Don't let anyone ever steal your dreams!

 CALL TO ACTION

Reflect on times that you shared a big dream with other people and they voiced skepticism to you about whether you could accomplish that dream.

What did you think? How did you feel? What did you do? If you could go back to those times, how would you respond differently? Learn from the past but do not stay trapped in what didn't work. Keep your dream in front of you, believe in it, and stay persistent!

During my time at Rochester, my entrepreneurial passions led me to open a private practice with four other psychiatric mental health nurse practitioners. We delivered mental health services to children and teens in five schools and hired a psychiatrist to be our collaborating physician who would consult with us on the most complex cases that we encountered. I also continued making the 2-hour trek to provide care to the children and teens at the Elmira Psychiatric Center and completed my post-master's psychiatric mental health nurse practitioner certificate while still serving as research dean and director of the PNP program. Many people said it was not possible to be successful at multiple roles, which included teaching, research, practice, and administration. I provided evidence that all things are possible when you have big dreams/purpose, passion, and perseverance.

CALL TO ACTION

How many times throughout your life and career have people told you what you can and cannot do? What was your response? Did those people slow you down in accomplishing your dreams? What will you do differently to respond to the skeptics in your life moving forward?

While I was associate dean for research and director of the Center for Research and Evidence-Based Practice at the University of Rochester School of Nursing, I was recruited to take the dean's position at the Arizona State University (ASU) College of Nursing and Health Innovation in 2004. As I was leaving Rochester, I founded another company with three other colleagues called *COPE for HOPE*, which became the venue for disseminating the evidence-based COPE programs I had innovated to improve outcomes for critically ill/hospitalized children, premature infants, and their parents. What is interesting about this COPE program is that for the longest time I struggled to get the program implemented, despite studies that showed its multiple benefits for children and their families, such as less emotional distress, improved parent–child interactions, and better child development. I had assumed hospitals would flock to the program because it dramatically improved these outcomes. However, that was not the case. The COPE program did not truly take off until I started to measure hard "so what" outcomes (i.e., length of hospital stay) and apply entrepreneurial principles to help get it adopted. Without showing the reduced length of stay for preemies whose parents received COPE in the neonatal intensive care unit (NICU) with its associated reductions in hospital costs, it would have been much harder to scale that program to hospitals throughout the United States and the globe. Once I better understood who were the key decision makers and their motivations to adopt new programs, magic happened. Suddenly, I had the attention of the C-suite in healthcare systems, and they were offering to pay for my program. Understanding who my true customer was, what mattered most to the customer, and being able to offer a competitive pricing package were key to getting my program implemented across the world.

No one ever mentored me in establishing an S-corp, so we had to do a lot of background work and obtain legal and expert consultation on how to start and run a successful company. That company is still in existence today as hospitals and healthcare systems throughout the United States and the globe continue to implement these evidence-based COPE programs.

> **Entrepreneurship Lesson Learned**
>
> If you are thinking about starting your own company, establish your niche in the market with hard evidence on outcomes whenever possible, including why the product or service is needed, how it is different than what already exists, and its return on investment (ROI).
> Get good advice from attorneys and other savvy successful entrepreneurs.
> Develop a solid business plan.

In my first 3 years of the dean's position at ASU, I recruited several new faculty to the college by building big dreams and providing support for our team to accomplish them. One of our big dreams was to build a beautiful new building for the college. Some of my alums were skeptical about whether all of these dreams could be accomplished and would say "that will happen when pigs fly!" After 4 years of dreaming, discovering (i.e., risk-taking), and delivering, several of our dreams and innovations came to fruition, including a beautiful new building for the college, large enrollment growth, and a terrific rise in *U.S. News and World Report* and NIH-funding rankings. The once skeptical alums came to see me with a beautiful oil painting of a pig flying across a lake saying, "Please forgive us; we now believe, pigs can indeed fly!"

> Never underestimate the power of a dream.

> If you don't know where you are going, you will end up someplace else.

During the sixth year of my deanship at ASU, I started to receive calls from The Ohio State University's search committee chair for a new dean of nursing. I told her that I was humbled that Ohio State thought of me for the dean's position, but that I had no intention of making a lateral move. However, I went on to say that if Ohio State would consider a joint role for me as dean of nursing and also its first Chief Wellness Officer (CWO) in which I would spearhead population health and well-being across the entire campus, I would be willing to talk with senior leadership about the opportunity. As background, I had been studying corporate wellness for a couple of years and could not understand why big companies across the United States understood the value and **ROI** (i.e., measures the gain or loss generated on an investment relative to the amount of money invested) of hiring CWOs to optimize employee health, yet no universities throughout the country had such a role. Therefore, it was my dream to be the first CWO at a big public university and spearhead population health and well-being across the entire campus. Shortly after the chair of the search committee informed the president and provost at Ohio State about my aspirations, I was invited to campus to discuss the opportunity. I was well equipped to present the best evidence for why a CWO position was necessary at universities throughout the country. When entering a new position, you must also negotiate well for resources because if you don't receive them initially, it will be harder to obtain them once in the position. The evidence presented to the top leaders at Ohio State was compelling and convincing enough that they were willing to have me enter this new joint position. Once again, my family and I moved across country so that I could pursue yet another dream.

Leadership Lessons Learned

Make a case for what you dream about using the best evidence.

The secret sauce to negotiation is solid data.

Use evidence to negotiate well for resources before agreeing to start a new position as it will be much harder to obtain them once you have accepted a new position.

Research has shown that people don't regret what they did in life; they regret what they didn't do.

CALL TO ACTION

Think about the times when you did not take a risk and share your dream.

Do you have regrets?

From now own, make a commitment that you will not only dream, but that you will take risks and put your dream out there when opportunities present themselves.

I am a big innovator and change agent. When I take on a new position and enter a brand-new organization, I look for people with a twinkle in their eye and a fire in their belly to create an exciting team dream and begin to execute a well-designed strategic plan. When entering a new position, you have 90 days to get off to a great start. In fact, there is a book called *The First 90 Days* by Michael Watkins (2013) that has a lot of golden nuggets regarding how to have a successful start in a new position. Remember, changing an organization is a highly emotional process. I often say that the few people who like change are babies with wet diapers. Most people do not like change—they fear it and often provide resistance. As a result, many leaders get discouraged with their change efforts and give up before they see their desired outcomes. Critical conversations must take place with the resisters; directly ask them about their fears. However, if you want to move organizational change quickly, follow Everett Rodgers's Diffusion of Innovation Theory and work with the innovators and early adopters first (Dearing & Cox, 2018). Once a critical mass of people joins your change effort, the culture will shift (see Chapter 7, Leading Organizational Change and Building Wellness Cultures for Maximum ROI and VOI, for more strategies on stimulating organizational/culture change). However, culture change often takes 5, 7, or even 10 years. Don't give up. Keep your team focused on your dreams, support and encourage them to innovate, and persist through the "character-builders!"

I was in Thailand several years ago to deliver the keynote presentation to an international pediatric research congress. After the conference, my family and I were on a long-tailed boat traveling to the floating market. We had a guide who was a retired philosophy professor who related that there was an Asian bamboo tree that gets planted in the ground there. It must be watered every single day for 5 years. After 5 years of watering, the seed breaks ground and grows 90 feet in 90 days. Did the tree grow 90 feet in 90 days or 5 years and 90 days? Of course, the answer is 5 years of daily watering and 90 days. However, most people give up on their dreams when they are working hard at a change effort and do not see immediate outcomes.

Leadership Lessons Learned

Be consistent and persistent in working toward your dreams.
   Be patient: Anything worth having is worth the daily effort required to achieve it.

 CALL TO ACTION

Think about a time in your life when you weren't seeing the outcome(s) of your efforts?
   What did you think? How did you feel? What did you do?
   Did you sustain the effort or give in a bit too prematurely?
   What will you do next time if you do not see the outcomes happening as quickly as you
expect them to happen?

It has now been 8 years since I entered my joint position at Ohio State and so many great outcomes have been achieved because of a terrific team who dreams big, has the courage to innovate and take risks, believe in those dreams, and persevere through character-builders. As far as the college is concerned, our *U.S. News and World Report* and NIH rankings have soared, enrollment has doubled, and new centers/institutes have been endowed.

Ten years earlier, I started to pitch an innovative dream for a national institute for EBP to the Helene Fuld Health Trust, located in New York City. Every year for 10 years, my wonderful colleague Laurel Van Dromme and I would visit the Trust and explain to the trustee why this new institute was desperately needed to improve healthcare in the United States. Finally, after 10 years, she looked at us and asked, "How much funding would you need to launch this national institute?" The largest gift the Trust had on record was $6 million. Because I am a competitive person, I said $6.5 million. She responded that she thought they could do it and invited me back to the Trust to make a presentation to her supervisors. In the spring of 2017, after 10 years of pitching this dream, we were awarded $6.5 million to establish the Helene Fuld Health Trust National Institute for Evidence-based Practice in Nursing and Healthcare (see https://fuld.nursing.osu.edu). What would have happened if I had given up on the dream for this national institute after 7, 8, or 9 years? It would have never come to fruition.

Leadership Lessons Learned

If the dream is important enough, you need to keep putting it in front of you and persist in following it.
   Anything worth having is worth the intense effort that goes into it.
Never, never, never, never, never, never, never quit!—Winston Churchill

Another dream of mine was to hold a national summit on building healthy academic communities. When 300 leaders from 93 universities across the country were convened to focus on improving population health outcomes in academia across the United States, this dream also came to fruition in 2013 amid skepticism from many people. Shortly after the summit, I founded the National Consortium for Building Healthy Academic Universities (BHAC) with 16 founding universities. This new national organization is thriving (see www.healthyacademics.org) with over 60 universities now represented. The fourth national BHAC Summit was held April 30–May 3, 2019, at Ohio State. Remember, anything is possible with a big dream, belief in that dream, and consistent execution.

With both of my moves across country for leadership positions, I anticipated working for my bosses for several years. However, in both situations, those individuals were removed from their positions within the first 2 years of my working in the new roles. Although you must be selective about the person whom you choose to work for in a new position, you also must remember that there is currently a lot of flux in administrative positions. You must always be prepared for change and therefore expect the unexpected and get comfortable with uncertainty. However, if you do a great job at what you do, outstanding opportunities will continue to present themselves.

I will now finish this first chapter with an inspiring story of Lou, an 88-year-old man, who came to see me when I was associate dean for research in Rochester. He told me that he had been home alone choking on a piece of hard candy a few months ago and almost died. Lou said he threw himself over a chair as a last attempt to dislodge the piece of candy that was obstructing his airway. With that chair maneuver, the piece of candy flew out of his throat and he survived. After this episode, Lou decided to invent a device so that if anyone was ever alone choking, they could use the device to perform a Heimlich maneuver. At that point, he reached into his briefcase and pulled out a very rudimentary looking apparatus. It consisted of a Styrofoam block that was taped to a piece of broom handle. Also taped to the broom handle were paper towel rolls. Lou showed me how the device would be used to perform a Heimlich maneuver if choking. It was his dream for this device to be in every household and assisted living center in the country. I could see how this device could work, yet I was curious as to why Lou had come to see me, so I asked him. Lou responded that he read all about me and my passion for evidence on the university's website. He said that he needed me to get him evidence to support his choking device. That was quite a tall request given I really did not have knowledge about what type of evidence the Heimlich maneuver had behind it. However, I was up for the challenge and, as a result, pulled a team of people together to first search for how the evidence behind the Heimlich maneuver was generated and then determine how we would gather evidence behind Lou's "save-a-life device," which is the name he had given his invention. After some months, I was recruited away to Arizona and left the project in my team's hands. I had forgotten about the project for 4 years until my assistant came into my office one day to inform me that a gentleman named Lou from Rochester was on the phone, insisting to talk with me. I was delighted to pick up the phone and hear Lou's voice. I was ecstatic that he was still alive. Lou said "Bern—do you remember my save-a-life device? I now have a patent on it and a manufacturer in China to mass produce it. Your team in Rochester never finished the project and I now need you to get me the evidence I need to support that this device works!" I flew Lou to Arizona at 92 years of age to meet with me and our university's technology commercialization team. He had a bigger twinkle in his eye and fire in his belly than most 30-, 40-, 50-, and 60-year-olds as his dream was coming to fruition.

I was telling Lou's story to a group of alums, two of whom were tearful in the back of the room. I went up to these two alumni after my talk and asked whether they would share why this story was so emotional for them. The two women said that they had a dream for a health-care company 15 years ago, which they believed would be successful. However, their spouses and their friends told them all the reasons why it would not work. Unfortunately, they listened to these "well-meaning people" and never started their company. They then went on to tell me that they now sit here 15 years later with many regrets. I asked the two women their ages; one replied 70 and the other said 71. I said, "Look at Lou! You have the rest of your lives. Put your dream on the front burner again and start executing." You see, the number one thing that research shows people regret the most in their lives is not what they did, but what they didn't do." Bottom line: Don't let anyone tell you what you can or can't accomplish in your life as you don't want to look back years from now with a lot of regrets. Although Lou has since passed, his device was sold on Amazon for many years—his dream came to fruition.

In **closing**, please do not move on to the next chapter unless you answer my final question, put a date on your answer, and place it where you can see it every single day. If I could be your fairy godmother and give you any wish you could accomplish:

What will you do in the next 5 to 10 years if you know you cannot fail?

Keep dreaming, discovering, and delivering!

KEY TAKEAWAY POINTS

- Don't let anyone discourage you from accomplishing your dreams; keep dreaming, discovering, and delivering!

- How you think affects how you feel and how you behave; changing your thinking can positively change your life.

- You cannot be your best as a leader, innovator, or entrepreneur if you do not take good care of yourself; prioritize your own well-being and take consistent action to optimize it.

- Focus on the important things daily, not the urgent that can detract you from accomplishing your dreams and goals.

- Create a culture in which innovation is the norm; make it easy for people to get excited about new ideas and ways to accomplish them.

- Persist through the "character-builders" until your dreams come to fruition!

REFERENCES

American Association of University Professors. (2017). *Tenure*. Washington, DC: Author. Retrieved from https://www.aaup.org/issues/tenure

Dearing, J. W., & Cox, J. G. (2018). Diffusion of innovations theory, principles and practice. *Health Affairs, 37*(2), 183–190. doi:10.1377/hlthaff.2017.1104

Dickerson, J. F., Lynch, F. L., Leo, M. C., DeBar, L. L., Pearson, J., & Clarke, G. N. (2018). Cost-effectiveness of cognitive behavioral therapy for depressed youth declining antidepressants. *Pediatrics, 141*(2), e20171969. doi:10.1542/peds.2017-1969

Hoying, J., Melnyk, B. M., & Arcoleo, K. (2016). Effects of the COPE cognitive behavioral skills building TEEN program on the healthy lifestyle behaviors and mental health of Appalachian early adolescents. *Journal of Pediatric Health Care, 30*(1), 65–72. doi:10.1016/j.pedhc.2015.02.005

Johnson, S. (2010). *The present: The gift for changing times.* New York, NY: Penguin Random House

Kozlowski, J., Lusk, P., & Melnyk, B. M. (2015). Pediatric nurse practitioner management of child anxiety in the rural primary care clinic with the evidence-based COPE. *Journal of Pediatric Health Care, 29*(3), 274–282. doi:10.1016/j.pedhc.2015.01.009

Lusk, P., & Melnyk, B. M. (2013). COPE for depressed and anxious teens: A brief cognitive-behavioral skills building intervention to increase access to timely, evidence-based treatment. *Journal of Child and Adolescent Psychiatric Nursing, 26*(1), 23–31. doi:10.1111/jcap.12017

Maxwell, J. C. (2009). *How successful people think: Change your thinking, change your life.* New York, NY: Center Street

Melnyk, B. M., Amaya, M., Szalacha, L. A., Hoying, J., Taylor, T., & Bowersox, K. (2015). Feasibility, acceptability and preliminary effects of the COPE on-line cognitive-behavioral skills building program on mental health outcomes and academic performance in freshmen college students: A randomized controlled pilot study. *Journal of Child and Adolescent Psychiatric Nursing, 28*(3), 147–154. doi:10.1111/jcap.12119

Melnyk, B. M., Fineout-Overholt, E., Giggle, M., & Choy, K. (2017). A test of the ARCC© model improves implementation of evidence-based practice, healthcare culture, and patient outcomes. *Worldviews on Evidence-Based Nursing, 14*(1), 5–9. doi:10.1111/wvn.12188

Melnyk, B. M., Jacobson, D., Kelly, S. A., Belyea, M. J., Shaibi, G. Q., Small, L., O'Haver, J. A., & Marsiglia, F. F. (2015). Twelve-month effects of the COPE healthy lifestyles TEEN program on overweight and depression in high school adolescents. *Journal of School Health, 85*(12), 861–870. doi:10.1111/josh.12342

Melnyk, B. M., Jacobson, D., Kelly, S., Belyea, M., Shaibi, G., Small, L., ... Marsiglia, F. F. (2013). Promoting healthy lifestyles in high school adolescents: A randomized controlled trial. *American Journal of Preventive Medicine, 45*(4), 407–415. doi:10.1016/j.amepre.2013.05.013

Melnyk, B. M., Kelly, S., Jacobson, D., Arcoleo, K., & Shaibi, G. (2013). Improving physical activity, mental health outcomes and academic retention of college students with freshman 5 to thrive: COPE/healthy lifestyles. *Journal of the American Academy of Nurse Practitioner, 26*(6), 314–322. doi:10.1002/2327-6924.12037

Merikangas, K., Jian-ping, H., Burstein, M., Swanson, S., Avenevoli, S., Cu, L., ... Swendsen, J. (2010). Lifetime prevalence of mental disorders in U.S. adolescents: Results from the National Comorbidity Survey Replication Adolescent Supplement (NCS-A). *Journal of the American Academy of Child and Adolescent Psychiatry, 49*(10), 980–989. doi:10.1016/j.jaac.2010.05.017

Peale, N. V. (1956). *The power of positive thinking*. Englewood Cliffs, N.J: Prentice-Hall.

Schwartz, D. J. (1987). *The magic of thinking big*. Marietta, GA: Fireside Printing.

Wang, Z., Whiteside, S. P. H., Sim, L., Farah, W., Morrow, A. S., Alsawas, M., ... Murad, M. H. (2017). Comparative effectiveness and safety of cognitive behavioral therapy and pharmacotherapy for childhood anxiety disorders: A systematic review and meta-analysis. *JAMA Pediatrics, 171*(11), 1049–1056. doi:10.1001/jamapediatrics.2017.3036

Watkins, M. D. (2013). *The first 90 days: Proven strategies for getting up to speed faster and smarter*. Boston: Harvard Business Review Press.

Weersing, V. R., Brent, D. A., Rozenman, M. S., Gonzalez, A., Jeffreys, M., Dickerson, J. F... Iyengar, S. (2017). Brief behavioral therapy for pediatric anxiety and depression in primary care: A randomized clinical trial. *JAMA Psychiatry, 74*(6), 571–578.

Understanding Yourself and Developing as a Leader

T. Scott Graham

"The most important single ingredient in the formula of success is knowing how to get along with people."—Theodore Roosevelt

LEARNING OBJECTIVES
- Gain an understanding of yourself as a leader.
- Take action to further develop yourself as a leader.
- Describe key strategies for becoming an effective leader.

INTRODUCTION

The title of this chapter suggests vital steps and insights that must be embraced to understand what it takes to lead and then to develop yourself into an effective leader. For everyone, this is a very personal, individual dive into the practice of leadership. First focus on self and develop personal skills before leading others. Further, understand yourself before engaging in self-development. According to the Center for Creative Leadership (2018), self-awareness serves as a foundation for strengthening all other leadership skills. However, you need to be more than self-aware. Once one is self-aware, the vital second step is doing something with that knowledge.

This chapter highlights several evidence-based and vital strategies you can use to gain a better understanding of yourself as a leader. It then provides strategies and techniques to develop leadership skills.

PEOPLE SKILLS

"I believe that you can get everything in life you want if you will just help enough other people get what they want."—Zig Zigler

The first and most vital skill for a leader is skill with people. Nearly everyone has heard a comment such as this at some point: "Boy, he/she could really use some work on his/her people skills," or "My boss is great. She has those special people skills that make you want to be a better employee, even a better person."

So, what are people talking about when they say "people skills"? They might mean *emotional and social intelligence (ESI)*. We have to be smart and skillful about how we bring our personalities, experiences, and unique way of connecting to others, and yes, our emotions, to our work environments.

The Center for Creative Leadership (Ruderman, Hannum, Leslie, & Steed, 2001) published a research-based paper that showed key leadership skills and perspectives are directly related to those vital people skills or ESI competencies. The research also demonstrated that the absence of ESI competencies is strongly connected to career derailment (i.e., falling off the success track).

Research conducted by one of the leading leadership research organizations in the world confirms the importance of ESI. Depending on which ESI expert you read and follow, the list of skills is different. The model that the Center for Creative Leadership supports is the Bar-On Emotional Quotient Inventory, or EQi (Stein & Book, 2011).

Table 3.1 lists the 15 people skills (competencies) you need to be successful at work and in life, along with a bit of information related to each:

TABLE 3.1 Emotional Quotient Inventory People Skills

People Skill	Definition
Emotional self-awareness	Understanding one's own feelings
Assertiveness	Expressing and standing up for oneself
Independence	Being self-directed and self-controlled
Self-regard	Accepting oneself as good
Self-actualization	Attaining one's full potential
Empathy	Being aware of, and understanding, others' feelings
Social responsibility	Being a cooperative and constructive member of one's social group
Interpersonal relationships	Establishing and maintaining mutually satisfying relationships
Problem-solving	Defining problems with effective solutions
Reality testing	Aligning the subjective emotional with the objective reality
Flexibility	Adjusting to changing situations
Stress tolerance	Coping successfully with adversity and strong emotions
Impulse control	Resisting or delaying an impulse, drive, or action
Happiness	Being happy and satisfied with one's life and oneself
Optimism	Having a positive attitude, especially during times of adversity

CALL TO ACTION

Assess yourself; then make copies of this assessment for others and have them provide input to see whether what you think about your skills aligns with what others observe.

People Skills Self-Assessment

These are the interpersonal and intrapersonal (people) competencies that research shows are vital for success. Rate yourself on how strongly you agree you have them (Exhibit 3.1; Graham, 2017).

EXHIBIT 3.1 **Self Rating Scale**

People Skills Self-Assessment Statement	Strongly Disagree 1	Disagree 2	Neutral/ Unsure 3	Agree 4	Strongly Agree 5
1. I understand my own feelings in most situations.					
2. I can express and stand up for myself.					
3. I am self-directed and self-controlled.					
4. I accept myself as good.					
5. I believe I have attained or can attain my full potential.					
6. I am aware of, and understand, others' feelings.					
7. I am a cooperative and constructive member of my social group.					
8. I establish and maintain mutually satisfying relationships.					
9. I can define problems and provide effective solutions.					
10. My subjective emotions are congruent with objective reality.					
11. I adjust well to changing situations.					
12. I cope successfully with adversity and strong emotions.					
13. I resist or delay any action that can be construed as impulsive.					
14. I get enjoyment and satisfaction from my life and myself.					
15. I have a positive attitude, especially during times of adversity.					

People Skills Assessment by Others

Exhibit 3.2 lists the interpersonal and intrapersonal (people) competencies that research shows are vital for success (Graham, 2017).

EXHIBIT 3.2 **Leader Rating Scale**

People Skills Assessment Statement	Strongly Disagree 1	Disagree 2	Neutral/ Unsure 3	Agree 4	Strongly Agree 5
1. My leader understands people's feelings in most situations.					
2. My leader can express and stand up for him- or herself.					
3. My leader is self-directed and self-controlled.					
4. My leader accepts him/herself as good.					
5. My leader believes she or he can attain her or his full potential.					
6. My leader is aware of, and understands others' feelings.					
7. My leader is a cooperative and constructive member of his or her social group.					
8. My leader establishes and maintains mutually satisfying relationships.					
9. My leader can define problems and provide effective solutions.					
10. My leader's subjective emotions are congruent with objective reality.					
11. My leader adjusts well to changing situations.					
12. My leader can cope successfully with adversity and strong emotions.					
13. My leader resists or delays any action that can be construed as impulsive.					
14. My leader gets enjoyment and satisfaction from his or her life and self.					
15. My leader has a positive attitude, especially during times of adversity.					

CALL TO ACTION

Rate how strongly your leader has the qualities listed in Exhibit 3.2.

Based on the assessment, what are this leader's top two people skills/strengths?

Based on the assessment, what are the top two areas related to people skills that this leader needs to improve?

What is the one big thing you wish this leader would stop doing, start doing, and/or change related to his or her people skills? Why did you choose that one?

Understanding and developing yourself as a leader is only partially covered with the competencies focused on with ESI. There are other vital areas that will need to be understood if one is to develop as a leader. Five of these come from *The Leadership Challenge* by Kouzes and Posner (2017).

Five Practices of Exemplary Leadership

"Leadership is everyone's business!"—James Kouzes and Barry Posner

For nearly three decades, researchers and authors Drs. Barry Posner and Jim Kouzes published their research findings in *The Leadership Challenge*, now in its sixth edition, highlighting the top four traits of exemplary leaders. These four traits have been the top vote getters when key decision makers examined an extensive list of traits they sought in team members: Honesty, competence, forward-looking, and inspiring (Kouzes & Posner, 2017). As Stephen Covey said in *The Seven Habits of Highly Effective People* (2013), to be effective and successful, one must begin with the end in mind. With these four traits in mind, one then needs to determine how to achieve these, and how to make these four traits become habits.

Posner and Kouzes offer five practices of exemplary leaders: Model the Way, Inspire a Shared Vision, Challenge the Process, Enable Others to Act, and Encourage the Heart. Each of these practices surfaced from the data collected over decades to make the concepts become real. The first practice being highlighted is Model the Way.

CALL TO ACTION

Look at the partial list of values given in Table 3.2 and pick three that are very important to you . . . that is, you value them so much they guide your words and actions each day. Then respond to these questions. Talk about these with those who would benefit from knowing this about you.

1. What do these values look like to others?
2. How would someone know these three guiding principles are important to you?
3. Give an example of how each played out in your life this past week.

TABLE 3.2 **List of Potential Values That Guide You**

Achievement	Fame	Peace
Adventure	Friendships	Pleasure
Authenticity	Fun	Poise
Authority	Growth	Popularity
Autonomy	Happiness	Recognition
Balance	Honesty	Religion
Beauty	Humor	Reputation
Boldness	Influence	Respect
Challenge	Inner harmony	Responsibility
Citizenship	Justice	Security
Community	Kindness	Self-respect
Compassion	Knowledge	Service
Competency	Leadership	Spirituality
Contribution	Learning	Stability
Creativity	Love	Status
Curiosity	Loyalty	Success
Determination	Meaningful work	Trustworthiness
Fairness	Openness	Wealth
Faith	Optimism	Wisdom

Modeling the Way means to model the behavior that is expected of others. As Eric Harvey says in *The Leadership Secrets of Santa Clause* (Harvey, 2015), one must behave his or her beliefs. Leaders must lead from what they believe, sometimes called *core values*, or *guiding principles*. People should know what a leader's core values are by watching and listening to him or her—in that order. Actions DO speak louder than words to others, but both are vitally important. Be aware, people follow the person, and then they follow the plan.

Inspiring a Shared Vision is dreaming of what can be accomplished with you and your team. It is having or gaining a desire to make something happen, change the way things are, and create something that no one else has ever created before. This clear image of the future keeps you moving forward and encourages others to follow you. Leadership is a dialogue, not a monologue. Be enthusiastic.

Challenging the Process means seeking and accepting challenges. Be a pioneer. Step into the unknown. Make it safe for others to experiment, when and where it makes sense. Freely admit your mistakes as you go. Break mind-sets. Give people choices. Also, do not forget to add fun to everyone's work.

Enabling Others to Act is evidenced by your use of the word "we" and how often it is used. Ask questions, listen, and take advice. At staff meetings, stop talking and start building relationships and safe conversation spaces. Create places and opportunities for informal interactions, creating a learning climate filled with lots of human moments.

Encourage the Heart by finding people doing things right, and rewarding and recognizing them in ways that work for *them*. Be creative about rewards, but also tailor them to the needs and interests of the recipients. Say "thank you" frequently. Provide feedback on the workplace-learning journey. Be positive and constructive. Show passion and compassion as you demonstrate caring by walking around. Care for others routinely!

As stated by the fishmongers of the Pike Place Fish Market in their popular book *Fish! Sticks* (Lundin, Christensen, & Paul, 2011), to make these habits stick, live the words every day. Then, commit to doing that action. Once these habits are formed, you owe it to others to coach them. With all you have learned and become, you now owe it to others to share your strengths and skills by helping them to become more competent and confident. Coaching the leadership practices and ESI competencies requires you to understand and develop your coaching skill set, which is the focus of the next section.

COACHING FOR SUCCESS

If we think of coaches and coaching, we typically think of the stern tough athletic coach who expertly motivates and inspires the team with passionate locker-room speeches. Coaching is a skill set that anyone who aspires to show leadership can learn, adapt, and adopt. Experience has highlighted a number of competencies that help a leader become a great leader/coach. Some of those mentioned most frequently in nearly three decades of leadership workshops follow (Graham, 2017).

Eleven Suggestions on Ways to Be an Effective Coach

1. **Communicate clear expectations to group members.** These are questions to help you know whether you are communicating clearly. If people are not clear on expectations, how can they do their jobs?

    Are my expectations crystal clear? (If yes, how do you know?) Have they received the training needed to do the job right? Do they understand why it is important to do the job correctly? Am I holding people accountable for their performance? Are there appropriate and consistent consequences for nonperformance? Do I recognize and reward positive performance? Have I given them the freedom to be successful? Are they facing any obstacles to performing as desired? How do I know? Are my expectations reasonable?

2. **Build relationships.** Find ways to connect with others and cultivate relationships and networks.

3. **Give feedback on areas that require specific improvement.** Do this in a timely, appropriate, helpful manner.

4. **Listen actively.** Be in the moment when you are talking and listening to another. Avoid distractions, including technology.

5. **Help remove obstacles.** What stands in individuals' ways to reach success? What can you do about it? What will you do about it?

6. **Give emotional support when and where needed.** Stress is all around us, and to listen and care may be all you can offer, and it may be all that is needed. It often is.

7. **Reflect content or meaning** to ensure that all involved understand the job, the communication's intent, and the definition of success.

8. **Give some gentle advice and guidance** when and where needed. Be there for your people. Often, it helps to ask for permission to offer advice.

9. **Allow for modeling of desired performance and behavior.** Give others the opportunity to try, and fail, where it makes sense and cannot harm anyone.

10. **Gain a commitment to change.** Understand what success looks like, and how your colleagues can get there from where they are.

11. **Applaud good results.** Determine whether the person prefers public or private recognition.

Focus on Strengths to Engage

"If human beings are perceived as potentials rather than problems, as possessing strengths instead of weaknesses, as unlimited rather that dull and unresponsive, then they thrive and grow to their capabilities."—Former First Lady Barbara Bush

The Gallup Organization has led much of the research into engagement, so it would be helpful to underscore the importance of engagement using Gallup's definitions of *engagement, disengagement,* and *active disengagement.*

Engaged employees work with passion and connect profoundly to their organization. They drive innovation and move the organization forward. They offer discretionary effort to do great work. Disengaged employees are essentially "checked out." They are sleepwalking through the workday, putting in time, but not energy or passion. The actively disengaged employee is not just unhappy at work; he or she is busy acting out that unhappiness. Every day, these workers undermine what their engaged coworkers attempt to successfully accomplish (O'Boyle & Harter, 2013).

A chapter on understanding and developing yourself as a leader must include information and research into the vital topic of engagement by focusing on one's strengths. To engage self and others, one must use more of what he or she is good at (your strengths) and use fewer weaknesses (Buckingham, 2015). Meanwhile, too often our strengths and talents get little attention as we assume they continue to be used and remain strong.

 CALL TO ACTION

Think of this example: You work in a job that requires an overabundance of detailed work with math, numbers, and spreadsheets. You hate that part of your job, but the few times you get a chance to organize a social event for the organization, you not only jump at this chance, you feel energized. The research shows that those who get to push themselves and to do more of what they love because they are talented at it and have the strengths in those key areas are vastly more likely to be engaged. In this example, if you never get a chance to use your strengths, but are asked day in and day out to "crunch numbers," you likely will be one of the 51% of the workforce who is actively seeking another job (Gallup, 2013).

If you do not understand your own strengths and cannot figure out a way to use more of them every day, you will constantly be disengaged, unhappy, unmotivated, and missing one of the main motivators in life. There is a saying in the popular literature: "If you do what you love, you'll never have to work a day in your life." Figure out what you are good at (your talents, your strengths) and find ways to put more of those skills into play each day. If you cannot put them into play, perhaps that is a key indicator you are in a job/career/profession that is not a good fit for you, and you should consider a career change.

CALL TO ACTION

Consider getting these resources: *Now Discover Your Strengths*, *StrengthsFinder 2.0*, and *Go Put Your Strengths to Work*. Read the first book and get the second book to take the assessment. Read over your results and share these with others who know you well to ensure they are an accurate picture of you. Then, get the third book in this list and make a plan to push yourself toward more use of your strengths each day.

CASE STUDY ON SELF-DEVELOPMENT

Jessica was a 42-year-old head nurse for a large health network in California. She was very successful in her career as a clinician, winning awards for her patient satisfaction scores and commitment to quality. She worked on a busy intercity ICU with more than 50 other highly skilled clinicians, staff members, and contract personnel, where she rose as high as she could in the organization without going into a management position. She often said in passing, "I would rather be fired than be promoted to management."

Her boss and the chief nursing officer, Daniele, took her aside one day and said, "I will be blunt. I see something in you that makes me think there is more in store for you in this organization. I want you to be my next ICU nurse manager."

It would mean a significant promotion, a pay raise, and a major change in her job function. This was *management* and that was something she said she would never do. Floored, Jessica asked, "Why me?"

Daniele replied that Jessica was detail-oriented, a good listener, a skilled problem solver, optimistic but with a realistic slant, a team player, and she cared about her teammates. These strengths all were a good match for the nurse management position.

Jessica said, "Daniele, I am flattered, but this is a gigantic career change for me. I need to give it some thought." Her role would change considerably. She needed to know that she would be able to use her intimate knowledge of the technical world to help her understand problems, but her major challenges would be dealing with, managing, leading, and caring for people. She would be supportive but would often have to make tough calls. Not everyone would love all of her decisions, and she would have to be okay with that.

Currently, Jessica was a team member. As a nurse manager, she would be the team's leader. She could be friendly but would need to ensure she was not showing favoritism. The skills she needed to bring to this new position were different.

Jessica called Daniele the next day to ask whether she would support Jessica attending a 2-week "Transition to Leadership" workshop offered by the local university. Enrollment in the workshop would gain Jessica her own leadership coach for 6 months to use as needed. Daniele supported that. Jessica talked to many of her team members, her networks, and her family, and decided to take the risk and accept the challenge.

Six months later, Jessica was delighted with her decision. She had learned a lot regarding how to be a more confident and competent leader. She also found a good mentor to help her with growth and development. In addition, Jessica enrolled in a graduate healthcare leadership and innovation program at a local, nationally regarded university.

Moral: Sometimes you must take a leap of faith and step into the unknown to challenge yourself. **Success comes from trying, failing, and succeeding, and trying some more.** Leadership is a series of successes and failures combined to help yourself, your team, your organization, and society. The best way to learn leadership is to volunteer to lead, but doing so with as much information and preparation as is practical given the situation and timing.

🔑 KEY TAKEAWAY POINTS

- *Get an accountability partner/coach.* Find someone who is very good at a people skill you wish to improve. This should be someone who can observe you in action versus someone at a great distance who cannot. Then, ask this person whether he or she will offer you tips and suggestions about what may work better for you in a particular area. You can have two or three of these type of people working with you at any one time. The timelier the feedback and suggestions, and the more frequent, the more likely you are to improve.

- *Be aware of your thoughts and feelings and the associated body language that shows those feelings.* Look in a mirror to see what your facial expressions may be "telling" others. Practice emotional expressions, in a mirror, by yourself. See whether a trusted friend or spouse will be able to guess the emotion you are trying to relay. This can be fun and funny and is worth the effort.

- *Just say no.* Learn to be assertive by being able to say no in a nice professionally acceptable way. Practice different ways, such as "My plate is simply too full right now to add more. I am sorry. I wish I could, but I would want to do a great job and I will not be able to give it my full effort." The backup plan is always "Let me look at my schedule and commitments and get back to you by (date/time)." This buys you time and allows you to avoid saying, "Okay, sure."

- *Listen to your self-talk.* Is it mired in harmful conversations, such as "What if I make a wrong decision? I may look foolish and feel humiliated. I will not be able to live with that type of embarrassment." Write down arguments against these self-talk statements, as well as arguments to overcome them with positive self-talk, such as "I know part of learning is taking risks. I am willing to do this so I can be a more confident, competent person." I may even have to tell folks, "I am trying to work on being more self-reliant, and it is kind of empowering."

- *Pay close attention to others' facial expressions and body language to try to understand their feelings.* Parrot back what you think others may be thinking and feeling based on those indicators. Seek verification of your assessment of the situation by asking people, "How does/did that make you feel?" In other words, do not be afraid of validating others' feelings.

- *Write down three worthwhile things/actions you can do to help others.* These may be family members, community organizations, coworkers, or even strangers. Pick items you are passionate about and know would help you feel like a more well-rounded person/team member. Commit to the actions. Have a timeline of when you will do them. Examples are getting coworkers to share one positive action they took at work, or asking what each person did that day to make a positive difference in someone's life.

■ *Try to be more sociable and socialize more.* People like and are more attracted to sociable people. Think about ways you can meet and network with people and what you can do with and for others. Make a real effort not to let friendships get cold. Try reconnecting with old friends or acquaintances you have not seen in a while. Use social media to reconnect, if appropriate. People will see you as more likable and will respond more positively to you.

■ *De-stress.* In our hectic world, it may help to divide larger tasks into smaller, more manageable chunks and concentrate only on those tasks that truly require your attention now. Exercise. Take a walk with someone. Move. Change your scenery. Take a break. Breathe deeply. Close your eyes and visualize a pleasant memory, place, or time.

■ *Fun, fun, fun.* What do you find that is fun in life? What makes you smile and brings you happiness? Seek ways to add more fun to your daily routine. See *fun* as a valuable and worthy goal in and of itself. When possible, surround yourself with happy people and avoid downers. Complain less; enjoy more. Identify what makes you unhappy, and minimize or eliminate it. Smile more; frown less. Look in a mirror if you cannot tell the difference!

■ *Focus on affirming others.* Give feedback that is more positive. Try to suppress your pessimistic self-talk. Find out what boosts others' morale. Everyone is unique. One size of morale boosting does not fit all (Graham, 2017).

CHAPTER BONUSES

The following areas are also vitally important in understanding and developing yourself as a leader. Given here are specific, tested strategies of self-development.

Chapter Bonus #1

How to Understand and Develop Self as a Leader: Leading Change

On Understanding and Developing the Ability to Change (Bridges & Bridges, 2017; Graham, 2017)

1. Explain the change and reasons for it. Do this repeatedly. Respond as quickly and clearly as you can. If you do not know the answer, *find out*. In the absence of good information, people plug the holes with misinformation, rumors, and lies.

2. Listen, listen, and listen. Do not try to talk your team members out of what they are feeling. If what they are feeling is based on bad information, help them with good information. Then listen some more.

3. Gently remind them of the reality. As they internally process the change, remind them of the change's realities, softly and gently, based on where they are with change.

4. Focus on Bridges' 4 Ps. Be clear on the *purpose* (reason) of the change by asking whether they understand it. Share their *part* in the new change. Share as much of the *plan* as you know and have permission to reveal. Explain what the *picture* of the new change will look like.

5. Promote supportive group events, interaction, and social time for all to be together. These are real people with real emotional needs. Often, informal gatherings (with refreshments to show you care) are good forums for people to vent, talk, laugh, cry, and just be human as they grasp the realities of life and work.

6. Acknowledge and sympathize with your team. You are not bargaining or telling them what they want to hear but acknowledging, "This is a difficult and challenging change for you, and for many of us. We have to do the best we can to get through how to make this work. I certainly know how difficult this must feel to you right now. I will be as supportive as I can to help the entire team be successful and confident in our success moving forward."

7. It takes time. Do not rush the team through its emotions. Do not expect members to embrace change overnight. Some adapt faster than others do. Those who "come aboard" early can be tremendous ambassadors for the change. Ask the early adopters to help you as you help everyone understand the *good* and *positive* parts of the change, especially early on.

8. Map out and celebrate small victories. As the change begins to take root, wherever and whenever there is success, highlight that to everyone. Find out why it was successful, and ask those who are embracing change to help those who seem challenged by the change.

9. Be honest and consistent. Tell the same story to all; be consistent with the message. As the message becomes clearer, continue to update people. Be honest. If you destroy the team's trust, they will never believe anything you have to say regarding the change.

10. Provide opportunities to practice and fail. Yes, some will likely fail at first. Ensure that plans are in place that factors this in. Safety is of paramount importance in instituting some changes, so failure may not be an option there. However, for most changes, expect a drop in productivity, morale, and goal attainment. It will take time for people to figure out what to do.

Chapter Bonus #2

How to Understand and Develop Self As a Leader: Communication Competencies

Top 10 Communication Areas for Leaders' Nonverbal Communication

- Pay attention to clues like eye contact, facial expressions, gestures, posture, body movements, and tone of voice (beyond the words).

- Match words with nonverbal cues; for example, he says he is happy, but is frowning, kicking the ground, and glaring at you.

- Listen to your tone of voice. Do you sound enthusiastic, uninterested, upset, or afraid?

- Make eye contact. Too little and you may appear to be evading or hiding something. Too much and it may intimidate and seem confrontational.

- Ask questions of clarification if you receive a nonverbal response, or mixed or confusing signals. You may say, "Is this what you are saying ...?"

- Match nonverbal signals and gestures with your words.
- Consider the context; is it formal or informal?
- Try not to misread signals. Do not assume, for example, a weak handshake means disinterest or no fortitude. It could simply mean the person has a muscular problem.
- Observe and practice. Watch who aligns verbal and nonverbal communication and is extremely effective at it. Take mental notes of what they do and how they do it.

  Then practice emulating that behavior … and practice it a lot (Graham, 2017).

One-on-Ones

- Choose words you believe the receiver will understand.
- Be courteous. Take turns. Do not interrupt.
- Be well read so you can speak on a number of topics and participate in conversations involving many interests.
- Be enthusiastic as a speaker and as a listener. If you are flat and dull, people will drift off or "log out."
- Be aware of your words, the tone of your voice, and your nonverbal language in this one-on-one environment.

One-on-Team

- Inspire others with a clear vision, or ideas to get behind. Know their passions and yours, and be able to merge the two with inspiring words. Listen. Your employees need to see how they fit into this vision and the role they play. They need a picture of what this will look and feel like.
- Surround yourself with engaged, focused people. You want to work with good listeners.
- Teach others how to see what you see for the team. If they see the meaning and purpose, they will catch the momentum and push the team along.
- Be aware of the signals you are sending. Ask those who know you best to tell you what signals you send to others. Be open to changing them if they present the wrong messages.

One-on-Organization (Giving a Public Address or Presentation to a Large Group)

- Breathe to relax. It is okay to pause.
- Make an outline and print it larger than usual. If on a stage, you can have note posters flat on the ground, where only *you* see them, to keep your thoughts flowing.
- Be confident. You are the expert; act like it. Own what you know (probably better than anyone else there).
- Make eye contact by slowly scanning the audience and looking for particular people, then look into their eyes.
- Practice in advance. Let others in a small group hear, watch, and provide specific, helpful feedback on what would make your presentation better (assessing the words and nonverbal cues).
- Take questions at the end.
- Do not worry too much about timing.

- Be aware of your nervous habits, such as saying "um"/"uh," flipping a pencil, jingling change in your pocket, or twiddling your thumbs.
- If you hear yourself say "um" or "uh," slow down, take a breath, and then speak.
- Bring a bottle of cool water to avoid cottonmouth.

Observe and Listen

- Stop talking. If you are talking, you are not listening. This is true with self-talk, too.
- Make space for listening, physical and mental space. Make room for focused listening, and let the noise die down so you can stay in that space.
- Pause for reactions. Take time to let what you hear sink in. Notice reactions, both verbal and nonverbal.
- Do not judge people. Wait. Give them an opportunity to speak.
- Focus by making eye contact, nodding affirmatively, leaning toward them, or encouraging them to go on. Do not interrupt or be a sentence finisher, ask open questions or summarize.
- Visualize what they are saying to you.
- Remember names. Repeat them, such as by saying, "Hi, Jason, nice to meet you." Fold their names into the conversation. Associate the person with something or someone you can visualize in order to recall names later.
- Use questions to show you are in the moment.
- Be in the moment. Force yourself to let go of competing thoughts.
- Look at the person you are talking to.
- Tune out extraneous noise.
- Repeat back key learning to ensure you heard it correctly.

Ask Questions

- Facts are instantly available on a smartphone, but questions require more thought and reflection.
- Challenge your own beliefs and assumptions. Open your mind to your subject's complexity. Before registering your opinion, allow your mind to slip into a state of not knowing. You let others feel ownership of decisions through questioning.
- "Whose decision is this?" If it is yours, ask questions of others to arrive at the best answer you can in the time you have. If it is someone else's decision, ask questions to help him or her. Help the decision maker gain ownership, which creates engagement, drive, and efficiency.
- If you do not trust others to make good decisions, mentor them so they learn how to do so. They will either rise to the challenge or not. If not, it may be time for training, or provide them an opportunity to seek their success elsewhere (i.e., fire them).
- It is easy to give others the solutions, right or wrong. It is hard to ask questions, especially if you *think* you know the answers. However, if you are open to the possibility that there might be better options in other people's heads, you will become even more effective.
- If people keep coming to you for answers, you need to keep coming back at them even harder with challenging, open-ended questions.

Give Feedback

- Make it about work performance (positive or negative).
- Communicate directly to that person; do not share with others and then tell that person later.
- Do it within 24 hours of the event.
- Choose a private place.
- Balance negative feedback with positive feedback, too. Not *all* feedback is or should be negative/corrective. Reread that statement.
- Show respect.
- Accept some of the responsibility as it makes it easier for the person to accept it.
- Be specific.
- Explain why this is a problem (if it is).
- Ask and listen.
- Be open and empathetic.
- Agree with what is going on. Solve the problem together. Get buy-in from the person on a workable, helpful solution.
- Be quiet. Let the person talk. Ask for feedback.
- Share your own personal stories, if and when they relate.
- Offer support.
- Be persistent. Agree to a date to review progress, and keep that date firm.
- Help others to learn how to give feedback to their peers. Coach this skill in them so not everyone feels the need to come to you.

Feedback Formula for Success:

Balanced start: "I like the way you …"
Explain what: "I've noticed when you … that …" Explain why: "I feel …" or "It is a problem because …"
Be specific: "Your handling of Customer X this morning, especially the way you soothed his nerves when he was irate, was perfect."
Check his or her view: "What do you think? Am I being reasonable?"
Work out change: "What solutions can we come up with together? What solutions have you thought of? How can we solve this? In the future, would you please …?"
Agree: "So we agree that … right?"
Ask for feedback: "Is there anything you think I should be doing differently?" Follow up. Make an appointment to meet again.

Persuasion

Being persuasive and influential are key skills for leaders. It is vital to get the support and co-operation of others to help leaders reach their goals and the organization's goals. Leaders need people.

- Enter their world; pretend you are in their place. What are they thinking? What would I do if I were they? What would my thoughts, feelings, and opinions be?

- Mirror their body language; observe how they act, speak, and think. Act like them. Mirror their speech for clarity and pace. Be careful not to come across as mocking. Be subtle and choosy about what you mimic.

- Be optimistic, cheerful, and nice. People gravitate to and like others who make their day brighter and lighter.

- Be sincere and trustworthy. Overdeliver on expectations. Make them feel you are the go-to person when something needs doing right. Be sincere with your compliments.

- Show evidence that your ideas are compelling and perhaps most effective. Use testimonials, focus-group results, before-and-after scenarios, and/or comparison data.

- Give them the WIIFT (What is in it for them?) answers. What do they want? What do you provide that satisfies this?

- Care about them. Focus on *their* interests, desires, needs, and expectations. This builds trust.

Self-Talk

- Usually the self-talk patterns start in childhood.

- Notice your patterns as they happen in your head (both positive and negative self-talk).

- Keep a journal; this helps you understand what you are hearing in your mind. Do this as you go along or at the day's end.

- Say "Stop!" aloud or loudly in your mind when negative thoughts take over.

- Put a rubber band on your wrist. When you have a negative thought about yourself, snap the band on your arm to get a negative feedback sting.

- Replace negative thoughts with positives, or use milder wording.

- Change "I hate" to "I really dislike" and "I am so mad" to "I am a bit upset." Make it milder and less over the top.

- Turn negatives (like a flight cancellation) into nonfactors or positives ("I can catch up on work, emails, calling friends …").

- Turn self-limiting statements into positive questions: from "I cannot do this" to "How can I find a way to do this?"

Technology and Communication

- Focus on how and what technology does to enhance the value you bring to the workplace. If you ask yourself at the end of each work period—"What did I accomplish today and did I earn my pay?"—and you feel good about your answer, that is a good thing. If you only can point to things that ate up your time but did not earn real results or positive outcomes, then that may be a red flag.

- Turn the technology off when you can. Most of us can; we simply do not. Develop empathy with face-to-face interactions. Some suggest this skill is eroding.

- Relationships cannot be forged on a deep level in an all-text world. If all I know about you comes from texting, and I know another person on a deeper, interpersonal level, who do you think will come to mind when I need someone or want to recommend someone for an opportunity?

- Do not use Facebook at work unless you need it for work (e.g., human resources personnel may use it to help screen potential job applicants). Do not check your personal email at work.

- When at work, turn off communication devices unless you have to have them to work. Keep them off.

- It is not enough to understand technology, its impact, and its connection to communication for leadership development. Knowledge is partial power. Taking action is what really matters once you understand it.

CONCLUSIONS

Before one can lead others, one must understand one's self. This chapter served as a starting point on the journey of leadership self-discovery. The focus covered ESI, five practices of exemplary leadership, strengths-based engagement, coaching, change, and communications. These are all areas that must be understood and developed to experience genuine connection to others.

Dr. Ken Blanchard sums up leadership best in a way that connects all of these competencies. According to Blanchard, leadership is *"the capacity to influence others by unleashing the potential and power of people and organizations for the greater good"* (2010, p. xvi).

 CALL TO ACTION

Commitment and Accountability

Putting Ideas Into Action on Self-Development
What one specific behavior will you commit to start doing, stop doing, and/or change how you do based on this chapter?

Specific Behavior That I Will Commit to	By When?	I Will Share This Commitment With ...

I (your name here) _____ commit to focus on the specific behavior outlined here for 6 months. I give my accountability partner (AP) my permission to ask me often what and how I am doing with this commitment.

Date: _____   Your Signature: _____

Date: _____   AP Signature: _____

> **CALLS TO ACTION**
> 1. Assess self using the 15-item self-assessment in Exhibit 3.1.
> 2. Assess self using the 15-item assessment in Exhibit 3.2 by asking AT LEAST THREE OTHERS (who know you well enough to provide feedback).
> 3. Come up with ONE action item to implement using this assessment, and find someone who will help to hold you accountable to work on your action item.

REFERENCES

Blanchard, K. (2010). *Leading at a higher level: Blanchard on how to be a high performing leader* (2nd ed.). Philadelphia, PA: Trans-Atlantic Publications.

Bridges, W., & Bridges, S. (2017). *Managing transitions: Making the most of change*. Boston, MA: Da Capo Press.

Buckingham, M. (2015). *StandOut 2.0: Assess your strengths, find your edge, win at work*. Boston, MA: Harvard Business Review Press.

Center for Creative Leadership. (2018). *4 sure-fire ways to boost your self-awareness*. Retrieved from www.ccl.org/articles/leading-effectively-articles/4-ways-boost-self-awareness/

Covey, S. R. (2013). *The 7 habits of highly effective people: Powerful lessons in personal change* (Anniversary Edition). New York, NY: Simon & Schuster.

Gallup. (2013). *State of the global workplace*. Washington, D. C.: Gallup Organization.

Graham, T. S. (2017). *Leadership boosters: How to make an immediate positive impact on those you lead*. Indianapolis, IN: Lulu Publishing.

Harvey, E. (2015). *Leadership secrets of Santa Claus: How to get big things done in YOUR "Workshop"… all year long*. Naperville, IL: Sourcebooks.

Kouzes, J. M., & Posner, B. Z. (2017). *The leadership challenge: How to make extraordinary things happen in organizations* (6th ed.). Hoboken, NJ: Jossey-Bass.

Lundin, S. C., Christensen, J., Lundin, S. C., Paul, H., & Christensen, J. (2011). *Fish! sticks: A remarkable way to adapt to changing times and keep your work fresh*. London, England: Hodder and Stoughton.

O'Boyle, E., & Harter, J. (2013). State of the American workplace: Employee engagement insights for US business leaders. Washington, DC: Gallup.

Ruderman, M., Hannum, K., Leslie, J. B., & Steed, J. L. (2001). Making the connection: Leadership skills and emotional intelligence. *LIA Center for Creative Leadership*, 21(5), 3–7.

Stein, S. J., & Book, H. E. (2011). *The EQ edge: Emotional intelligence and your success*. Ontario, Canada: John Wiley & Sons.

Key Strategies for Optimizing Personal Health and Well-Being: A Necessity for Effective Leadership

Bernadette Mazurek Melnyk and Susan Neale

"You cannot take good care of others unless you prioritize yourself and your own self-care!"—Bernadette Melnyk

LEARNING OBJECTIVES

- Describe each of the nine dimensions of wellness.
- Discuss how the nine dimensions interrelate for optimal well-being.
- Identify key strategies for improving your well-being in each area.
- Create a plan to improve at least two dimensions of personal well-being.

INTRODUCTION

Although nurses, other clinicians, and healthcare leaders take great care of others, they often do not prioritize their own self-care. As a result, the effects of burnout, compassion fatigue, depression, and suicide have become a major public health problem across the United States for healthcare professionals and leaders. Burnout and depression now affect over 50% of clinicians in the United States (Dzau, Kirch, & Nasca, 2018; McHugh, Kutney-Lee, Cimiotti, Sloane, & Aiken, 2011; Melnyk et al., 2018; Shanafelt et al., 2015) and compromise the quality and safety of healthcare, as nurses and physicians who are experiencing poor mental and physical health are at greater risk of making medical errors. A recent national study of over 2,300 nurses from 19 healthcare systems throughout the country found that depression was the leading cause of medical errors (Melnyk et al., 2018). In this study, nurses who reported poor mental or physical health had a 26% to 71% higher likelihood of making medical errors. Further, most nursing leaders experience fatigue (Steege, Pinekenstein, Arsenault Knudsen, & Rainbow, 2017) and findings from research support that a leader's stress and emotional well-being affect those on his or her staff (Skakon, Neilsen, Borg, & Guzman, 2010). Therefore, it is critical that healthcare leaders and clinicians prioritize their own self-care so that they can achieve optimal health and well-being for themselves, support a high level of wellness in their staff, and deliver the highest quality of safe care to others.

One out of two individuals in the United States has a chronic condition and one out of four has multiple chronic conditions, yet 80% of chronic disease can be prevented with healthy lifestyle behaviors, such as 30 minutes of physical activity 5 days a week, consumption of five fruits and vegetables per day, not smoking, limiting alcohol intake, and regularly engaging in stress-reduction activities (Ford, Zhao, Tsai, & Li, 2011). Healthcare providers who engage in these healthy behaviors themselves are more likely to counsel their patients on healthy lifestyles (Oberg & Frank, 2011). Although registered nurses comprise the largest healthcare workforce in the United States, they have fewer healthy lifestyle behaviors, higher levels of depression, and poorer health than physicians and the general population (Bass & McGeeney, 2012).

To raise attention on the adverse effects of clinician burnout and depression, the National Academy of Medicine (NAM) launched an Action Collaborative on Clinician Well-Being and Resilience in 2017. This coalition is developing evidence-based solutions to tackle this public health epidemic that negatively impacts healthcare quality, safety, and patient outcomes (Dzau et al., 2018; https://nam.edu/initiatives/clinician-resilience-and-well-being).

This chapter describes the nine dimensions of wellness and highlights strategies to enhance self-care for optimal health, well-being, and effectiveness. Calls to action include time for self-reflection and goal setting to optimize personal health and well-being.

 CALL TO ACTION

What, specifically, are you doing now every week to prioritize your own self-care?
How often during the week are you building time into your schedule to enhance your own well-being?

KEY STRATEGIES FOR OPTIMIZING PERSONAL HEALTH AND WELL-BEING

Taking time each day to monitor and attend to your own well-being can have multiple rewards for you, from physical to emotional and financial health and well-being. Presented here is an overview of the nine dimensions of wellness, designed to start you on your journey toward optimal well-being. Each dimension of wellness is vital and interconnected. Continue to learn about them and grow in your practice of caring for yourself. Just as you are told by a flight attendant to place an oxygen mask on yourself first before you put one on your child, you cannot take good care of your family, your staff, or your patients unless you first prioritize your own health and well-being and engage in good self-care.

THE NINE DIMENSIONS OF WELL-BEING

Physical Wellness

Physical wellness is not just limited to exercise; it includes healthy eating, engaging in regular preventive care and health screening as recommended by the United States Preventive Services Task Force (see www.uspreventiveservicestaskforce.org/Page/Name/recommendations), proactively taking care of health issues that arise, and sustaining healthy lifestyle practices on a daily basis. Focusing on self-care now will have lasting positive effects on your long-term health and well-being.

Heart disease remains the number one cause of death in both men and women, and can be present with no symptoms. The new American Heart Association (AHA) guidelines define normal blood pressure (BP) as less than 120/80 mmHg, and recommend BP checks at every healthcare provider visit, or at least once every 2 years if BP is normal. Unfortunately, half of the people who have high BP do not have it under control, which places them at great risk for a heart attack or stroke. Fortunately, approximately 80% of cardiovascular disease and other chronic diseases are preventable with healthy lifestyle behaviors.

Four healthy behaviors for better health. Research has shown that people who engage in the following four healthy lifestyle behaviors have 45% less heart disease, 66% less diabetes, 93% less depression, 45% less back pain, and 74% less stress:

- Engage in 30 minutes of physical activity at least 5 days a week.
- Limit alcohol intake if you drink to one drink a day for women, two for men.
- Don't smoke.
- Eat at least five fruits and vegetables a day (Ford et al., 2011).

Risk for chronic disease can be reduced even further by practicing daily stress reduction, sleeping at least 7 hours a night, and avoiding long periods of sitting (Melnyk & Neale, 2018). One recent study found that prolonged sitting (i.e., 6 or more hours a day vs. less than 3 hours/day) was associated with higher risk of mortality from all causes, including cardiovascular disease (coronary heart disease and stroke-specific mortality), cancer, diabetes, kidney disease, suicide, chronic obstructive pulmonary disease, pneumonitis due to solids and liquids, liver, peptic ulcer and other digestive disease, Parkinson's disease, Alzheimer's disease, nervous disorders, and musculoskeletal disorders (Patel, Maliniak, Rees-Punia, Matthews, & Gapstur, 2018). Sitting is also the biggest zapper of your energy.

The bottom line is: Reduce your sedentary time! Sit less and move/stand more.

Have standing or walking meetings instead of sitting meetings—in addition to being good for your cardiovascular health, you will get through meetings much faster when you are standing rather than sitting. In addition to the evidence-based recommendation of 30 minutes of physical activity 5 days a week (U.S. Department of Health and Human Services, 2018), engage in strength training at least twice a week. Resistance bands are a portable inexpensive piece of exercise equipment used for strength training that provide multiple benefits, including increased muscle mass, increased bone strength, better stability, and lower BP. You can travel with a resistance band in your suitcase and keep one at your desk or by your television for use. Many websites (e.g., https://greatist.com/fitness/resistance-band-exercises) offer band workouts.

Even a relatively small weight loss in overweight/obese people—just 5% of body weight—can lower diabetes and heart disease risk as well as improve metabolic function (Magkos et al., 2016). There are numerous weight loss plans advertised, so if you are considering participating in one, read the evidence on the various programs carefully and choose the one that is best for you and your lifestyle. Simply substituting vegetables and fruits for some carbohydrates throughout your day as well as increasing your level of physical activity can result in slow weight loss that is more likely to be sustained rather than losing pounds rapidly through some type of fad diet. Also, don't forget to limit your sodium intake to ideally less than 1,500 mg/day and drink plenty of water; the recommended amount is approximately 15.5 cups for men and 11.5 cups a day for women. In addition to staying well hydrated, you will feel less fatigued.

Emotional Wellness

Emotional wellness includes the ability to identify, express, and manage the full range of your feelings. It also includes practicing techniques to deal with stress, depression and anxiety, and seeking help when your feelings become overwhelming or interfere with everyday functioning.

A little stress is good for the body and mind to grow and to build resilience, but without regular stress management and acknowledgment of emotions, any amount of stress can build to overload. Even if you cannot control negative events and stressors in your working or home environments, you can harness healthy ways to cope with them.

COGNITIVE BEHAVIORAL SKILLS-BUILDING

Evidence shows that a lot of our emotions come as reactions to our thoughts. Negative thoughts are often followed by feelings of anxiety, stress, and depression. Negative thinking can also lead to unhealthy or unhelpful behaviors. This pattern is often referred to as the *thinking, feeling, and behaving triangle*. The first step in cognitive behavioral skills-building is to learn to catch your automatic negative thoughts. When you feel your mood change for the worse, or when you feel physical symptoms of anxiety, such as rapid heartbeat, headache, stomachache, and sweating, ask yourself, "What was I just thinking?" Many negative thoughts become automatic or habitual. Next, learn to recognize trigger or activating events. When you notice negative automatic thoughts in response to stressful events, you can change the negative thought to a positive one by rewriting it. Try keeping a journal of negative thoughts, patterns, and the emotions that came with them, and choose how you would rather react the next time. With time and practice, you can actually change your thinking in response to the stressors in your life, and that will change how you feel (Melnyk & Neale, 2018).

Other tactics, such as the following, can help to optimize your emotional wellness too.

- Engage in some physical activity each day (even small amounts of physical activity have positive benefits).
- Keep a journal of what causes you stress and activities that help to reduce it.

- Get at least 7 hours of sleep a night to avoid excess cortisol from being released, which has many negative effects on multiple body systems. Lack of sleep also contributes to fatigue, mental dullness, and depression.

- Learn about and practice mindfulness—the ability to stay in the present moment, which will help you to worry less and feel less guilty about things that have happened in the past. Worry and guilt are two of our most wasted emotions because most of what is worried about never happens and you cannot go back and change something that happened in the past for which you feel guilty. As a mindfulness exercise, chew a piece of gum and count the number of chews it takes before it runs out of flavor. Another way to practice mindfulness is to focus on your breathing; concentrate on the air moving in and out. Acknowledge thoughts as they arise and then let them go without exploring anxieties about the future or regrets about the past. A few minutes of mindfulness practice a day allows you to relax, de-stress, and recharge. Meditation and yoga are other ways to immerse yourself in mindfulness. Just like anything else, daily practice is important to form a new habit. Many free apps, such as Headspace and Calm, can help you quickly ease into mindfulness. Other tactics to improve emotional well-being include:

  - Manage your energy by taking short recovery breaks throughout the day (even a few minutes of activity every hour can increase your level of energy).

  - Read a positive-thinking book of your choice 5 minutes every morning to elevate your mood and protect yourself against negativity that can arise each day.

  - When stressed, take just five slow deep breaths in and out—this works to decrease stress and lower BP. As you breathe in say, "I am calm." As you breathe out say, "I am blowing all stress out."

  - Help others and be kind; compassion for others will help you to feel good, too.

  - Talk to someone you trust about how you feel.

  - Resolve to keep your workplace positive.

  - Cultivate a daily attitude of gratitude.

 CALL TO ACTION

Name three people or things for which you are grateful.
Make gratitude a daily habit and watch your mood and level of happiness improve!

If symptoms of anxiety, stress, or depression persist for more than 2 weeks and interfere with your daily functioning, do not wait; seek help from a qualified therapist or your healthcare provider. Emotional wellness includes seeking help when needed.

Financial Wellness

Financial well-being includes being fully aware of your financial state and budget, and managing your money to achieve realistic goals. When you analyze, plan well, and take control of your spending, you can make significant changes in how you save, spend, and feel. Almost three in four Americans surveyed in a recent American Psychological Association (APA) study (2015) said they experience financial stress. Financial stress can affect your physical and emotional well-being. According to the APA, high levels of financial stress are associated with an increased risk for ulcers, migraines, heart attacks, depression, anxiety, and sleep disturbance, and may lead to unhealthy coping mechanisms, such as binge drinking, smoking, and overeating. By analyzing, planning, and managing your spending, you can take small steps that lead to significant changes. Try these tactics:

Set aside time to evaluate your finances. Make a series of financial dates with yourself (and your spouse or partner) to plan for how and on what you will spend your finances. Schedule monthly checkups to stay on track.

Analyze money in, money out. Three months' worth of credit card and bank statements should give you a clear picture of income and expenses. Identify how much money you have coming in each month. Then, identify your fixed expenses, such as car payments, mortgage, student loans and utility bills, and your variable expenses, such as money spent on food, clothing, vacations, emergencies, and health. Variable expenses may present opportunities to cut back or save, and fixed expenses can sometimes be renegotiated.

Prioritize. Decide where you want your money to go each month and draw up a budget you can live by. Online resources like Quicken, YNAB (You Need a Budget), and Moneydance can help.

CALL TO ACTION

Analyze the last 3 months of your credit card and bank statements to see where you are spending your money. Prioritize where you want to spend your money and write down a plan to cut back on one or two expenses if you are under financial stress.

Save rather than borrow. Money you invest earns you more money, and money you borrow costs you money. As financial analyst Trent Hamm of The Simple Dollar explains, three $4 lattes a week for 40 years cost a total of $24,960, but invest that $12 a week in a fund earning 5% interest and in 40 years, it will yield $79,772. It pays to save to buy something rather than borrow for it.

Protect yourself from big loss. Reduce worry about financial emergencies by saving a cushion of at least 6 months' pay.

Find help. A certified financial planner (CFP) can help you evaluate your current situation and show you ways to pay off debt and invest in your future. Look for fee-based CFPs, who charge a one-time fee rather than taking a percentage of your investments' earnings.

Find healthy outlets for your stress that cost nothing. Physical activity and taking care of yourself can reduce your overall stress, which will help you to think more clearly and get a better handle on your finances.

Intellectual Wellness

Just as a flexible body indicates physical health, a flexible mind indicates intellectual health. When a person is intellectually healthy, he or she has a value for lifelong learning; fosters critical thinking; develops moral reasoning; expands worldviews; and engages in education for the pursuit of knowledge. Any time you learn a new skill or concept, attempt to understand a different viewpoint or exercise your mind with puzzles and games, you are building intellectual well-being. Studies show that intellectual exercise may improve the physical structure of your brain to help prevent cognitive decline.

Intellectual well-being—keeping your mind flexible, informed, and engaged—is as important as maintaining physical health. Also, intellectual well-being is more than just a concept: it actually improves the physical structure of your brain. Research shows that physical and mental exercise support the growth of new neurons, whereas stress and depression can hinder it (Barry, 2011). Challenging your brain also helps existing neurons form new connections. Combining intellectual growth and relaxing mindfulness can boost your brain's health and prevent mental decline as you age.

Try some of these techniques to keep your mind active:

Read. Spend 5 to 10 minutes at the start of each day reading a book about positive thinking to elevate your mood and to protect you from negativity. Spend another 5 to 10 minutes each day either reading the news to stay informed about the world or reading nonfiction to learn about a new subject.

Practice short periods of quiet time every day. Relax and recharge your brain regularly throughout the day with just a few minutes of quiet time.

Do not multitask; focus on one task at a time. Multitasking is the enemy of being able to fully engage and concentrate.

Disrupt your routine. Any time you step out of your normal routine, your brain has to work a little harder as it adjusts, processes new information, and finds creative solutions and new stimuli. Try driving home using a different route, eating at a new restaurant, or rearranging your furniture. In addition to finding new things to enjoy, stepping outside of your comfort zone improves your brain's neuroplasticity. Engaging in lifelong learning, challenging your mind, and following your curiosity sets the stage for a vibrant, centered, and mentally active life.

Career Wellness

Engaging in work that provides personal satisfaction and enrichment and is consistent with your values, goals, and lifestyle will keep you professionally healthy. After sleep, we spend most of our time at work, so ask yourself if your work motivates you and lets you use your strengths or abilities to their full potential. Burnout, stress, and dissatisfaction at work should prompt an evaluation of your career wellness.

  CALL TO ACTION

What would you do in the next 5 to 10 years if you knew you could not fail?
Are you aligned with your dream(s)/purpose/passion at your work?
If you are, you probably wake up in the morning excited about going to work.
If you are not, how can you become more aligned at work with your dream(s) or passion(s)?
If you decide that you cannot fulfill your dream(s) or purpose in your current role, maybe it is time to reflect upon and make plans for a work or career change.

Even if you cannot change where you work right now, you can change your approach to the stressors and challenges you face at work. Several on-the-job strategies can help you reevaluate your career, cope with change and stress, and reenergize your work life.

Mindfulness on the job. Practicing mindfulness on the job can help you keep a clear head so that you can respond, rather than react, to situations. Research supports that mindfulness can increase on-the-job resiliency and improve effectiveness and safety.

Cultivate a positive mind-set. Leadership experts Tim and Brian Kight of Focus 3 explain that one of the distinguishing characteristics of successful people is not only their ability to generate a positive, productive mind-set, but to sustain it. You will find a lot of power in keeping yourself positive and remembering that every event's outcome is tempered by your response to it.

Multitask less, monotask more. Multitasking can drain your energy. Cultivate long periods of focus. Try becoming more aware of when you are distracted and picture a stop sign. Then, give your all to just one task.

Purpose, pleasure, and pride. Author and founder of Blue Zones, Dan Buettner, who has researched happiness and longevity, says purpose, pleasure, and pride are important to a long and happy life. Design your workplace to increase each of these. Friendship at work is important. Buettner (2017) found that one of the most powerful indicators of work satisfaction and productivity was agreement with the statement, "I have a best friend at work." Finding a job that fits your talents and gives you good feedback can create a great deal of satisfaction. Also, evaluate your work hours and include time you spend commuting in that count. If you cannot cut your commuting time, try making use of drive time to listen to audiobooks or positive music.

Social Wellness

Social wellness can be defined as our ability to effectively interact with people around us and to create a support system that includes family and friends. Evidence shows that social connections not only help us deal with stress but also keep us healthy.

If you are feeling socially disconnected, you can learn ways to improve the relationships you have, build your support network, and make new connections. Even if you already have a large social circle, there are many skills to learn: conflict management, setting boundaries, communication skills, assertiveness, respect for others, and the ability to balance your time between social and personal needs are all part of maintaining healthy relationships. In other words, much of social wellness is learned behavior, and we can all improve on these skills.

Loneliness. Research into the impact of loneliness on physical and mental health is alarming. Loneliness has been found to cause inflammation and raise stress hormone levels, which can increase the risk of heart disease, arthritis, type 2 diabetes, depression, pain, fatigue, and dementia (Jaremka et al., 2014). Jaremka et al. (2013) also found that people who are lonely may have suppressed immune systems, brought on by stress. Social isolation or being alone does not necessarily mean one is lonely, though. Psychology researchers Holt-Lunstad and Smith (2016), who studied the links of loneliness and social isolation to cardiovascular disease, define *loneliness* as the discrepancy between one's desired and actual level of social connection. That means that if being alone does not bother us, we are not lonely; only when we notice the lack of social connection do we feel the stress of loneliness.

Steps to improve social wellness include disconnecting from technology to take time to communicate with others, improving communication skills, evaluating emotional intelligence, cultivating a positive attitude, and taking time to celebrate with and compliment friends and family members. Show respect for others by being on time, and make an action plan for spending more time with others.

Conflict management. It is alright to disagree as long as disagreements are handled respectfully. Disrespectful arguing includes criticizing the other's character, being defensive or blaming, showing contempt, threatening to withdraw from the argument, or ignoring the other. Successful arguing uses respectful language, focuses on "now" and not previous arguments or unrelated incidents, and may include brief breaks to cool down. Have perspective and remember to value respect over being "right."

Creative Wellness

A review of more than 100 studies of the benefits of the arts (music, visual arts, dance, and writing) found that creative expression has a powerful impact on health and well-being among various patient populations (Jacobs, 2015). Most studies agree that engagement in the arts decreases depressive symptoms, increases positive emotions, reduces stress, and, in some cases, improves immune system functioning.

Creative wellness means valuing and participating in a diverse range of arts and cultural experiences to understand and appreciate your surrounding world. Expressing your emotions and views through the arts can be a great way to relieve stress. Do not let self-judgment or perfectionism get in the way. Allow yourself creative freedom without worrying about whether you are doing it well, and take time to appreciate the creative efforts of others.

If you do not currently have any creative pursuits, give yourself permission to be a beginner and try a new creative outlet. *The Artist's Way* by Julia Cameron can help you get started. Join an art or pottery class, give yourself a photography assignment you can shoot with your phone, join a singing group or local choir. Try doodling in a blank journal to relieve stress, or try a free doodling app like Doodle Buddy and You Doodle. Freewriting, journaling, and writing poetry and stories can be cathartic and healing. If you are looking for a way to increase your social wellness at the same time, join a play production or gather with friends to read through a play script, or take a trip with your family to a local art museum.

Creativity doesn't have to mean creating great art. It can include cooking, gardening, redecorating your home or office, and more. Studies show that creative pursuits also boost intellectual wellness and may delay cognitive decline in older people.

Environmental Wellness

Increasing awareness of your surroundings can improve overall well-being. Being environmentally well means recognizing the responsibility to preserve, protect, and improve the environment, and to appreciate your connection to nature. Environmental wellness intersects with social wellness when you work to conserve the environment for future generations and improve conditions for others around the world.

Research has demonstrated that green space, such as parks, forests, and river corridors, is good for our physical and mental health (World Health Organization, 2016). Your environment is not limited to the great outdoors though; it also includes everything that surrounds you—your home, your car, your workplace, the food you eat, and the people with whom you interact.

Pay attention to your environment at work, since our surroundings can have a profound effect on how we feel and function. Studies show that we thrive better when surrounded by people who support our goals and want to help us succeed. We cannot usually choose the people with whom we work, but we can support an environment of workplace civility, and choose to spend more time with those who support and uplift us. Also, we can contribute to making our physical surroundings healthier, from recycling to creating a culture of respect and gratitude.

You can improve your environment by taking steps to be conscious about how you use natural resources: reuse and recycle, turn off water or electric appliances and lights when not in use, save gas by walking, biking, or taking public transportation instead of driving, and support your colleagues' efforts to recycle at the office. When you show respect for the natural environment, you show respect for others, too, and for future generations.

Spiritual Wellness

Spiritual wellness is largely about your purpose, not religion. You can seek spiritual wellness in many ways, including quiet self-reflection, reading, and open dialogue with others. A spiritually well person might explore the depth of human purpose, ponder human connectedness, and seek answers to questions like, "Why are we here?" Spiritual wellness includes being open to exploring your own beliefs and respecting the beliefs of others.

Barbara Dossey (2015), a pioneer in the holistic nursing movement, writes that our spirituality involves a sense of connection outside ourselves and includes our values, meaning, and purpose. Your spiritual well-being is not what you own, your job, or even your physical health. It is about what inspires you, what gives you hope, and what you feel strongly about. Your spirit is the seat of your deepest values and character. Whether or not you practice a religion, you can recognize that a part of you exists beyond the analytical thinking of your intellect; it is the part of you that feels, makes value judgments, and wonders about your connection to others, to your moral values, and to the world.

Although religion and spirituality can be connected, they are different. A faith community or organized religion can give you an outlet for your spirituality, but religion is not spirituality's only expression. Hope, love, joy, meaning, purpose, connection, appreciation of beauty, and caring and compassion for others are associated with spiritual well-being.

Our purpose, our reason for living on this planet, is at the foundation of our spiritual nature. If you are feeling disconnected from your values and purpose, try these ways to reconnect with your spiritual nature:

- Set aside some retreat time with yourself to consider your purpose and whether you are living it out. Identify what you need to do to adjust. Ask yourself what you would do in the next 5 years if you knew you could not fail. Take stock periodically to keep yourself on track with your purpose.

- Ramp up your positive outlook. Actively seek ways to increase positivity, such as keeping a gratitude journal, celebrating your strengths, and recognizing and practicing small acts of kindness daily.

- Adopt a meditative practice. Traditional forms of meditation can include prayer or sitting in stillness with a quiet mind. Some people prefer physical action that incorporates meditation, such as yoga, tai chi, or walking. Experiment and find what works for you.

TAKE ACTION TO PROTECT AND CULTIVATE YOUR HEALTH AND WELL-BEING

If it is difficult for you to prioritize your own self-care, think about doing it for the people who love you—who want you to be around for a very long time. I (Bern Melnyk) lost my mom suddenly when I was 15 years old and home alone with her when she sneezed and had a stroke. I did not have a mother to see me graduate from high school, become a nurse, and go on to have my three beautiful daughters. When I do not feel like exercising, I think about my three daughters and two small grandsons who provide the motivation for me to continue to lead a healthy lifestyle. Who will be your motivator(s) as you make a commitment to engage in a higher degree of healthy lifestyle behaviors?

Now that you are thinking about your own well-being, take time to start a journal about your health and wellness. Awareness is the first step toward action.

> **CALL TO ACTION**
>
> Write down how you are feeling physically, the stressors in your life and how you can proactively deal with them, what you would like to accomplish, and how you would like to feel in a week, 6 months, and a year from now?

Changing your wellness habits is not easy; **it typically takes 30 to 60 days to make or break a new habit.** Setting goals for your well-being can make a significant positive difference in your life and in the lives of others. When trying to make changes, set SMART goals: goals that are Specific, Measurable, Achievable, Realistic, and Time-bound. Most people are not successful with their health and wellness objectives because they set goals that are unrealistic. For example, if you only exercise for 15 minutes, twice a week, do not set a goal to exercise for 30 minutes 5 days a week. A more realistic goal is 15 minutes three times a week or 20 minutes twice a week.

> **CALL TO ACTION**
>
> Write down one new wellness goal and place it where you can see it every day. Stretch yourself a little but do not make it very difficult. Take one small step at a time.
> What barriers might interfere with you being able to achieve your goal? What might facilitate it? It also helps to tell someone about your goal to increase your accountability to achieve it. If you fall off the wagon one day, just get back on and start again. You and your well-being are definitely worth it!

The steps you take today to safeguard and improve your well-being can lead you on a journey to optimal health, well-being, self-discovery, connectedness, and satisfaction. Great leaders engage in good self-care and model wellness behaviors for others. They also see to it that their workplaces encourage and provide resources for their employees' well-being. Chapter 7, Leading Organizational Change and Building Wellness Cultures for Maximum ROI and VOI, will provide evidence-based strategies to build and sustain cultures in which organizations and people within them thrive, which includes assisting them to attain their highest level of well-being.

> **CALL TO ACTION**
>
> Choose two of the nine wellness dimensions that you will prioritize in the next 6 months? Create a 30-, 60-, 90-, and 180-day plan with specific goals and action tactics that you will implement to achieve them.

🔑 KEY TAKEAWAY POINTS

- ◼ You can't be a great leader, innovator, or entrepreneur and take terrific care of others unless you take good care of yourself.

- ◼ If you say you don't have the time to take good self-care now, you will have to make time for illness later.

- ◼ There are nine dimensions of wellness which are necessary for optimal well-being.

- ◼ Eighty percent of chronic disease can be prevented with healthy lifestyle behaviors, including physical activity, healthy eating, not smoking, sleeping at least 7 hours per night, and regularly implementing stress reduction strategies.

- ◼ If stress, anxiety, or depression is interfering with your functioning, don't wait—get help!

ACKNOWLEDGMENTS

Special thanks to the *American Nurse Today* "9 Dimensions of Wellness" by Bernadette Mazurek Melnyk and Susan Neale with Brenda C. Buffington, EdD, NBC-HWC, EP-C, David Hrabe PhD, RN, NC-BC, and Laura Newpoff. Excerpts from this series were adapted for this chapter.

REFERENCES

American Psychological Association. (2015, February 4). American Psychological Association survey shows money stress weighing on Americans' health nationwide. Retrieved from https://www.apa.org/news/press/releases/2015/02/money-stress

Barry, S. R. (2011). How to grow new neurons in your brain. *Psychology Today*. Retrieved from https://www.psychologytoday.com/intl/blog/eyes-the-brain/201101/how-grow-new-neurons-in-your-brain

Bass, K., & McGeeney, K. (2012). Physicians set good health example: Physicians in better health than nurses and employed adult population. *Gallop polls*. Retrieved from https://news.gallup.com/poll/157859/physicians-set-good-health-example.aspx

Blake, H., & Chambers, D. (2011). Supporting nurse health champions: Developing a new generation' of health improvement facilitators. *Health Education Journal, 71*(2), 205–210. doi:10.1177/0017896910396767

Buettner, D. (2017). *The blue zones of happiness: Lessons from the world's happiest people.* Washington, DC: National Geographic Partners.

Dossey, B. M. (2015). Integrative health and wellness assessment. In B. M. Dossey, S. Luck, & B. S. Schaub (Eds.), *Nurse coaching: Integrative approaches for health and well–being* (pp. 109–121). North Miami, FL: International Nurse Coach Association.

Dzau, V. J., Kirch, D. G., & Nasca, T. J. (2018). To care is human—Collectively confronting the clinician-burnout crisis. *New England Journal of Medicine, 378*(4), 312–314. doi:10.1056/NEJMp1715127

Ford, E. S., Zhao, G., Tsai, J., & Li, C. (2011). Low-risk lifestyle behaviors and all-cause mortality: Findings from the national health and nutrition examination survey III mortality study. *American Journal of Public Health, 101,* 1922–1929. doi:10.2105/AJPH.2011.300167

Holt-Lunstad, J., & Smith, T. B. (2016). Loneliness and social isolation as risk factors for CVD: Implications for evidence-based patient care and scientific inquiry. *Heart, 102*(13), 987–989. doi:10.1136/heartjnl-2015-309242

Jacobs, T. (2015, April 8). Making art tied to fewer cognitive problems in old age. *Pacific Standard*. Retrieved from https://psmag.com/social-justice/making-art-tied-to-fewer-cognitive-problems-in-old-age

Jaremka, L. M., Andridge, R. R., Fagundes, C. P., Alfano, C. M., Povoski, S. P., Lipari, A. M., … Kiecolt-Glaser, J. K. (2014). Pain, depression, and fatigue: Loneliness as a longitudinal risk factor. *Health Psychology, 33*(9), 948–957. doi:10.1037/a0034012

Jaremka, L. M., Fagundes, C. P., Peng, J., Bennett, J. M., Glaser, R., Malarkey, W. B., & Kiecolt-Glaser, J. K. (2013). Loneliness promotes inflammation during acute stress. *Psychology Science, 24*(7), 1089–1097. doi:10.1177/0956797612464059

Magkos, F., Fraterrigo, G., Yoshino, J., Luecking, C., Kirbach, K., Kelly, S. C., … Klein, S. (2016). Effects of moderate and subsequent progressive weight loss on metabolic function and adipose tissue biology in humans with obesity. *Cell Metabolism, 23*(4), 591–601. doi:10.1016/j.cmet.2016.02.005

McHugh, M. D., Kutney-Lee, A., Cimiotti, J. P., Sloane, D. M., & Aiken, L. H. (2011). Nurses' job dissatisfaction, burnout, and frustration with health benefits signal problems for patient care. *Health Affairs, 30*(2), 202–210. doi:10.1377/hlthaff.2010.0100

Melnyk, B. M., & Neale, S. (2018). 9 dimensions of wellness. Evidence-based tactics for optimizing your health and well-being. Columbus, OH: The Ohio State University.

Melnyk, B. M., Orsolini, L., Tan, A., Arslanian-Engoren, C., Melkus, G. D., Dunbar-Jacob, J., Rice, V. H., … Lewis, L. M. (2018). A national study links nurses' physical and mental health to medical errors and perceived worksite wellness. *Journal of Occupational and Environmental Medicine, 60*(2), 126–131. doi:10.1097/JOM.0000000000001198

Oberg, E. B., & Frank, E. (2011). Physicians' heath practices strongly influence patient health practices. *J R College Physicians Edinburgh, 39*(4), 290–301. doi:10.4997/JRCPE.2009.422

Patel, A. V., Maliniak, M. L., Rees-Punia, E., Matthews, C. E., & Gapstur, S. M. (2018). Prolonged leisure time spent sitting in relation to cause-specific mortality in a large US cohort. *American Journal of Epidemiology, 187*(10), 2151–2158. doi:10.1093/aje/kwy125

Shanafelt, T. D., Hasan, O., Dyrbye, L. N., Sinsky, C., Satele, D., Sloan, J., & West, C. P. (2015). Changes in burnout and satisfaction with work-life balance in physicians and the general US working population between 2011 and 2014. *Mayo Clinic Proceedings, 90*(12), 1600–1613. doi:10.1016/j.mayocp.2015.08.023

Skakon, J., Nielsen, K., Borg, V., & Guzman, J. (2010). Are leaders' well-being, behaviours and style associated with the affective well-being of their employees? A systematic review of three decades of research. *Work and Stress, 24*, 107–139. doi:10.1080/02678373.2010.495262

Steege, L. M., Pinekenstein, B. J., Arsenault Knudsen, E., & Rainbow, J. G. (2017). Exploring nurse leader fatigue: A mixed methods study. *Journal of Nursing Management, 25*(4), 276–272. doi:10.1111/jonm.12464

U. S. Department of Health and Human Services. (2018). *Physical activity guidelines for Americans* (2nd ed.). Washington, DC: Author.

World Health Organization. (2016). Urban green spaces and health: A review of evidence. Geneva, Switzerland: Author.

5

Learning From a History of Great Leaders

T. Scott Graham

"A leader is one who knows the way, goes the way, and shows the way."—John C. Maxwell

LEARNING OBJECTIVES

- Describe the strengths of two leaders highlighted in this chapter in terms of their greatest exemplary leadership practice.

- Identify which of the five exemplary leadership practices you will work toward achieving in the next 90 days.

- Discuss how you will encourage the heart of others from this day forward.

INTRODUCTION

The process of identifying leaders to include in a chapter on lessons learned from great leaders appeared daunting, subjective, inexact, and close to impossible at first. Who determines what is "great"? Scholars? Other famous leaders? Authors? It is like trying to define *success*. Who gets to define it? Once there is identification of a research-based, widely regarded set of criteria against which to measure greatness, finding examples of each of the criteria is that next step.

The research-based resource used here is Kouzes and Posner's (2017) *The Leadership Challenge*. Based on thousands of cases studies, focus groups, interviews, and observations over three decades, the authors identified five practices of exemplary leaders, including:

- Challenge the process.

- Inspire a shared vision.

- Model the way.

- Enable others to act.

- Encourage the heart.

These five practices were described in detail in Chapter 3: Understanding and Developing Yourself as a Leader. From this chapter title's perspective, the word *great* is synonymous with *exemplary*. Each of the 10 identified leaders in this chapter are examined under the lens of one or more of these five exemplary evidence-based practices. For each historical leader in this chapter, a notable quote is shared and a brief overview of who the person is and the key leadership lessons he or she embodies is described along with some of his or her inspirational and insightful words of leadership wisdom. Each leader identified in this chapter could have been an example of a person who embodied all of the five exemplary leadership practices. However, each is presented through the lens of one particular practice. The master list is included here.

THE LIST

1. Pope Francis
2. Dr. Martin Luther King, Jr.
3. Bill Gates
4. Dr. Loretta Ford
5. Sir Winston Churchill
6. Senator John Glenn
7. President Barack Obama
8. Oprah Winfrey
9. Mother Teresa
10. Coach Mike Krzyzewski

CHALLENGE THE PROCESS

Pope Francis—Servant, Inspiration, Spiritual Leader

A Pioneer Willing to Challenge the Status Quo

> *"The most important thing in the life of every man and every woman is not that they should never fall along the way. The important thing is always to get back up, not to stay on the ground licking your wounds"*—Pope Francis

Born in Buenos Aires, Argentina, on December 17, 1936, Jorge Mario Bergoglio became Pope Francis on March 13, 2013, when he was named the 266th pope of the Roman Catholic Church. Bergoglio, the first pope from the Americas, took his papal title after St. Francis of Assisi of Italy. Prior to his election as pope, Bergoglio served as archbishop of Buenos Aires from 1998 to 2013 (succeeding Antonio Quarracino), as cardinal of the Roman Catholic Church of Argentina from 2001 to 2013, and as president of the Bishops' Conference of Argentina from 2005 to 2011. Named Person of the Year by *Time* magazine in 2013, Pope Francis has embarked on a tenure characterized by humility and outspoken support of the world's poor and marginalized people, and has been involved actively in areas of political diplomacy and environmental advocacy (Fortune, 2014).

Since he became pope in 2013, the leader of the Catholic Church, Pope Francis, has electrified the Church and attracted legions of non-Catholic admirers by energetically setting a new direction for the Church. He has refused to occupy the palatial papal apartments, has washed the feet of female Muslim prisoners, is driven around Rome in a Ford Focus, and famously asked, "Who am I to judge?" with regard to the Church's view of gay members. He created a group of eight cardinals to advise him on reform, which a Church historian calls one of the most significant events in the life of the Church. Francis recently asked the world to stop treating him as a rock star. He knows that although revolutionary, his actions so far have mostly reflected a new tone and intention. His hardest work lies ahead (Fortune, 2014).

Here is an inspiring insight into leadership from Pope Francis:

"Even if you feel your life has been a disaster, even if it has been destroyed by vices, drugs, or anything else—God is in your life. You can, you must, try to seek God in every human life. Although the life of each of us is a land full of thorns and weeds, there is always a space in which the good seed can grow. You have to trust God. Situations can change; people can change. Be the first to seek to bring good. Do not grow accustomed to evil, but defeat it with good." —Pope Francis

Dr. Martin Luther King, Jr.—Pastor, Evangelist, Ambassador, Visionary, Spiritual Leader

Sought to Accept Overwhelming Challenges, Change Mind-Sets, and Stepped Into the Unknown to Make the World a Better Place

"The ultimate measure of a [person] is not where he/she stands in moments of comfort and convenience, but where he/she stands at times of challenge and controversy."
—Dr. Martin Luther King, Jr.

During the less than 13 years of Dr. Martin Luther King, Jr.'s leadership of the modern American Civil Rights Movement, from December 1955 until April 1968, African Americans achieved more genuine progress toward racial equality in America than the previous 350 years had produced. Dr. King is widely regarded as America's preeminent advocate of nonviolence and one of the greatest nonviolent leaders in world history.

Drawing inspiration from both his Christian faith and the peaceful teachings of Mahatma Gandhi, Dr. King led a nonviolent movement in the late 1950s and 1960s to achieve legal equality for African Americans in the United States. While others were advocating for freedom by "any means necessary," including violence, Martin Luther King, Jr. used the power of words and acts of nonviolent resistance, such as protests, grassroots organizing, and civil disobedience to achieve seemingly impossible goals. He went on to lead similar campaigns against poverty and international conflict, always maintaining fidelity to his principles that men and women everywhere, regardless of color or creed, are equal members of the human family.

Dr. King's "I Have a Dream" speech, Nobel Peace Prize lecture, and "Letter from a Birmingham Jail" are among the most revered orations and writings in the English language. His accomplishments are now taught to American children of all races, and his teachings are studied by scholars and students worldwide. He is the only nonpresident to have a national holiday dedicated in his honor, and is the only nonpresident memorialized on the Great Mall in the nation's capital. He is memorialized in hundreds of statues, parks, streets, squares, churches, and other public facilities around the world as a leader whose teachings are increasingly relevant to the progress of humankind (The King Center, 2018).

Inspiring Leadership Insights From This Leader

Here is an inspiring insight into leadership from Dr. King:

> *"You must develop and maintain the capacity to forgive. If you are devoid of the power to forgive then you are devoid of the power to love. Know this … there is some good in the worst of us, and some evil in the best of us. When we discover this, and embrace this truth … we are much less prone to hate our enemies, and much less likely to think so highly of ourselves that we value ourselves above any and all others."*
> —Dr. Martin Luther King, Jr.

INSPIRE A SHARED VISION

Bill Gates—Business Mogul, Visionary, Entrepreneur, Philanthropist

Dreamed of What Could Be, Created Something Unique With Abounding Enthusiasm

> *"Success is a lousy teacher. It seduces smart people into thinking they can't lose."*
> —Bill Gates

Bill Gates is the richest person on the planet, but he did not start his life with riches. He is a totally self-made genius who envisioned the future of our world relying on computing power. His vision could not have been more right. As a young boy, he was extremely intelligent and industrious. He had several jobs that involved exploring computer code and figuring out how computers worked. When he became bored figuring out how computers worked, he went on to even more substantial mental challenges by figuring out how humans could use them to work.

Bill Gates certainly can be described as intelligent. He scored a near perfect 1,590 out of 1,600 on the college entrance Scholastic Aptitude Test. Harvard, of course, accepted him. While at Harvard University, he met another brilliant entrepreneur and they worked on many projects together. This person was Paul Allen. Though Paul graduated from Harvard, Bill Gates decided, with his parents' blessing, to pursue his dream and left Harvard rather than waiting to pursue his passion after graduation. He and Paul started what would become one of the world's most influential and vital companies—Microsoft. So, a keen and unwavering vision, along with the ability to inspire other bright minds to embrace his vision join with him, is what set this entrepreneur apart.

Not only is Bill Gates extremely wealthy, visionary, and influential, he is also philanthropic. He and his wife, Melinda, began the Bill and Melinda Gates Foundation, which aims to eradicate polio from the planet, and raised over $10 billion to ensure vaccines were available to the poorest countries. He no longer runs Microsoft as his philanthropic work has taken his time and energy since 2010, but he still serves as the visionary on the board of directors.

Walt Whitman, in *Leaves of Grass*, once penned these words: "The powerful play goes on and you may contribute a verse" (Whitman, 2015, p. 111) So, when Bill Gates spoke at a commencement address at Harvard several years ago, he shared these lessons and contributed this verse:

"Be committed and passionate, be proud of who you are, be humble always, love learning, and share your success with others as you did not get there alone."

One can say that due to his vision, Bill Gates has given the planet the Windows to the world.

Dr. Loretta Ford—Pioneer, Nurse Leader, Educator, Champion, Servant

Had a Clear Image of the Future, Magnetized Others to Follow, and Changed the Way Things Are

"Advance practice is dynamic ... it moves with every new bit of knowledge and technology. We cannot run and ask for permission every time we want to do something new. What other profession does that?"—Loretta Ford

Dr. Loretta Ford is considered the founder of the nurse practitioner (NP) movement. Many decades ago, Dr. Ford predicted that the NP would someday be working in all settings. She later said, "The profession has expanded beyond my wildest dreams." Although the specialty is only a little over 40 years old, there are now more than 270,000 licensed NPs in the United States, and that number continues to swell. The needs are great, their roles are expanding, and even Dr. Ford's early vision may not have been this expansive.

Ford has graduate degrees in nursing and a doctorate in education from the University of Colorado, and she is a certified public health nurse. In the 1960s, with a regional shortage of family care physicians and pediatricians hampering healthcare delivery to rural and underserved areas, Ford saw the need for an innovative solution. With a small seed grant from her university, she created a demonstration project, focusing on extending the role of the nurse in the community. The published findings later evolved into an educational curriculum for NPs. The NP movement was born, and she and her vision gave it life.

Ford shares the message that nurse practitioners touch all parts of our healthcare system. These professional healthcare team members are required to have a master's degree and there is a movement to prepare all NPs with a doctor of nursing practice (DNP) degree by 2025. The current rise of the DNP is an evolutionary growth of the NP role in our world.

Dr. Ford offers this insight into leadership:

"Do what's right, and don't ever give up."—Loretta Ford

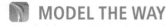 MODEL THE WAY

Sir Winston Churchill—Prime Minister, Statesman, Patriot, Visionary

Led From His Beliefs and Aligned His Words and Actions at All Times

"Kites rise highest against the wind—not with it."—Winston Churchill

Sir Winston Churchill (1874–1965) was a British politician, military officer, and writer who served as the prime minister of Great Britain from 1940 to 1945 and from 1951 to 1955. Born to an aristocratic family in 1874, Churchill served in the British Army and worked as a writer before his election to Parliament in 1900. After becoming prime minister in 1940, Churchill helped lead a successful Allied strategy with the United States and Soviet Union during World War II to defeat the Axis powers and craft postwar peace. Elected prime minister again in 1951, he introduced key domestic reforms.

It was his resolve and his ability to rally the entire country to his bold and maverick plan of victory at all costs that put Churchill at the top of the list of some of the most admired leaders of all time. When many in Parliament thought it best to negotiate with Hitler, he did not. He knew this strategy would signal the end of the British Empire. His radio interviews inspired hope, and his tenacity and bulldog spirit kept this hope alive in the people of England, even as Hitler bombed Britain mercilessly. Churchill was a skilled negotiator able to gain the support of Stalin and Roosevelt to assist with supplies and materials. He helped to convince his allies that this war against the greatest aggressor the world had ever known could be won. His oratorical skills and knowledge of battlefield tactics combined to make him someone that his people would willingly follow into hell.

Here is an inspirational insight into leadership from Winston Churchill:

"Are you an optimist or a pessimist? People want to be around positive thinkers. Here is how you can tell which you are. A pessimist sees the difficulty in every opportunity; an optimist sees the opportunity in every difficulty."—Winston Churchill

John Glenn—Astronaut, Senator, Statesman, Philanthropist, Political Leader

Lived His Solid and Unwavering Core Values at All Times

"We are more fulfilled when we are involved in something bigger than ourselves."
—John Glenn

Colonel John Herschel Glenn, Jr. was a U.S. Marine Corps aviator, engineer, astronaut, and a U.S. Senator from Ohio. In 1962, he became the first American to orbit the Earth, circling it three times.

Before joining the National Aeronautics and Space Administration (NASA), Glenn was a distinguished fighter pilot during World War II, as well as in China and Korea. He shot down three MiG-15 aircraft, and was awarded six Distinguished Flying Crosses and 18 Air Medals. In 1957, he made the first supersonic transcontinental flight across the United States. His onboard camera took the first continuous, panoramic photograph of the United States.

He was one of the Mercury Seven, military test pilots selected in 1959 by NASA as the United States' first astronauts. On February 20, 1962, Glenn flew the *Friendship 7* mission, becoming the first American to orbit the Earth, and the fifth person and third American in space. He received the NASA Distinguished Service Medal in 1962 and the Congressional Space Medal of Honor in 1978, was inducted into the U.S. Astronaut Hall of Fame in 1990, and was the last surviving member of the Mercury Seven.

Glenn resigned from NASA in January 1964. He planned to run for a U.S. Senate seat from Ohio, but an injury in February 1964 forced his withdrawal. He retired from the Marine Corps the following year. He lost a close primary election in 1970. A member of the Democratic Party, Glenn first won election to the Senate in 1974 and served for 24 years until January 1999. In 1998, while still a sitting senator, Glenn became the oldest person to fly in space as a crew member of the *Discovery* space shuttle and the only person to fly in both the Mercury and Space Shuttle programs. He received the Presidential Medal of Freedom in 2012 (Wikipedia, 2018).

ENABLE OTHERS TO ACT

Barack Obama—Senator, First Black President, Nobel-Prize Winner, Devoted Husband and Father

Yes, We Can! Listened Intently, Took Advice, and Built Relationships

> *"There is not a liberal America and a conservative America—there is the United States of America. There is not a black America and a white America and Latino America and Asian America—there's the United States of America."*—Barack Obama

Barack Obama, in full Barack Hussein Obama II (born August 4, 1961, Honolulu, Hawaii, USA), was the 44th president of the United States (2009–2017), and the first African American to hold the office. Before winning the presidency, Obama represented Illinois in the U.S. Senate (2005–2008). He was the third African American to be elected to that body since the end of Reconstruction (1877). In 2009, he was awarded the Nobel Peace Prize "for his extraordinary efforts to strengthen international diplomacy and cooperation between peoples" (Nobelprize.org, 2019).

After receiving his law degree, Obama moved to Chicago and became active in the Democratic Party. He organized Project Vote, a drive that registered tens of thousands of African Americans on voting rolls and that is credited with helping Democrat Bill Clinton win Illinois and capture the presidency in 1992. The effort also helped make Carol Moseley Braun, an Illinois state legislator, the first African American woman elected to the U.S. Senate. During this period, Obama wrote his first book and saw it published. The memoir, *Dreams from My Father* (1995), is the story of Obama's search for his biracial identity by tracing the lives of his now-deceased father and his extended family in Kenya. Obama lectured on constitutional law at the University of Chicago and worked as an attorney on civil rights issues.

Per the *Washington Monthly* journal, these are the Top 10 accomplishments of Obama during his 8 years as President of the United States (Glastris & LeTourneau, 2017):

1. Passed Health Care Reform to provide healthcare to millions of uninsured
2. Rescued the economy
3. Passed Wall Street reform
4. Negotiated a deal to block a nuclear Iran
5. Secured U.S. commitment to a global agreement on climate change
6. Located and Eliminated Osama Bin Laden
7. Ended U.S. combat missions in Iraq and Afghanistan

8. Turned around U.S. auto industry
9. Repealed "Don't Ask, Don't Tell"
10. Supported federal recognition of same-sex marriages

Here is an insight into leadership from President Obama:

"We cannot know, for certain, how long we have here. We cannot foresee the trials or misfortunes that will test us along the way. We cannot know God's plan for us. What we can do is to live out our lives as best we can with purpose, love, and joy. We can use each day to show those who are closest to us how much we care about them, and treat others with the kindness and respect that we wish for ourselves. We can learn from our mistakes and grow from our failures. And, we can strive at all costs to make a better world, so that someday, if we are blessed with the chance to look back on our time here, we can know that we spent it well; that we made a difference; that our fleeting presence had a lasting impact on the lives of other human beings."—Barack Obama

Oprah Winfrey—Entertainer, Pioneer, Visionary, Actress, Philanthropist
Ask Great Questions, and Listen for Answers

"I've come to believe that each of us has a personal calling that's as unique as a fingerprint—and that the best way to succeed is to discover what you love and then find a way to offer it to others in the form of service, working hard, and also allowing the energy of the universe to lead you." —Oprah Winfrey

Oprah Winfrey was born in Mississippi in 1954, and moved to Baltimore in 1976, where she entered the television business by hosting a chat show. She was recognized as a talent and brought to Chicago to host a TV show soon thereafter. The network saw superstardom in her ability to interview and share interesting insights and news stories, and she was given her own TV show, The *Oprah Winfrey Show*, which aired for 25 years. Upon leaving that show, she launched her own television network. Oprah Winfrey is one of the richest persons in the world, yet remains very popular and altruistic due to her liberal donations to worthy causes around our planet.

ENCOURAGE THE HEART

Mother Teresa—Nun, Missionary, Servant Leader
Passion and Compassion, Cared for All Others Over Self

"Life is an opportunity, benefit from it. Life is a beauty, admire it. Life is a dream, realize it. Life is a challenge, meet it. Life is a duty, complete it. Life is a game, play it. Life is a promise, fulfill it. Life is sorrow, overcome it. Life is a song, sing it. Life is a struggle, accept it. Life is a tragedy, confront it. Life is an adventure, dare it. Life is luck, make it. Life is life, fight for it!"—Mother Teresa

Nun and missionary Mother Teresa experienced her call to serve our world in 1946. The order of nuns to which she belonged established a hospice; began centers for the blind, aged, and disabled; and began a leper colony. In 1979, she received the Nobel Peace Prize for her humanitarian work. In 2015, Pope Francis recognized a second miracle attributed to Mother Teresa, and she was canonized in 2016. Mother Teresa is recognized as one of the greatest humanitarians of the 20th century. She embodied empathy and servant leadership even after her death. Her charities touched and aided millions of lives, and continues to do so (Biography, 2018).

Coach Mike Krzyzewski ("Coach K")—Head Basketball Coach, Mentor, Friend, Humanitarian

Relationship Builder Who Rewards and Recognizes Others for Doing Things Right

"People have to be given the freedom to show the heart they possess. I think it is a leader's responsibility to provide that type of freedom. In addition, I believe it can be done through relationships and family. Because if a team is a real family, its members want to show you their hearts." —Coach K

Coach K is an American college basketball coach and former player. Since 1980, he has served as the head men's basketball coach at Duke University, where he has led the Blue Devils to five National Collegiate Athletic Association (NCAA) championships, 12 Final Fours, 12 Atlantic Coast Conference (ACC) regular-season titles, and 14 ACC tournament championships. Among men's college basketball coaches, only the University of California at Los Angeles's (UCLA) John Wooden, with 10, has won more NCAA championships. Krzyzewski was also the coach of the U.S.A. Basketball Men's National Team, which he has led to three gold medals at the 2008 Summer Olympics, 2012 Summer Olympics, and 2016 Summer Olympics. He also served as the head coach of the American team that won gold medals at the 2010 and the 2014 FIBA (Fédération Internationale de Basketball Amateur) Basketball World Cup. He was also an assistant coach for the 1992 USA Dream Team, which won a gold medal at the summer Olympics. The College Basketball Hall of Fame inducted Coach K in 2006, and the United States Olympic Hall of Fame inducted him in 2009 (with the Dream Team).

In 2006, Krzyzewski and his family founded the Emily Krzyzewski Center, a nonprofit organization based in Durham, North Carolina, named in honor of Krzyzewski's mother. Its mission is to inspire students from kindergarten to high school to dream big, act with character and purpose, and reach their potential as leaders in their community. The Center's K to College Model serves academically focused students in out-of-school programming designed to help them achieve success in school, gain entry to college, and break the cycle of poverty in their families.

Here is an inspiring insight into leadership from Coach K:

"There are five fundamental qualities that make every team great: communication, trust, collective responsibility, caring and pride. I like to think of each as a separate finger on the fist. Any one individually is important. But all of them together are unbeatable."
—Coach K

CONCLUSIONS

We all should, and can, learn a great deal from looking back for examples of how to lead and how not to lead. As with any leadership lesson, one can learn a great deal from our predecessors' and role models' successes and failures. History is a great teacher. The 10 leaders named in this chapter have been and, in some cases, continue to be, great teachers of leadership. These 10 leaders embody exemplary practices of leadership—through a lifetime of work, service, and caring. In this brief chapter, their words have been quoted, their lifetime of gifts to the world covered in an abridged fashion, and some advice shared as to what they would have us carry forward.

🔑 KEY TAKEAWAY POINTS

- The five practices of exemplary leaders include: (a) challenging the process, (b) inspiring a shared vision, (c) modeling the way, (d) enabling others to act, and (e) encouraging the heart.

- People want to be around leaders who are positive.

- Show others how much you care about them and treat people with kindness.

- There are five ingredients that make a great team: communication, trust, collective responsibility, caring, and pride.

CALL TO ACTION

1. Pick one of the five practices of exemplary leadership for which you feel you have the most strengths, based on the explanation of that practice within this chapter. How do you feel you are similar to one or both of the leaders highlighted in that section? How can you show that practice each day in your work?

2. Focus on the "Encourage the Heart" section of this chapter. Explore the quotes and the advice from each leader. What can you model, behavior-wise, from either or both leaders?

3. Pick one lesson from one leader and tell another person you work with what that lesson is and how you will make that lesson "come alive" each day at work. Let that person be your accountability partner (AP).

4. Examine each of the pieces of advice at the end of the description of each leader highlighted within this chapter. Which five are the most relevant/compelling to you? Pick one, and focus on that one for the next 2 weeks. Then, pick another, and focus on that one for 2 weeks. Then choose another.

   Find three colleagues from your workplace. They will be your leadership APs. Each of the four of you reads this chapter. Each of you will pick one skill that he or she commits to working on based on examples from these 10 impactful leaders. Have each person share the skill he or she has chosen and tell the others how they will know whether he or she is improving.

   Ask each other at least once each week for 3 months these five questions:

   - How are you working on your skill now?

   - How do you know?

   - How are you working to continually improve your skill?

   - How do you know it is improving?

   - How are you sharing your best practices and lessons learned with others?

REFERENCES

Biography. (2018). Mother Teresa. Retrieved from https://www.biography.com/people/mother-teresa-9504160

Fortune. (2014). The world's 50 greatest leaders (2014). Retrieved from www.fortune.com/2014/03/20/worlds-50-greatest-leaders

Glastris, P., & LeTourneau, N. (2017, January/February). Obama's top 50 accomplishments, revisited. *Washington Monthly*. Retrieved from https://washingtonmonthly.com/magazine/januaryfebruary-2017/obamas-top-50-accomplishments-revisited/

The King Center. (2018). About Dr. King: Overview. Retrieved from www.thekingcenter.org/about-dr-king

Kouzes, J. M., & Posner, B. Z. (2017). *A coach's guide to developing exemplary leaders: Making the most of the leadership challenge and the leadership practices inventory (LPI)*. San Francisco, CA: John Wiley & Sons.

Nobelprize.org. (2019). The Nobel Peace Prize 2009. Retrieved from https://www.nobelprize.org/prizes/peace/2009/summary/

Whitman, W. (2015). *The complete writings of Walt Whitman, Leaves of Grass*. New York, NY: Andesite Press

Forming and Leading a High-Performing Team

Bernadette Mazurek Melnyk, Dianne Morrison-Beedy, and Robert Smith

"Teamwork is the ability to work together toward a common vision. The ability to direct individual accomplishments toward organizational objectives. It is the fuel that allows common people to attain uncommon results."—Andrew Carnegie

LEARNING OBJECTIVES

- Discuss the rationale for building and leading a high-performing team.
- Define various approaches to interviewing when selecting team members.
- Describe important strategies for building and sustaining effective teams.
- Identify stages of a team's life cycle.
- Apply concepts of team building in football to building effective teams in organizations.

INTRODUCTION

Helen Keller once said, "Alone we can do so little, together we can do so much." **Team** means together, everyone accomplishes more. A key to moving from good to great and achieving organizational goals is to build and lead high-performing teams. Team building works. It helps members to build on their strengths and minimize their limitations in order to reach their goals. Further, team-building interventions have been found to consistently result in improvements in team effectiveness (Beauchamp, McEwan, & Waldhauser, 2017). In healthcare, interprofessional teams composed of members from different disciplines who are working together toward a common goal produce better outcomes. An effective and high-performing team is often the key differentiator in organizations that successfully accomplish their vision and those that do not. This chapter discusses the rationale for building and leading a high-performing team, describes two models that portray a team's life cycle, and identifies key strategies for building and sustaining high-performing diverse and inclusive teams.

WHY BUILD A TEAM?

A *team* is defined as a group of individuals working together for a common purpose, who rely on each other to achieve mutually defined results. The team's mission is driven by the organization's vision, which must be communicated to all team members in order to inspire them and gain their buy-in. When the team becomes stronger than the sum of all its individual members, it achieves synergy, which may be the single most important key to building effective teams. The most success-ful teams achieve their best results by using optimal contributions of all its team members. Find-ings from research have supported that interprofessional teams demonstrate higher healthcare quality and better outcomes than individual professions functioning in silos (Institute of Medicine, 2013). For team effectiveness, it is essential to build trust and respect among team members. Building a team encourages members to manage their differences together and promotes a better understanding among individuals. Actions for building relationships within a team include:

- Clarify work expectations and assignments.
- Listen actively.
- Use candor/managing conflict in healthy ways.
- Recognize effort.
- Facilitate participation.
- Reflect on each other's values.
- Collaborate.

 CALL TO ACTION

Think about a team of which you are currently a member.
Are you clear about the team's mission and goals as well as how they relate to the organiza-tion's vision and goals?
Is there trust and respect among the team members? If not, how could they be further built?

FORMING AN EFFECTIVE TEAM

Select a strong team to accomplish your vision and goals. Understand your own personality style and strengths to form an effective team, as the team members you choose should comple-ment your attributes (see Chapter 3, Understanding and Developing Yourself As a Leader). For example, if a leader has a predominantly **D personality** style that encompasses dreaming (big-picture vision), discovery or risk-taking, and fast-paced action, he or she may specifically want to balance the team out with an individual who is high on **C personality** traits who will be more focused on details of the strategic plan and the implementation process. Because the U.S. Census Bureau predicts the population of the United States will be mostly non-White within the next 30 years, increasing diversity and inclusion when forming a team is a strategic necessity (Hegwer, 2016).

CALL TO ACTION

Reflect on your predominant personality style traits. If you were to select individuals to be on your team to accomplish a specific project, what types of people would you look for to complement your own strengths and enhance your limitations?

Conducting an Effective Interview for Team Members

Why is interviewing so important? Interviewing is about the triple aim of details, match, and fit. A leader can gain further insight into the information that was provided in the individual's application and résumé or curriculum vitae (CV) and determine whether the individual's skills, abilities, and experiences are a good match for the organization and the position that is to be filled. Conducting an effective interview also helps to assess the candidate's fit with the organization's culture, vision, and mission.

As you try to build an effective team, you will most likely gravitate toward finding true high performers—isn't everyone? You are looking beyond employees who have the skills and experiences that are required in the job, but beyond those qualities, you are looking for candidates who have a positive attitude and passion for the role that really makes them stand out from other applicants. Successful leaders often hire for attitude as skills can be taught and built. Identifying how eager the person actually is to do the job and how self-motivated he or she is to make a difference in your organization is the key to good hiring. An interview allows you to gain insight on questions such as, "Can the person overcome obstacles he or she might encounter? Is he or she passionate about the role and the work? Does he or she seem to fit with the culture in the way he or she wants to function in the position?" Asking the right questions during an interview can help to determine whether you have a candidate who is willing to go the extra yard to attain solutions, even in tough situations, as you want a candidate who will not give up and will try to make things work.

There are various approaches to interviewing applicants for positions in your organization, including open-ended unstructured interviews, using more structured behavioral-interviewing approaches, and motivationally based interviewing. Each type of interview has its advantages and disadvantages, but no matter how you approach the interview, remember that your time to gather information to assist you in decision-making is short, so do not waste your time asking questions that are irrelevant to the job, superficial, and do not provide additional information that expands on what is already in the written application, or that would be considered offensive or illegal.

UNSTRUCTURED INTERVIEWS

An unstructured approach to interviewing can seem less time intensive because these types of interviews are more conversational with no set of predetermined questions to use, although the interviewer has specific topics in mind that he or she would like to cover. The interviewer must be both purposeful and directive. He or she must keep the applicant focused and steer him or her to relevant topics rather than to let the conversation drift away to discussions of pets, travel, and people they might jointly know.

Unstructured interviews take a skilled interviewer and, if many different interviewers are used, cross-training is especially important. Otherwise, candidates might not get a fair shake if there are many applicants being assessed because the conversations in each interview went off in very different directions. This loss of reliability can make this type of interviewing a challenge. Unstructured interviewing allows for spontaneity and probing questions are asked based on the direction provided by the applicant's prior answers. This type of interview does allow the chance for the interviewer to see behind the screen of the applicant's stage presence, which can occur during interviews.

 ## BEHAVIORAL INTERVIEWS

Behavioral interviewing requires more preparation prior to the actual interview because questions focus on past exemplar circumstances or situations. Past behavior can often indicate future behavior, so behavioral interviews could help to determine the applicant's potential to handle similar situations in your organization. Behavioral-interview questions are structured and probes are often used to provide additional information. Within behavioral interviewing, a specific set of relevant questions is asked about the position and predetermined rating scales are used to evaluate all candidates so that they are interviewed under the same types of conditions. This makes it easier for you as the interviewer to evaluate and compare the candidates in a fair manner, reducing bias and ambiguity. Try to ask each candidate the questions using the same wording, in the same order, and using the same scoring system. It is not surprising that it takes considerable time and effort to prepare for these types of interviews. Your organization will need to first identify the critical competencies needed for the posted position. In this process, really think about what knowledge, skills, abilities, and other characteristics are critical for success in the position. Examples of questions would be to ask about a situation, for example, "Tell me about a time when you had to lead a team of people with diverse opinions and capabilities" or "Tell me about a time when you had to make a change in your organization that you did not fully support." Interviewers should insert pertinent situations connected to the specific position into the questions. Similarly, determining what actions a candidate took to accomplish certain tasks ("What did you do when you had to make a change in a project at the last minute and did not have sufficient resources?") and outcomes ("What were the results of those actions? How did it turn out?") are all useful interview probes.

It is necessary to create rating scales for each question in behavioral interviewing. These ratings can range from relatively simple dichotomous yes/no, acceptable/unacceptable or satisfactory/unsatisfactory responses to more complex Likert-type scales for scoring such as, "far exceeds requirements/exceeds requirements/ meets requirements/ below requirements/significant gap." The latter usually provides better differentiation among candidates.

Following all the extensive scale development and identification of required competencies with applicable questions and probes, your next step is determining who will interview candidates. Your interviewers should represent a diverse cross-section of people in your organization who will be involved with this role. These interviewers should have a thorough understanding of the job so that they can assess for important behavioral and technical competencies as well as being able to put interviewees at ease so they will feel comfortable and provide sufficient information to make a decision regarding hiring. The interviewee also needs to be able to assess the fit of the applicant with the organizational cultural. Thus, it often requires extensive training for behavioral interviewing for all the people who will be interviewing applicants. Instead of using a task-oriented approach with candidates, reviewing what might be on their résumés, the behavioral interviewer facilitates applicants in telling a short story on what they have accomplished and how they accomplished it as well as positive and negative reactions to the situation.

MOTIVATIONALLY BASED INTERVIEWS

Whether individuals are intrinsically or extrinsically motivated will impact your organization's results. Individuals who are intrinsically motivated select opportunities because of how rewarding the opportunity is to them personally or they find it satisfying, whereas those who are driven by external factors, such as money, employment security, titles, or other rewards, are more extrinsically motivated. Interview questions will encompass not job-initiative competencies, but rather motivation competencies such as drive and energy, commitment, resilience, and service.

Asking more motivationally based interview questions can help determine whether the applicant will continue to be motivated in the constraints of the role (e.g., set salary, no independent decision-making, pressing deadlines). Each position is unique and might have a different balance of possible intrinsic and extrinsic rewards associated with it. You can assess commitment by asking, "Tell me about a time on the job when you went the extra mile." Similarly, if you ask the candidate to "Describe a time when your enthusiasm for a project dwindled," or "Have you ever worked hard on getting a project ready, only to have it be canceled? How did you react?" can be helpful in assessing resilience. In general, motivation can be assessed by asking applicants to "Describe the work environment where you are happiest and most productive. Can you give me an example of when you were the most motivated at work, what was the experience like and what was it that got you so energized?" Try to prompt the candidate to provide not only details about the situation and his or her behavior or actions taken but also the impact or outcomes as a result.

INTERVIEWING SUMMARY

Ultimately, interviewing should identify applicants with the position IQ and experience needed to function in the role. In addition, assessment of internal integrity is critical as no leader wants a new hire to become a detriment to the organization. Determining whether the applicant has the energy to persevere through adversity to find answers and reach solutions is key to a successful hire. Passion for the position cannot be taught and is a primary driver of successful hires. When building your team, you may choose to incorporate aspects of all types of interviewing styles depending on the type of position, level of leadership required, number of positions available, and number of applicants. There is no right or wrong choice when it comes to an approach, but as previously mentioned, there are more effective and less effective ways to carry out the interview. Choose team members wisely because when people who are not a good fit are hired, adverse outcomes to the leader and organization are very costly.

STRATEGIES FOR BUILDING AND SUSTAINING HIGH-PERFORMING TEAMS

There are some very key tactics for building and sustaining high-performing teams, including:

1. Establish an exciting team vision and mission.

   Having a vision and mission that all team members have contributed to will enhance buy-in and provide motivation to the team, especially when "character-builders" arise along the course of the team's journey. If a team does not know where it is going, it will end up someplace else. If you find the team's work is slowing down, place the vision and purpose in front of team members again to reignite their enthusiasm for the mission.

2. Establish strong leaders or coleaders for the team.

   Match individuals with strong leadership characteristics to spearhead the effort. Do not discard "informal" leaders as they can be more effective at times than leaders who have formal titles (Melnyk & Fineout-Overholt, 2019).

3. Determine team values.

   Ask the team what values are important to them (e.g., honesty, transparency, promptness) and come to a consensus on which values are most important to all team members. These become the core values of the team.

4. Establish team norms.

   Team norms are the principles that guide certain behaviors (e.g., being on time for meetings, maintaining confidentiality, allowing everyone on the team to have an opportunity for input without judgment, having crucial conversations).

5. Assess commitment to team norms.

   The team will function effectively if all team members are committed to the norms.

6. Establish team goals.

   Team goals should be SMART (specific and easily understood, measurable, attainable, relevant [congruent with the vision and mission] and time bound).

7. Set clear priorities and expectations.

   Uncertainty regarding priorities and expectations is often a source of anxiety for team members. Also, having clear expectations facilitates effective team performance.

8. Match individual team member's roles and responsibilities to his or her strengths.

   When people have an opportunity to be matched in a role or position that builds on their strengths or what they do best, they and their outcomes soar. StrengthsFinder assessment is an outstanding strategy to use to identify each team member's strengths based on 34 themes of talent (e.g., achiever, activator, arranger, developer, learner, maximizer, includer, relator, strategic, futuristic) and is a very worthwhile exercise for team members to complete before roles and responsibilities are assigned (Rath, 2007).

9. Build trust in the team.

   With trust comes teamwork and collaboration. Have integrity and be transparent, that is, willing to disclose information on a regular basis. Follow through on what you say. Tell the team you believe in them and their ability to accomplish their goals. Listen carefully to team members and act on some of the suggestions offered by the group. Hold people accountable for their behaviors. Have a "no secrets" policy. Be fair: Don't show favoritism. Manage conflict effectively—learn how to have crucial conversations. Give credit to your team when members deserve it.

   "Create a large "trust bank" with your team that will not be drained the first time that you make a mistake."—Stephen Covey

10. Conduct effective regular team meetings.

    Determine how often the team believes it is necessary to meet. Send out an agenda prior to the meeting to ensure that meetings are productive and goals are accomplished. Keep discussion focused during the meeting to ensure the meeting concludes on time. Encourage team members to stand for portions of the meetings. In addition to being good for cardiovascular health, you get through meetings more quickly when everyone stands versus sits! If serving snacks for the meeting, ensure that they are healthy.

11. Monitor outcomes regularly.

    One or two team members should be charged with the responsibility of monitoring outcomes to ensure that progress is made in accomplishing the SMART goals established.

12. Recognize team members' contributions regularly.

    Recognition and appreciation are terrific motivators. Remember to thank and recognize team members for their contributions on a regular basis.

13. Conduct celebrations for successes along the journey.

    The best way to prevent team fatigue is to create short-term wins and celebrate accomplishments/achieved goals.

LIFE CYCLE OF A TEAM

The **life cycle of a team** is based on group dynamics theory and captures the distinct phases of team development. Leaders must know what to anticipate in terms of the life cycle of a team so that they do not get discouraged when they observe the characteristics that typically happen in the second "storming" stage of development (Table 6.1). In the "storming" stage of a team's life cycle, leaders need to keep the team focused, plan for early and frequent successes, resolve individual differences, have candor in communication, and treat mistakes as opportunities for growth. In the "norming" stage, leaders should continue open and frequent communication, encourage autonomy and shared leadership, review and continue to build relationships, and address issues forthrightly and civilly as necessary. After a team meets its goals and if it is to be disbanded, leaders must recognize the need for team members to express their feelings and concerns, pointing out all of the impactful outcomes that resulted from the team's efforts, reflecting on the positive experience, thanking and recognizing team members for their commitment and work, and celebrating accomplishments.

TABLE 6.1 **Stages of Team Development**

Stage	Description	Characteristics
Forming	A group of individuals transitions into a functioning team	• Anxiety • Excitement • Exploration • High motivation • Testing • Trust
Storming	Team members experience tension and negativity when they realize the amount of responsibility and work that lies ahead	• Attitude changes • Competitiveness • Defensiveness • Disunity • Resistance to varying approaches
Norming	Team members acclimate to working cooperatively with each other, thereby increasing satisfaction	• Collaborative decision-making • Constructive feedback trust and respect • Shared responsibilities
Performing	Team matures and is extremely productive	• Confidence • High interaction • Increased performance • Optimism

Source: Adapted from Egolf, D. B., & Chester, S. L. (2013). *Forming, storming, norming & performing. Successful communication in groups and teams* (3rd ed.). Bloomington, IN: iUniverserve.

LESSONS IN BUILDING PROFESSIONAL FOOTBALL TEAMS BY ROBERT SMITH

(*Note:* Robert Smith is a former running back who played college football at The Ohio State University and played professionally with the Minnesota Vikings of the National Football League [NFL]).

Teamwork is the foundation of success in football, which is the ultimate team sport. The team is composed of multiple units—with some units operating on the field together to achieve a task on a particular play and some units working independently as other units watch from the sideline. Each unit has a different task and each unit must properly prepare to execute its task efficiently so that the overall team has the greatest chance for success—a win. A football team is said to be working at its best when all three "phases" are operating efficiently. These phases are referred to as *offense, defense*, and *special team* units. Each phase is on the field independently while the others are on the sideline watching their teammates perform. The best teams realize that overall success (wins and losses) depends on both individual and collective effort. The best teams are inspired to work for their teammates and work to inspire their teammates. They know that for a team, success never happens alone.

Building a football team begins months before games are ever played. Offseason conditioning is about more than conditioning the bodies of individual players. Players are asked to train together in the offseason because it inspires them to work harder when they are in groups—a healthy peer pressure. Getting up at 5 a.m. to run until you are nauseated may not sound like a lot of fun and it is not meant to be. People work harder when they feel their efforts are a part of something bigger than themselves. They push harder when their teammates are watching and they begin to trust each other more when they see that they can rely on their teammates to push themselves.

I was initially surprised that the training-camp lodging was the same in the NFL as it had been in college. It was back to dorm room life for everyone. Simple wire-frame beds and thin mattresses and roommates for everyone, whether your salary was six, seven, or even eight figures! Why bring the players together like this right before the season? My NFL coach, Denny Green, referred to it as the "rarefied air" of training camp. Special conditions arranged to reinforce the notion that everyone on a team should think of himself as part of the collective group. No one gets special accommodations because everyone is expected to have to deal with the same discomforts because the real focus should be on getting better as a team. What does that mean in football? It means that you should be studying to become a better player. That means understanding your responsibilities as well as the responsibilities of your teammates on given plays. It means understanding how your performance can affect your teammates and how their performance can affect yours.

My running-back coach with the Minnesota Vikings was Tyrone Willingham. He is one of the most detail-oriented individuals I have ever met. The day after I was drafted, he sat me down to watch a film of me playing in college. It was a run to the far left side of the line of scrimmage. He stopped the film at a point where I could have turned the ball upfield toward the goal line instead of continuing on my path further to the outside. He said "if you made this cut [*cut* refers to a sharp turn when running with the football] here, you could have gained eight more yards on this play. You have to do a better job of reading your blocks [a *block* is one player getting in the way of another player to keep him from making a tackle]." He was right; my lineman was doing his job the way he was supposed to do. If I did a better job of studying what he was trying to do on a given play, I would have a better chance of anticipating it and reacting to it. My performance would improve, which meant the results for the team would be better. As a result, we would have a better chance at success if I studied my job better to better understand what I was supposed to do at every level of detail. Your individual performance was always closely examined, but this was always done in a way to emphasize the impact of your play on the overall goals and actions of the team.

Days in the locker room always started the same way: Our head coach, Denny Green, would stand in front of the large meeting room and address the entire team. No one dared to be late or tried to carry on another conversation while the head man was talking to us. He played drums in his spare time (he had a set in one of the rooms of the football facility) and often talked about the importance of drums to music—they set the beat of the entire band—and related this to his role as the head of the team. Like a drummer, he set the tempo and we followed along, always keeping in mind the importance of how what we did as individual players affected the overall performance of the team. He also noted the importance of acknowledging players' different backgrounds and interests while placing the goals of the team first. We were encouraged to spend time together and to get to know each other because stronger bonds between teammates translated into greater accountability to each other.

After the team meeting, we would split into meetings as an entire offense and defense and then as smaller position units. There was very little that was ever done on an individual basis. People often ask me if I miss playing. You certainly miss competing and the excitement, but, more than anything else, most former players miss the camaraderie of the locker room. We spent a great deal of time studying, practicing, and playing together, but we also spent time sharing stories and laughing together. The best teams I was ever a part of truly enjoyed being around each other. It wasn't that we were all the same or always got along perfectly. Differences were understood, embraced, and even celebrated. We were like family. Like any big office or other working group, there are always some people who you will be closer to than others, but the strongest teams have the most bonds, so individuals should always look to reach out and make more connections. We would go out to dinner together or go to movies together—all time spent strengthening the bonds that were so important to performing our jobs on game day.

You need to be able to trust your teammates in football. It's a physical game that involves violent collisions and, when someone fails to do his job properly, it could mean the possibility of serious injury for a teammate. This is why trusting that your teammate takes the proper step or uses the proper technique is so important in football. It is also why players are encouraged and even expected to call each other out if they feel that their teammates are not studying or working the way they should. This needs to be handled the right way, but teammates who respect each other also respect their opinions and constructive criticism that is meant to encourage, not demean. It is all about ensuring that everyone helps pull his own weight.

There is nothing like the feeling in the locker room after a victory. After all the hours of study and practice, after a hard-fought battle on game day—a win! Denny would stand in the locker room and address the team. The exhaustion and soreness always felt a little better after a successful outing on the field. He was always sure to mention the preparation that led up to the day and the teamwork that led to the day's result. Everyone had a job to do and because we did it individually the way we were supposed to, the team as a whole was successful. He would often remind us of the importance of selflessness on game day: "Know your role, accept your role, and be the best at your role!" We went in with confidence in our preparation and each other, and we all looked forward to the post-victory speech when Denny would remind us: "When we play together like we play, when we play our best, no one can touch us!" There's nothing like the feeling of winning with the team you love.

🔑 KEY TAKEAWAY POINTS

- The most successful teams achieve their best results by using optimal contributions of all team members.

- Building trust and respect among team members is essential for team effectiveness.

- When team members contribute to a vision and goals, they are more likely to sustain the motivation to reach them.

- Learn to conduct great interviewers to hire team members who will be a good match for your organization or project.

- Match team members' strengths to their roles/responsibilities for maximum outcomes.

- Know the stages of a team's life cycle (i.e., forming, storming, norming, and performing) and what strategies are helpful for optimal performance in each of the stages.

CALL TO ACTION

You are the director of eight medical–surgical units in a large healthcare system in the northeastern region of the United States. The CEO of your organization calls on you to solve the problem as to why there has been an increase in the number of falls in patients on your units. She asks you to put a team together to implement solutions to reduce the number of falls as not only are these incidents distressing for the patients and families, they are costly for the healthcare system. You take on this challenge with enthusiasm, but at the first meeting of all of the individual unit managers to discuss the situation, it is obvious that they have differing opinions regarding who should be on the team to address the issue and how this project should be implemented. How would you go about putting a terrific team together to take on this initiative? Outline the specific action steps you would take once the team members were identified at the beginning to the successful completion of the initiative.

REFERENCES

Beauchamp, M. R., McEwan, D., & Waldhauser, K. J. (2017). Team building: Conceptual, methodological, and applied considerations. *Current Opinion in Psychology, 16*, 114–117. doi:10.1016/j.copsyc.2017.02.031

Egolf, D. B., & Chester, S. L. (2013). Forming, storming, norming & performing. *Successful communication in groups and teams* (3rd ed.). Bloomington, IN: iUniverserve.

Hegwer, L. R. (2016). Building high-performing, highly diverse teams and organizations. *Healthcare Executive, 31*(6), 10–16, 18–19.

Institute of Medicine. (2013). *Interprofessional education for collaboration: Learning how to improve health from interprofessional models across the continuum of education to practice: Workshop summary.* Washington, DC: National Academies Press.

Melnyk, B. M., & Fineout-Overholt, E. (2019). Creating a vision and motivating a change to evidence-based practice in individuals, teams, and organizations. In B. M. Melnyk & E. Fineout-Overholt (Eds.), *Evidence-based practice in nursing and healthcare. A guide to best practice* (4th ed., pp. 428–444). Philadelphia, PA: Wolters Kluwer.

Rath, T. (2007). *StrengthsFinder 2.0.* New York, NY: Gallup Press.

Leading Organizational Change and Building Wellness Cultures for Maximum ROI and VOI

Bernadette Mazurek Melnyk and Sharon Tucker

"Maintaining an effective culture is so important that it, in fact, trumps even strategy."—Howard Stevenson, Professor Emeritus, Harvard University

LEARNING OBJECTIVES

- Discuss the importance of an exciting team vision for successful organizational change.

- Describe three organizational change conceptual models.

- Identify key steps in leading and sustaining organizational change initiatives.

- Describe barriers and facilitators of system-wide change in an organization.

- Discuss strategies in building a wellness culture, including return on investment (ROI) and value of investment (VOI).

INTRODUCTION

Many healthcare systems across the country desperately need change to improve healthcare quality, safety, and population health outcomes and to reduce costs. Yet change is typically a "character-building" process, as systems are often steeped in tradition or have a culture of "that is the way things are done here." Creating organizational change is often necessary for improved outcomes, but it is a complex and lengthy process. Cultures often take many years to change.

No successful change takes place without strong leadership. Unfortunately, many leaders leave their positions before they see the outcome of their years of intense efforts. Although leaders need to realize that change efforts fail about 50% of the time and culture change efforts have an average success rate of only 19% (Gibbons, 2015), they must keep their eyes on an exciting vision in order not to get discouraged if progress is slow. There are general principles of organizational change that accelerate the process of change when an exciting vision is created and a well-delineated strategic plan is carefully executed (Melnyk & Fineout-Overholt, 2019).

Vision + Strategic Execution = Outcomes

Most organizational change theories tend to be conceptual rather than evidence based (Gibbons, 2015). As a result, leaders are often left with making decisions about strategy without solid evidence to guide their planning. In addition, many organizational change initiatives fail because leaders and teams lose sight of their vision, get deterred by barriers that are challenging to overcome, and forget the stages of organizational change that are a normal part of the change process, which can lead to abandoning a change initiative before completion.

This chapter discusses critical principles and steps for leading and sustaining change in organizations, including common barriers and facilitators. Several change models are described. Strategies for building wellness cultures to maximize ROI and of VOI are also highlighted.

CREATING AN EXCITING VISION FOR ORGANIZATIONAL CHANGE AND INITIAL ACTION TACTICS

A key initial strategy for sparking organizational change is an exciting vision created by the leader and his or her leadership team. According to Carl Sandberg, "Nothing happens unless first a dream." A compelling vision that resonates with people keeps them excited about an organizational change effort. Achieving buy-in to the vision from the grassroots of an organization accelerates the change process, so invest time in holding focus groups/meetings with the people who will be implementing a system-wide change. Communicate the vision clearly with "heartfelt messages" that appeal to people's emotions, motivating them to engage in the change effort (Kotter & Cohen, 2012) because knowledge with facts does not typically lead to a change in behavior. To gain clarity and buy-in to a vision, a leader should ask his or her team the following question:

"What can we do in the next 5 to 10 years if we know we cannot fail?"—Bern Melnyk

Keep an exciting vision in front of the team at all times, especially when barriers and fears arise, or the team is experiencing fatigue. The first 90 days after a new leader enters a system is a critical period for assessment of the organization's structure, culture, and environment as well as for action. During this time, form a strong leadership team and create an exciting team vision. Leaders often forget how essential this team vision is and tend to focus on outlining specific details of a strategic plan. Understand that although you need a well-defined strategic plan and execution, *the lack of an exciting team vision is a fatal flaw in organizational change.* Further, autocratic dictates from a leader are counterproductive to establishing buy-in and creating sustained organizational change.

Dr. William DeVries, the chief surgeon who inserted the first artificial heart in a human patient, spoke about his vision of performing this procedure for years. DeVries rehearsed that procedure in his mind repeatedly in terms of exactly how he was going to perform it so that when the opportunity finally presented itself, he was ready for successful execution.

Mark Spitz dreamed of becoming an Olympic gold medalist for several years. He trained for the Olympics by getting up early every morning and swimming many hours a day looking at a black line on the bottom of the pool. Spitz contended that what kept him practicing day in and day out for multiple hours was that as he swam and looked at the black line, he kept the vision of standing on the Olympic platform and receiving an Olympic gold medal around his neck. It was this Olympic dream that kept him going and persisting through many character-building days of relentless practice.

Establish a strong leadership team that will spearhead organizational change. When a team of leaders shares a common vision for which everyone has had the opportunity for input, there is greater ownership and investment among the team members to facilitate organizational change. A leader should be keenly aware of his or her own personality style and strengths, and the team members chosen should complement these assets. Chapter 6, Forming and Leading a High-Performing Team, describes strategies for forming and sustaining effective teams.

If a leader enters an organization and finds that the leadership team in place is not effective or does not complement his or her strengths, changes to the team must be made early. Although it can be very difficult to remove people from their positions, organizational change will be accomplished faster with a leadership team that is "in sync" with the leader and committed to achieving the common vision.

CALL TO ACTION

What is the vision of your current organization? Do you buy into that vision?
Think about the leadership team in your current organization.
Is it effective? If yes, why? If not, why not?

Once you establish the vision and leadership team, identify clearly defined goals with deadline dates. Goals should be **SMART** (i.e., **s**pecific, **m**easurable, **a**ttainable, **r**elevant, and **t**ime bound [Feldman, 2016]). The established goals also should be high enough to facilitate growth in the organization, but not unrealistically high so that people get easily frustrated by their inability to reach them.

Next, form a well-defined and written strategic plan for successful change. Many initiatives fail because individuals and teams do not carefully outline implementation strategies for each established goal and do not implement a process for regularly monitoring their progress. As part of the strategic planning process, conduct a **SCOT** (**S**trengths, **C**haracter-builders or **Ch**allenges, **O**pportunities, and **T**hreats) analysis, including:

- Assess and identify the current strengths in the system that will facilitate the success of a new project.

- Assess and identify the internal character-builders or challenges in the system that may hinder the initiative, with strategies to overcome them.

- Outline the opportunities for success.

- Delineate the external threats or barriers to the project's completion, with strategies to overcome them.

As part of the SCOT analysis, perform an assessment of resources in the organization and the level of readiness for system-wide change.

Change efforts often fail because of a lack of persistence and patience as well as problems with execution, especially when challenges are encountered or the results of persistent action are not yet obvious. An analogy to this scenario may be seen in the giant bamboo Asian tree. This tree has a particularly hard seed. The seed is very difficult to grow; it must be watered and fertilized every day for 5 years before any portion of it breaks the soil. At the end of the fifth year of watering, the tree breaks ground and grows 4 feet a day to a height of 90 feet in less than a month. The question people often ask is: Did the tree grow 90 feet in under a month or did it grow to its height over the 5 years? Of course, the answer is that it took 5 years to grow. Persist until the dream or vision and outcomes are realized, even if not seeing observable changes in the early course of implementation.

MODELS OF ORGANIZATIONAL CHANGE

Healthcare organizations today need change to improve healthcare quality and safety and reduce costs. In creating and promoting a change vision that is exciting and that results in organization of a strong leadership team, leaders must contend with a number of work settings and workforce factors that make change challenging. These include advanced technology and global networking; a changing workforce, not only demographically but also how and where individuals expect and wish to work; economic swings; competitive pressures; and globalization (Stouten, Rousseau, & Cremer, 2018). Strategies and processes necessary to support change as seamlessly and efficiently as possible are thus strongly desired and needed by organization leaders and executives. To guide organizational change, numerous models, theories, and frameworks have emerged, and thousands of books, articles, webinars, and training programs can be found on the use of these models and theories. Select models and theories from popular and scholarly literature are described, followed by a recommended 10-step process of leading organizational change.

"There is nothing more practical than a good theory."—Kurt Lewin

Organizational theories and models have been developed in several sectors, including business, academia, industry, and healthcare. Many have overlapping principles and steps of change. The most well-known and widely used models are largely not evidence based, but rather are conceptual, drawn from experiences and the literature and often published in books (rather than peer-reviewed articles) by senior-level executives or leaders (Stouten et al., 2018). Although many have written on organizational transformation, little is clear about what specific transformational processes are most effective to guide organizations and policy makers in sustained transformational change (Lee, Weiner, Harrison, & Belden, 2012). Ultimately, the process is highly complex and influenced by numerous factors.

Despite the limited evidence base for the popularized organizational models, there are a number of similar steps in the various models that are grounded in evidence of their effectiveness. Five of these models that are widely used to guide organizational change are reviewed. In addition, two models from the more recently developed field of implementation science, which emerged to identify what factors and strategies influence or inhibit the uptake of evidence-based practice change, are presented as resources for leading organizational change. Last, the conceptualization of de-implementation is highlighted.

Lewin's Three-Phase Change Management Model. Lewin (1947, 1948) introduced a theory in the 1950s that grew out of field theory, group dynamics, action research, and his three phases of change: unfreezing, changing, and refreezing. In the unfreezing phase, the goal is to determine a vision related to a needed change, to solicit support from senior management, to create a need for change, and to manage the ensuing concerns. In phase two, the work centers around communication, clarifying miscommunication and wrong information, empowering action, including modifying existing systems to accommodate the change, and involving the people in the process. In the final phase, the goal is to connect the changes within the culture and infrastructure, develop strategies to sustain the change, provide necessary support and training, and celebrate achievements.

Kotter's Eight-Step Change Management Theory. Kotter, a Harvard Business School professor, developed an eight-step model for change management that is easy to follow and primarily proposes accepting change and preparing for it (Kotter, 1996). This model's first step involves creating a sense of urgency among the people to be affected by the change so as to motivate them to move forward toward objectives. Build a team with the right people who have a mix of skills, knowledge, and commitment; create a vision with emotional connection and objectives; communicate this vision; obtain support, remove roadblocks, and implement feedback; focus on short-term goals; and remain persistent with integration into the organizational infrastructure.

However, the creation of a sense of urgency is not supported by research and has been contested by several authors, including Stouten et al. (2018), who argued that this can create stress that goes beyond cognitive bandwidth, reduces adaptive coping, and may reduce credibility when introduced as everyday occurrences.

Beer's Six-Step Change Management Model. Another Harvard Business School faculty member, Beer, developed the popular six-step change management model (Beer, 1980, 2009). It begins with emphasizing the importance of diagnosing the problem accurately as a basis for mobilizing change commitment. As with Kotter and Lewin, Beer developed a change vision that includes roles and responsibilities and involves key stakeholders who will support and communicate the vision. This leads to the final three phases of implementing and spreading the change, institutionalizing the change through integration into formal structures and processes, and then ensuring ongoing monitoring and revision of the implementation plan as needed.

Appreciative Inquiry (AI). AI is a growing change model that builds on a strengths-based model. Pioneered in the 1980s by Cooperrider and Srivastva, two professors at the Weatherhead School of Management at Case Western Reserve University, AI is conceptualized as a way of being and seeing and is both a worldview and a process for facilitating positive change in human systems (e.g., organizations, groups, and communities; Cooperrider & Srivastva, 1987). It addresses change from a positive perspective and promotes the idea that all human systems have strengths that lead to successes. Stages in AI are discover, dream, design, and destiny. Movement begins with identifying the positives, then getting to ideals that can make the organization better, planning for the change or dream, and then executing the dream. Use of this model involves grounding in the five original principles of constructionist, simultaneity, anticipatory, poetic, and positive. In addition, participation of change recipients is a key thread in this model.

Hiatt's ADKAR Model. A newer model, developed by Hiatt, is ADKAR (**A**wareness, **D**esire, **K**nowledge, **A**bility, and **R**einforcement; Hiatt, 2006), a goal-oriented model that builds sequentially. The first stage is to spread employee awareness that change is needed, followed by developing and communicating a vision. The implementation stage empowers employees with knowledge and skills-building to promote participation. As with other models, the final stage involves reinforcement of the change and integrating the change into the infrastructure of the organization's structure and processes. Employees are recognized as ambassadors of change through recognition of individual needs and the consequences of the change for them.

Rogers's Diffusion of Innovation Theory. Rogers (2003) developed the diffusion of innovation theory, which is widely used today for promoting the spread and adoption of new ideas. It describes the process of communicating messages about an innovation in a social system. There are five main stages: knowledge, persuasion, decision, implementation, and confirmation. Rogers identified the characteristics of individuals, the internal organizational structure, and the external environment as being associated with an organization's level of innovation. Those considering adopting an innovation (change) evaluate the innovation with reference to its relative advantage, compatibility, complexity, ability to be tested, and observability. The more positively these are rated, the more likely the change or innovation can be expedited and adopted. In addition, Rogers emphasized that the types of adopters (innovators, early adopters, early majority, late majority, and laggards) influence the rate and success of adoption of a new idea. Once about 35% of individuals are ready to adopt or have adopted the innovation, the speed of adoption accelerates, thereby encouraging leaders to focus on the first three groups of individuals to promote successful change.

The RE-AIM Framework. The RE-AIM framework (**R**each, **E**ffectiveness, **A**doption, **I**mplementation, and **M**aintenance), now about 20 years old, was developed by Glascow and colleagues and first published in 1999. The model "grew out of the need for improved reporting on key issues related to implementation and external validity of health promotion and health care research literature" (Gaglio, Shoup, & Glascow, 2013, p. 38). The model aimed to provide a framework for evaluating real-world application of research evidence, rather than optimal settings that did not mirror the realities of real-world clinical practices, and to provide an alternative to the gold standard of optimal settings for randomized clinical trials. The RE-AIM framework focuses on factors that can affect successful implementation and that can be considered prior to a practice change or in evaluation of a practice change.

De-implementation. A final approach to change that has very recently emerged in the implementation science literature is de-implementation, defined as "reducing or stopping the use of a health service or practice provided to patients by healthcare practitioners and systems" (Norton, Kennedy, & Chambers, 2017, p. 1). De-implementation of a routine practice can be as challenging as implementation of a new evidence-based practice (EBP). As with EBP implementation, although the empirical evidence from well-designed studies should be sufficient to stop a practice deemed ineffective, and perhaps even harmful, other factors also influence the stopping of the practice "such as inertia, financial and professional conflicts, cultural and societal values, knowledge brokering, and lobbying" (Prasad & Ioannidis, 2014, p. 1). De-implementation of a practice should be considered when an effective alternative strategy has been identified so as to avoid the use of ineffective practices and to reduce inefficiencies and unnecessary costs in healthcare.

This problem of de-implementation is far more common than most clinicians realize. Prasad and Ioannidis (2014) contended that there are likely at least 150 potentially ineffective or unsafe practices, and most likely more. They discussed the 2007 COURAGE trial, which revealed that for patients with cardiovascular disease and stable angina, an initial trial of medical treatment was as effective as routine percutaneous coronary intervention (PCI). Although PCI procedures declined after the initial report was released, by 2010, the procedure numbers were back to those that existed prior to the release of the study finding. They recommended that all unproven practices be subjected to systematic evaluations. Priority testing should be given to the following practices: those with the weakest evidence and those with significant financial burden on health payers, those that have alternative evidence-based options, those that have proven cases of harm, those for which the cost of testing is less than that of continuing the practice, those in which there are proponents to support the change, and those that can provide valuable information through testing.

In sum, select models for organizational change and integration of best practices can guide the processes and help facilitate change for healthcare leaders. Step-by-step processes have been recommended in these models, and we next recommend a hybrid 12-step approach to organizational change that builds on these models, the research literature, and our experiences.

TUCKER AND MELNYK'S 12-STEP MODEL FOR LEADING AND SUSTAINING ORGANIZATIONAL CHANGE

As emphasized earlier, key steps for leading organizational change are the creation of an exciting and compelling vision that is supported and that will be executed by a strong leadership team along with the creation of a clear and detailed strategic plan.

In a recent publication, Stouten et al. (2018) presented a strong, thoughtful critique and review of the widely used practitioner-oriented organizational change models together with an extensive review of scholarly literature. Their purpose was to develop an integrative summary of the available evidence and identify what is contested and underutilized in change management. They identified 10 steps in managing planned organizational change that we build on and combine with other literature, as well as our own research programs and real-world experiences in leading organizational change. As scholars in EBP for healthcare settings, we also integrate findings from implementation science related to effective strategies for promoting and sustaining uptake of EBP changes.

Box 7.1 presents our hybrid 12-step approach to successfully leading organizational change. The *first step* is to *be clear about the reason(s) for the change* with compelling data and the rationale for key stakeholder involvement and for ultimately getting buy-in from those who will be recipients of the change. Some of the models reviewed, such as AI, emphasize the importance of participant involvement from the beginning. Talking with employees might be part of the data gathering to define the problem.

The *second step* is to *assess the organization's readiness for change*. Many organizational change models, such as the model by Beer as well as implementation models, highlight this process. The assessment should include the existing organizational change culture and environment, leadership model and competencies to lead the change, staff morale, previous success from change projects, financial status, capacity of the organization and its members to take on demands of the change, level of stress of employees, and stakeholder composition. Grimshaw, Eccles, Lavis, Hill, and Squires (2012) stressed that, for healthcare professionals and consumers, the choice of translation strategy is more likely to be successful if it is informed by an assessment

Box 7.1	Tucker and Melnyk's 12-Step Model of Leading and Sustaining Successful Organizational Change

12 Steps in Leading and Sustaining Successful Organizational Change
1. Identify whether and why change is needed with compelling data and rationales.
2. Assess the organization's readiness for change along with its strengths and potential barriers.
3. Create a compelling and exciting vision for change that is clearly communicated to all key stakeholders and staff.
4. Solicit input on the vision from all key stakeholders and staff.
5. Convene specific leadership teams to develop a detailed strategic plan with SMART* goals, identifying barriers and strategies to overcome them.
6. Provide effective change training for leaders and education for all staff along with the needed tools and resources to succeed.
7. Leverage social networks, change champions, opinion leaders in the grassroots of the organization, and mentors.
8. Use evidence-based implementation strategies to promote and sustain the change.
9. Engage in small steps of change for quick small wins that are celebrated.
10. Provide regular recognition/appreciation of individuals and teams for their implementation efforts.
11. Evaluate outcomes by monitoring progress over time, modifying the strategic plan as indicated.
12. Disseminate progress/outcomes to stakeholders and staff, celebrating goals that are accomplished.

*SMART (Specific, Measurable, Attainable, Relevant, and Timely).

Source: Tucker and Melnyk, copyright 2019.

of the likely barriers and facilitators. There are multiple standardized organizational readiness assessments available that can be considered to help guide this assessment (Gagnon et al., 2014).

The *third and fourth steps involve development and communication of the change vision.* These steps can be seen as iterative to allow the shaping of the vision to be influenced by the people involved and their voices. The main need for change can be put forward in a vision draft, shared with the relevant people who may be impacted by the change, and their input integrated to refine and strengthen the vision. A vision must also reflect a goal that will have broad appeal among those with whom it will be shared. The vision should be communicated through multiple channels (media, meetings, one-on-one sessions) and should be repeated regularly. Being transparent, compassionate, and honest about the consequences of the vision also matters in helping employees, especially those who may experience negative consequences of the vision (Stouten et al., 2018).

The *fifth step involves convening key stakeholders and leaders to promote the change vision and help develop the comprehensive strategic plan* to achieve the change. Some literature suggests that internal and external consultants are important in developing the strategic plan (Stouten et al., 2018). Those who will be most affected by the change should be involved as they can help identify alternative strategies to support the change. Coaching, a strong evidence-based strategy, can help guide people in behavior change. Leverage internal staff with expertise in coaching or training staff in coaching to possibly expedite the change. Celebrating small wins and offering incentives and rewards to move change along are additional evidence-based strategies. Regularly recognize individuals for their change efforts.

The *sixth and seventh steps are tactical in nature and involve leader training needs and leveraging informal leaders.* Leaders are often not equipped with the knowledge and competencies to be successful in leading change. Senior leaders should be aware of this issue and should properly assess training needs for themselves, their managers, and other staff by training staff on leading change and on the aspects of the specific change being implemented. The evidence is pretty solid that social networks, opinion leaders, change agents, and mentors can all influence change. Leveraging their skills, attitudes, competencies, influence, and personalities can be key to bringing along others less excited about change. Rogers's theory of innovation especially highlights the importance of using innovators and early adopters for early change success.

The *eighth step involves using evidence-based implementation strategies to promote and sustain the change* such as leadership, coaching, communication, reinforcements, recognition, measurement, and reporting. Coaching was mentioned in step five but is also highlighted here along with education strategies, audit and feedback, and use of reminders. Consider using computer systems as part of your strategy for a successful change. Leverage internal staff with expertise in coaching or train staff in coaching to help expedite the change. Continue to recognize and appreciate individual and team efforts.

Institute systematic reviews to identify effective change tactics and strategies. There are numerous resources on best implementation strategies published today. Li, Jeffs, Barwick, and Stevens (2018) recently published a systematic review on organizational contextual features that influence the implementation of EBPs across healthcare settings. They found that organizational culture, networks and communication, leadership, resources (financial, staffing and workload, time, and education and training), evaluation, monitoring and feedback, and champions were essential to EBP success. Factors in combination were more influential than a single factor, reflecting the importance of a multistrategy tool kit.

Step nine involves small tests of change to identify and achieve small wins that can propel staff forward. This notion is consistent with self-efficacy theory (Bandura, 1986), which involves one's judgment or confidence in one's ability to achieve a specific task. Self-efficacy has repeatedly been shown to predict performance. The most powerful source of self-efficacy is mastery that comes with practice and seeing one succeed. Thus, providing staff with small opportunities to practice and achieve success can build their self-efficacy and momentum to continue to change. Show staff the gains and how they are positively affecting the organization and themselves.

Step 10 involves providing regular recognition and appreciation of individuals and teams involved in the change effort. This is one of the best and most successful strategies for change fatigue.

Step 11 includes the ongoing monitoring and evaluation of outcomes essential to sustain success, modifying the road map, identifying alternative tactics, and providing feedback to individuals about their performance. A highly effective implementation strategy is auditing and feedback in real time, giving immediate feedback when compliance or struggles are identified, as well as positive feedback for success in order to continue to build team and individual performance for successful change.

Step 12 involves dissemination of progress and outcomes to stakeholders and staff. Celebrating the goals accomplished is part of this final step.

These 12 steps can help leaders achieve transformational change. Attend to these steps with a continual focus on the vision and execution of the strategic plan with strong leaders. In addition, be ready to overcome specific barriers and enhance facilitators of change (reviewed next) to prepare for successful organizational change.

BARRIERS TO AND FACILITATORS OF ORGANIZATIONAL CHANGE

People who resist (i.e., resistors) are a huge barrier to change. Early on, when a change is introduced, especially if people do not buy into the vision or see the benefit to themselves, they often resist the change. They typically have fears and anxiety about the change. Therefore, when you sense resistance, have direct forthright conversations with these individuals and ask them to share their fears, skepticism, or uncertainties regarding the change. Often, a transparent discussion about the vision and the benefit to them or their patients will overcome their fears or anxieties and facilitate "buy-in." If this type of conversation is not successful and resistance continues, you must not spend a large amount of time and energy on these individuals. You must roll with the resistance and invest time in individuals who are innovators or early adopters who are ready to embrace and assist with the organizational change effort. In the initial phase of change, people's emotions rise and productivity often drops temporarily. Be patient and reassured during this time, and keep moving forward with the initiative, reminding people of the exciting vision and informing them that you believe they have the ability to succeed with the change effort.

Not recognizing when individuals are becoming fatigued as part of the process also stymies change. Regular recognition and appreciation of efforts prevent fatigue during an organizational change effort.

A strategic planning process that is too short or too long or that lacks a detailed strategic plan and regular monitoring of outcomes can complicate the way to success. People will often get excited about a potential change, but if it is not acted on in a relatively short time, enthusiasm will wane, and it will be difficult to garner excitement for it again. Conversely, if the strategic plan is not well thought out and acted upon in haste without including strategies to overcome barriers, the change effort will most likely fail.

Although Kotter and Cohen (2012) contend that a key facilitator in successful organizational change is to create a sense of urgency, this is disputed by some involved in change efforts. Creating a sense of urgency can be especially helpful when individuals in an organization have been in a rut or complacent for some time.

Find opinion leaders across the organization who are supportive of the change (Kotter & Cohen, 2012). Opinion leaders are people who show enthusiasm for the change and can influence others. Informal leaders without titles can be more influential than formal leaders with titles, so identify these individuals and work with them to effect the change. Look out for middle managers for "buy-in" and support because if they are not in sync and supportive of the plan, their staff are not likely to back it either.

Form teams that consist of individuals from multiple disciplines to further accelerate the change effort and facilitate a higher quality of safe patient-centered care. Studies have found that interprofessional teams demonstrate a higher quality of patient care and better outcomes than individual professions functioning in silos (Institute of Medicine, 2013).

BUILDING WELLNESS CULTURES FOR MAXIMUM ROI AND VOI

There is currently an epidemic of clinician burnout, compassion fatigue, depression, and suicide among healthcare providers that is negatively impacting healthcare quality, safety, and patient outcomes. Symptoms of burnout and depression now affect over 50% of clinicians in the United States (Dzau, Kirch, & Nasca, 2018; Melnyk, Orsolini, et al., 2018; Shanafelt et al., 2015). In addition to having such adverse effects on the personal health and well-being outcomes of clinicians and their families, practicing nurses and physicians who are experiencing poor mental and physical health are at greater risk of making medical errors.

In a national study of over 2,300 nurses from 19 healthcare systems throughout the country, Melnyk, Orsolini, et al. (2018) found that depression was the leading cause of medical errors. The longer the shift work of the nurses, the poorer was their health and the greater their probability of making medical errors (Melnyk, Orsolini, et al., 2018). As a result, the National Academy of Medicine launched an action collaborative on clinician well-being and resilience in 2017 to raise visibility on this public health epidemic and create evidence-based solutions to improve the situation (see nam.edu/initiatives/clinician-resilience-and-well-being). The NAM action collaborative is calling for healthcare systems across the nation to hire chief wellness officers (CWOs) who can lead strategic implementation efforts to build a thriving wellness culture and a healthier workforce, which ultimately leads to higher quality and safety of care (Kishore et al., 2018). CWOs should be positioned within the C-suite to elevate the importance of the position. These wellness leaders are responsible for driving evidence-based improvements in healthcare systems and building cultures that facilitate optimal well-being in clinicians because those who are healthy and satisfied in their roles will have deeper levels of engagement and a higher level of productivity and deliver a higher quality of care than those without optimal well-being.

A comprehensive multicomponent integrative strategy similar to the one that has been executed across The Ohio State University needs to be implemented in order to improve the population health outcomes. At Ohio State, nine dimensions of wellness are promoted, including physical, emotional, financial, intellectual, career, social, creative, environmental, and spiritual, and a major thrust is given to creating and sustaining a culture of well-being that makes healthy behaviors the norm or default choice (Melnyk & Neale, 2018; Melnyk, Szalacha, & Amaya, 2018). Ohio State was the first university in the country to appoint a CWO, in 2011, who provides strategic vision and planning direction to the development, implementation, and evaluation of initiatives to improve population health and wellness outcomes at OSU and surrounding communities; oversees the successful design of multiple initiatives and business plan development for implementation and delivery of programs and services; directs the implementation of innovative wellness offerings to a range of university constituents such as students, staff, faculty, alumni, and neighboring communities, ensuring that respective constituents' needs are met; evaluates programs for cost-effectiveness and optimal health and wellness outcomes for individuals and groups as well as healthier communities; works collaboratively with other leaders of the university, consults with constituents to deliver health services that provide lasting value; and supervises and spearheads related grant and contract proposals, reports, articles, and educational materials for publication.

Ohio State uses the socioecological framework to guide evidence-based interventions that are targeted to individual clinicians, their social and family networks, the worksite culture, and organizational policies (Figure 7.1; Melnyk et al., 2016). At OSU, a comprehensive integrative approach to wellness is used that promotes nine dimensions of wellness: physical, emotional, financial, intellectual, career, social, creative, environmental, and spiritual. The wellness culture at OSU is one that makes healthy options and behaviors the norm or easy to choose. A One University Health and Wellness Council, led by the CWO and composed of leaders from all areas who have a wellness focus, as well as faculty, staff and student leaders, formulates

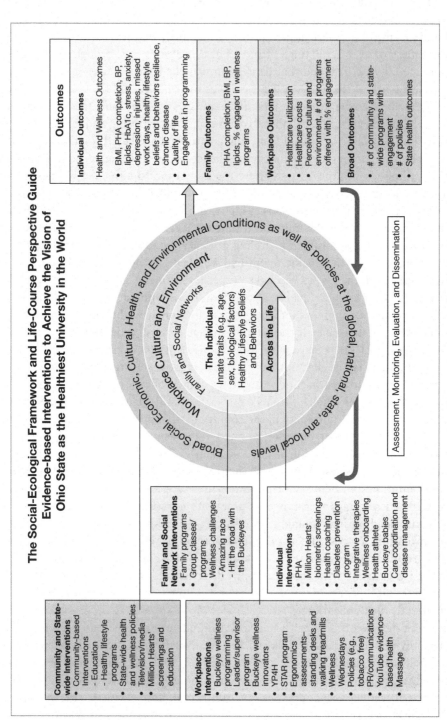

Figure 7.1 Framework for Ohio State's comprehensive and integrative strategy for health and wellness.

BMI, body mass index; BP, blood pressure; PHA, periodic health assessment; PR, public relations; STAR, Stress Trauma And Resilience program; YP4H, Your Plan 4 Health.

Source: Adapted from Model to Achieve Healthy People 2020 overarching goals. *Secretary's advisory committee on health promotion and disease prevention objectives for 2020* (2008, p. 7). Bernadette Mazurek Melnyk and Megan Amaya, copyright 2017.

the wellness strategic plan for the university, oversees its implementation, and regularly monitors its outcomes (see Figure 7.2 for the council's structure). Subcouncils that focus on alignment, faculty/staff, the medical center, outcomes, and students exist under the overall council (Figure 7.2).

Recognizing that culture consistently eats strategy for breakfast, lunch, and dinner, it is important to build a culture that makes healthy choices the easy choices for clinicians to make. Leaders must invest in wellness and "walk the talk." If leaders and supervisors do not role model and support wellness, it is unlikely that their employees will engage in healthy behaviors. Grassroots efforts, such as wellness innovators or champions used at OSU, are a low-cost but extremely effective strategy in helping to create a culture of well-being throughout an organization (Amaya, Melnyk, Buffington, & Battista, 2017). OSU has 600 wellness innovators who work with the CWO's Buckeye Wellness team in helping to build a culture of wellness at the grassroots of the organization. Formal programming is offered to the wellness innovators, and they are provided with the opportunity to apply for small grants to enhance their wellness initiatives in their colleges, departments, and hospital units (Amaya et al., 2017).

Health systems should conduct annual personalized wellness assessments and biometric screenings, including using valid and reliable assessment tools for depression, anxiety, and stress. For those clinicians with elevated symptoms, early interventions, such as cognitive behavioral therapy/skills-building and individual counseling, should be offered (Melnyk, Orsolini, et al., 2018). A menu of options that facilitate clinician engagement in wellness programming should also be available because not all clinicians will be motivated by the same activities or programs. Because one-time incentives do not typically result in sustained behavior change, incentives should be offered for consistent engagement with tiered incentives for long-term goal achievement. System solutions to problems, such as the time clinicians spend on documentation or in activities that waste clinician time versus devoting quality time to patient care and interaction, also need urgent action. Shanafelt and Noseworthy (2017) outline the following nine health system strategies to reduce burnout and improve clinician engagement:

- Acknowledge and assess the problem.
- Harness the power of leadership.
- Develop and implement targeted work unit interventions.
- Cultivate community at work.
- Use rewards and incentives wisely.
- Align values and strengthen culture.
- Promote flexibility and work–life integration.
- Provide resources to promote resilience and self-care.
- Facilitate and fund organizational science.

Many self-care and self-healing tools are of low cost and can significantly and positively affect the work environment. Leaders should incorporate self-care into meetings by using stretching exercises, mindful minutes, walking and standing meetings, or other techniques and set aside a tranquility room where staff can find calm. Provide rewards for wellness activities and self-healing behaviors to further encourage staff to engage in good self-care.

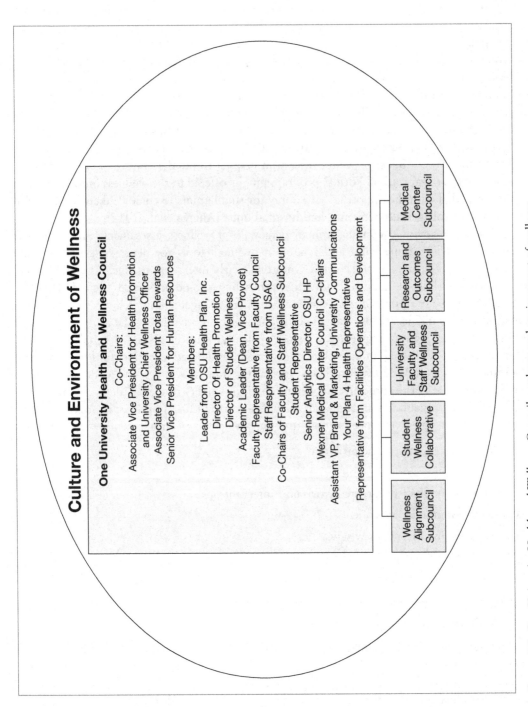

Figure 7.2 One University Health and Wellness Council—culture and environment of wellness.
OSU, The Ohio State University; OSU HP, Ohio State University Health Plan; VP, vice president; USAC, University Staff Advisory Council.

Return on Investment (ROI) and Value of Investment (VOI). Findings from multiple studies have indicated that, for every dollar invested in wellness, the typical ROI is $3.00 to $4.00 (Baicker, Cutler, & Song, 2010; Melnyk, Szalacha, et al., 2018; Sparling, 2010). Besides ROI, there is improved **VOI** with investment in wellness that includes better morale, higher job satisfaction, less "presenteeism" (coming to work but not being engaged) and less absenteeism, and higher patient satisfaction. Since the appointment of Ohio State's CWO, population cardiovascular health has improved by 7% and the university has been in a negative healthcare spend for 3 consecutive years, whereas other institutions have been experiencing upward trends of 4% to 6% annually in healthcare spending for their employees (Melnyk, Amaya, et al., 2018).

In summary, to eliminate error 2 in which clinician burnout, depression, and adverse health outcomes are resulting in compromises to healthcare quality and safety, leaders need to place priority on creating cultures of well-being and implementing programming and initiatives that can facilitate the highest level of well-being in their clinicians. Clinicians who are mentally and physically healthy will assist healthcare organizations in reaching the Quadruple Aim in healthcare (i.e., improved patient experience, which includes healthcare quality and safety, improved population health outcomes, reduced costs, and clinicians who are engaged and empowered).

KEY TAKEAWAY POINTS

- The first steps in sparking organizational change are to create an exciting team vision and formulate a strong leadership team that will lead the effort.

- Assessment of readiness for change with a SCOT analysis that identifies strengths, character-builders or challenges, opportunities, and threats with strategies to overcome the challenges is critical.

- Formulation of SMART goals and a detailed strategic plan with an outcomes evaluation is essential.

- Sharing small successes and recognizing efforts regularly will prevent change fatigue.

- Vision plus strategic execution yields success.

- Investing in a chief wellness officer and system-wide wellness culture will not only improve the quality and safety of care, but also have a substantial ROI and VOI.

- Persistence through the "character-builders" is necessary for success, so do not give up on the vision/dream.

CALL TO ACTION

You are the new CEO of a 350-bed hospital in the Midwest. In reviewing your hospital's outcome data, you see that the fall rate of patients throughout the hospital is costing you $2 million per year in unnecessary expenditures. In reviewing the policies for your hospital, you note that there is no system-wide organizational policy for the prevention of falls. While assessing the current situation, you also find that there is no consistent practice throughout the hospital for staff to follow in order to prevent patient falls. Outline the steps that you would take to lead a reduction in falls throughout your hospital.

REFERENCES

Amaya, M., Melnyk, B. M., Buffington, B., & Battista, L. (2017). Workplace wellness champions: Lessons learned and implications for future programming. *Building Healthy Academic Communities Journal, 1*(1), 59–67. doi:10.18061/bhac.v1i1.5744

Baicker, K., Cutler, D., & Song, Z. (2010). Workplace wellness programs can generate savings. *Health Affairs, 29*(2), 304–311. doi:10.1377/hlthaff.2009.0626

Bandura, A. (1986). *Social foundations of thought and action: A social cognitive theory*. Englewood Cliffs, NJ: Prentice Hall.

Beer, M. (1980). *Organization change and development: A systems view*. Santa Monica, CA: Goodyear.

Beer, M. (2009). Sustain organizational performance through continuous learning, change and realignment. In E. A. Locke (Ed.), *Handbook of principles of organizational behavior* (2nd ed., pp. 537–555). Malden, MA: Blackwell.

Cooperrider, D. L., & Srivastva, S. (1987). Appreciative inquiry in organizational life. In R. W. Woodman & W. A. Pasmore (Eds.), *Research in organizational change and development* (pp. 129–169). Greenwich, CT: JAI.

Dzau, V. J., Kirch, D. G., & Nasca, T. J. (2018). To care is human—Collectively confronting the clinician-burnout crisis. *New England Journal of Medicine, 378*(4), 312–314. doi:10.1056/NEJMp1715127

Feldman, S. (2016). *Smart goal setting. How to set smart goals*. Scotts Valley, CA: CreateSpace Independent Publishing Platform.

Gaglio, B., Shoup, J. A., & Glasgow, R. E. (2013). The RE-AIM framework: A systematic review of use over time. *American Journal of Public Health, 103*(6), e38–e46. doi:10.2105/AJPH.2013.301299

Gagnon, M. P., Attieh, R., Ghandour, E. K., Legare, F., Ouimet, M., Estabrooks, C., & Gibbons, P. (2015). *The science of successful organizational change. How leaders set strategy, change behavior, and create an agile culture*. New York, NY: Pearson Education.

Grimshaw, J. (2014). A systematic review of instruments to assess organizational readiness for knowledge translation in health care. *PLoS One, 9*(20), 1–35. doi:10.1371/journal.pone.0114338

Grimshaw, J. M., Eccles, M. P., Lavis, J. N., Hill, S. J., & Squires, J. E. (2012). Knowledge translation of research findings. *Implementation Science, 7*(1), 50. doi:10.1186/1748-5908-7-50

Hiatt, J. M. (2006). *ADKAR: A model for change in business, government and our community: How to implement successful change in our personal lives and professional careers*. Loveland, CO: Prosci Research.

Institute of Medicine. (2013). *Interprofessional education for collaboration: Learning how to improve health from interprofessional models across the continuum of education to practice: Workshop summary*. Washington, DC: National Academies Press.

Kishore, S., Ripp, J., Shanafelt, T., Melnyk, B., Rodgers, D., Brigham, T., & Dzau, V. (2018, October 26). Making the case for the chief wellness officer in America's Health Systems: A call to action. *Health Affairs Blog*. doi:10.1377/hblog20181025.308059

Kotter, J. P. (1996). *Leading change*. Cambridge, MA: Harvard Business Press.

Kotter, J. P., & Cohen, D. S. (2012). *The heart of change: Real-life stories of how people change their organizations*. Boston, MA: Harvard Business School Press.

Lee, S. Y., Weiner, B. J., Harrison, M. I, & Belden, C. M. (2013). Organizational transformation: A systematic review of empirical research in health care and other industries. *Medical Care Research and Review, 70*(2), 115–142.

Lewin, K. (1947). Frontiers in group dynamics. *Human Relations, 1*, 5–41. doi:10.1177/001872674700100103

Lewin, K. (1948). *Resolving social conflicts: Selected papers on group dynamics*. New York, NY: Harper.

Li, S., Jeffs, L., Barwick, M., & Stevens, B. (2018). Organizational contextual features that influence the implementation of evidence-based practices across healthcare settings: A systematic integrative review. *Systematic Reviews, 7*(1), 72. doi:10.1186/s13643-018-0734-5

Melnyk, B. M., Amaya, M., Gascon, G. M., & Mehta, L. S. (2018). A comprehensive approach to university wellness emphasizing Million Hearts® demonstrates improvement in population cardiovascular risk. *Building Healthy Academic Communities Journal, 2*(2), 6–11. doi:10.18061/bhac.v2i2.6555

Melnyk, B. M., Amaya, M., Szalacha, L. A., & Hoying, J. (2016). Relationships among perceived wellness culture, healthy lifestyle beliefs, and healthy behaviors in university faculty and staff: Implications for practice and future research. *Western Journal of Nursing Research, 38*(3), 308–324. doi:10.1177/0193945915615238

Melnyk, B. M., & Fineout-Overholt, B. M. (2019). *Evidence-based practice in nursing and healthcare. A guide to best practice* (4th ed.). Philadelphia, PA: Wolters Kluwer.

Melnyk, B. M., & Neale, S. (2018). *9 dimensions of wellness. Evidence-based strategies for optimal well-being*. Columbus: The Ohio State University.

Melnyk, B. M., Orsolini, L., Tan, A., Arslanian-Engoren, C., Melkus, G. D., Dunbar-Jacob, J., ... Lewis, L. M. (2018). A national study links nurses' physical and mental health to medical errors and perceived worksite wellness. *Journal of Occupational & Environmental Medicine, 60*(2), 126–131. doi:10.1097/JOM.0000000000001198

Melnyk, B. M., Szalacha, L. A., & Amaya, M. (2018). Psychometric properties of the perceived wellness culture and environment scale. *American Journal of Health Promotion, 32*(4), 1021–1027. doi:10.1177/0890117117737676

Norton, W. E., Kennedy, A. E., & Chambers, D. A. (2017). Studying de-implementation in health: An analysis of funded research grants. *Implementation Science, 12*(1), 144. doi:10.1186/s13012-017-0655-z

Prasad, V., & Ioannidis, P. (2014). Evidence-based de-implementation for contradicted, unproven, and aspiring healthcare practices. *Implementation Science, 9*(1), 1–5. doi:10.1186/1748-5908-9-1

Rogers, E. M. (2003). *Diffusion of innovations* (5th ed.). New York, NY: Simon & Schuster.

Shanafelt, T. D., Hasan, O., Dyrbye, L. N., Sinsky, C., Satele, D., Sloan, J., & West, C. P. (2015). Changes in burnout and satisfaction with work-life balance in physicians and the general US working population between 2011 and 2014. *Mayo Clinic Proceedings, 90*(12), 1600–1613. doi:10.1016/j.mayocp.2015.08.023

Shanafelt, T. D., & Noseworthy, J. H. (2017). Executive leadership and physician well-being. Nine organizational strategies to promote engagement and reduce burnout. *Mayo Clinic Proceedings, 92*(1), 129–146. doi:10.1016/j.mayocp.2016.10.004

Sparling, P. B. (2010). Worksite health promotion: Principles, resources, and challenges. *Preventing Chronic Disease, 7*(1), A25.

Stouten, J., Rousseau, D. M., & De Cremer, D. (2018). Successful organizational change: Integrating the management practice and scholarly literatures. *Academy of Management Annals, 12*(2), 752–788. doi:10.5465/annals.2016.0095

Achieving the Quadruple Aim in Healthcare With Evidence-Based Practice: A Necessary Leadership Strategy for Improving Quality, Safety, Patient Outcomes, and Cost Reductions

Bernadette Mazurek Melnyk and Lynn Gallagher-Ford

"If your actions inspire others to dream more, learn more, do more and become more, you are a leader."—John Quincy Adams

LEARNING OBJECTIVES

- Discuss the importance of evidence-based practice (EBP) in achieving the Quadruple Aim in healthcare.
- Describe the current state of EBP in healthcare, including EBP competencies.
- Identify the barriers and facilitators of EBP.
- Discuss the key leadership strategies to ignite and sustain EBP in healthcare.

EBP AND THE QUADRUPLE AIM IN HEALTHCARE

EBP is a seven-step problem-solving approach to the delivery of healthcare that integrates the best evidence from well-designed studies with a clinician's expertise and the values/preferences of the patient/family (Melnyk & Fineout-Overholt, 2019; Box 8.1). When delivered in a context of care within an organizational culture that supports it, EBP leads to the best clinical decisions, which ultimately lead to the highest quality of healthcare, improved patient outcomes, and reduced costs (Figure 8.1).

The Tiple Aim in healthcare was a concept/framework first described by the Institute for Healthcare Improvement, an independent nonprofit organization that is a leading innovator,

Box 8.1	The Seven Steps of EBP

STEP #0. Cultivate a spirit of inquiry within an EBP culture and environment.

STEP #1. Ask the burning clinical question in PICO(T) format (Patient/population, Intervention/area of interest, Comparison, Outcome(s), Time).

STEP #2. Search for and collect the most relevant best evidence.

STEP #3. Critically appraise the evidence (i.e., rapid critical appraisal, evaluation, and synthesis).

STEP #4. Integrate the best evidence with one's clinical expertise and patient/family preferences and values when making a practice decision or change.

STEP #5. Evaluate outcomes of the practice decision or change based on evidence.

STEP #6. Disseminate the outcomes of the EBP decision or change.

Source: Copyright 2019 Bernadette Mazurek Melnyk.

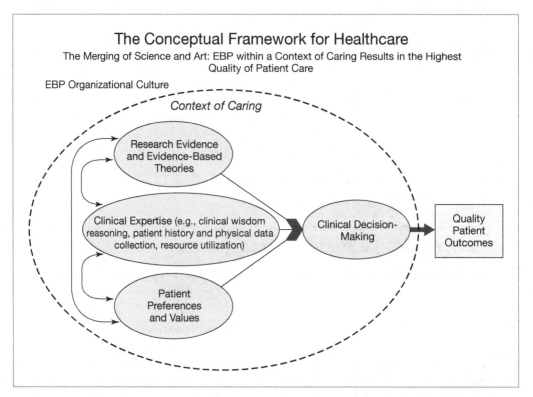

Figure 8.1 EBP in a context of care and an organizational culture that supports it leads to the best outcomes.

EBP, evidence-based practice.

Source: Copyright 2003 Bernadette Mazurek Melnyk & Ellen Fineout-Overholt.

convener, and driver of healthcare improvement worldwide, to optimize health system perfor-mance (Berwick, Nolan, & Whittington, 2008). This framework was conceptualized to stimulate healthcare organizations to implement programming that (a) improves the patient care experience, which includes quality and safety; (b) enhances the health of populations; and (c) reduces the per capita cost of healthcare. Years later, Bodenheimer and Sinsky (2014) contended that there should be a fourth aim added to the Triple Aim, that of improving the work life and well-being of clini-cians because of escalating high rates of burnout and job dissatisfaction, which adversely impacts healthcare quality and safety. The four aims are now known as the *Quadruple Aim in healthcare*.

Preventable medical errors are now the third leading cause of death in America (Makary & Daniel, 2016) and the United States is the worst country in the Western world in which to give birth with 700 women dying annually, many because healthcare providers are not following best practices (GBD 2015 Maternal Mortality Collaborators, 2016). Clinician burnout con-tributes to approximately 400,000 unintended deaths that occur annually in the United States (Johnson et al., 2017; Makary & Daniel, 2016; Shanafelt et al., 2015). Given that burnout affects more than 50% of healthcare providers, it is now considered a public health epidemic. Studies have shown that when clinicians are experiencing burnout or are in poor mental or physical health, they report making more medical errors (Melnyk, Orsolini et al., 2018; Tawfik et al., 2018). A recent national study with nearly 2,000 practicing nurses found that approxi-mately 25% of them were depressed and that depression was a leading cause of medical errors (Melnyk, Orsolini et al., 2018). In an attempt to address this public health issue by enhancing resiliency in clinicians and providing evidence-based solutions for healthcare systems, the Na-tional Academy of Medicine launched the Action Collaborative on Clinician Well-Being and Resilience (see https://nam.edu/initiatives/clinician-resilience-and-well-being).

Findings from numerous studies have indicated that implementation of EBP results in higher quality and reliability (safety) of care, improved population health outcomes, and reduced costs (Levin, Fineout-Overholt, Melnyk, Barnes, & Vetter, 2011; McGinty & Anderson, 2008;

 CALL TO ACTION

Reflect on your own situation.
Overall, based on your definition of *burnout*, how would you rate your level of burnout?"

1. = *I enjoy my work. I have no symptoms of burnout.*

2. = *Occasionally I am under stress, and I don't always have as much energy as I once did, but I don't feel burned out.*

3. = *I am definitely burning out and have one or more symptoms of burnout, such as physi-cal and emotional exhaustion.*

4. = *The symptoms of burnout that I'm experiencing won't go away. I think about frustra-tion at work a lot.*

5. = *I feel completely burned out and often wonder if I can go on. I am at the point where I may need some changes or may need to seek some sort of help.*

If you answered with a 3, 4, or 5, you are experiencing one or more symptoms of burn-out and should talk with someone regarding how you are feeling.

Melnyk, Fineout-Overholt, Giggleman, & Choy, 2017). In addition, EBP reduces geographic variation in the delivery of care (Dotson et al., 2014). Research also has supported that when clinicians implement EBP, they feel more empowered and satisfied in their roles (Fridman & Frederickson, 2014; Kim et al., 2016, 2017; Melnyk & Fineout-Overholt, 2019). Therefore, EBP is a critical and necessary strategy in reaching the Quadruple Aim in healthcare.

EBP = the Quadruple Aim in Healthcare

 ## THE CURRENT STATE OF EBP IN HEALTHCARE

The United States spends more money on healthcare than any country in the Western world, yet it ranks 37th in world health outcomes (Kaiser Family Foundation, 2017). A large contributor to this alarming situation is insufficient implementation of evidence-based care. Many practices that are routinely implemented in healthcare do not have a solid body of evidence to support them. Some even have data that support the claim that they promote adverse outcomes, including 12-hour shifts for nurses, double checking of pediatric medications, assessing nasogastric tube placement with air, and taking vital signs every 2 or 4 hours for stable hospitalized patients. These practices, which are steeped in tradition instead of best evidence, result in less than optimum care, poor outcomes, and wasteful healthcare spending.

There has been an explosion of scientific evidence to guide health professionals in their clinical decision-making over the past few decades. Even though this evidence is readily available and the National Academy of Medicine (formerly the Institute of Medicine) set the goal that, by the year 2020, 90% of clinical decisions would be supported by accurate, timely, and up-to-date information that is based on the best available evidence (McClellan, McGinnis, Nable, & Olsen, 2007), the implementation of evidence-based care is still not the norm in many healthcare systems across the United States and the globe. Although gold standard evidence-based guidelines and recommendations are available through venues such as the ECRI Guidelines Trust and the United States Preventive Services Task Force, adherence to rigorously produced guidelines is often poor (Vlada et al., 2013). The translation of research evidence into clinical practice remains painstakingly slow, often taking numerous years to decades (Melnyk & Fineout-Overholt, 2019). Further, the current U.S. healthcare system is plagued with multiple problems, including the continuation of practices that are steeped in tradition instead of those based on sound evidence, unnecessary screening for conditions when it is not indicated, inadequate reimbursement for best practices, and issues with the electronic health record that have resulted in clinicians spending less than 25% of their time providing patient care. Although quality and/or process improvement programs that utilize a systematic process, such as a plan, do, study, act (PDSA) model, are well established in hospitals and healthcare systems across the nation to improve the quality, safety, and outcomes of healthcare (Shirey et al., 2011), they are predominantly focused on improving and streamlining processes and they neglect to include a component to ensure that the accrual practice of concern is the best practice. Only by integrating a systematic search for and critical appraisal of evidence, to ensure the best practice is in place before improving the process (evidence-based quality improvement; Melnyk, Buck, & Gallagher-Ford, 2015) will outcomes actually improve and be sustained. All quality-improvement initiatives should be evidence based.

In 2014, research-based EBP competencies for practicing nurses were published in *Evidence-Based Practice Competencies for Practicing Registered Nurses and Advanced Practice Nurses in Real-World Clinical Settings* (Melnyk, Gallagher-Ford, Long, & Fineout-Overholt, 2014). Developed through a national consensus panel followed by a Delphi study with EBP experts throughout the United States, these competencies can assist institutions in achieving high-value, low-cost evidence-based healthcare (Beckett & Melnyk, 2018). There are 13 competencies for practicing nurses and an additional 11 for advanced practice nurses (Melnyk et al., 2014; Exhibit 8.1). The 24 competencies support the seven-step EBP process outlined by Melnyk and Fineout-Overholt (2019). Although initially designed for practicing nurses and APRNs, the competencies can be applied to other healthcare professionals as they encompass the seven-step EBP process, which should be embraced by healthcare providers from all professions.

In the first national study of the EBP competencies, which sampled 2,344 nurses from 19 hospitals and healthcare systems throughout the United States, nurses reported needing

EXHIBIT 8.1 EBP Competencies for Practicing RNs and APRNs in Real-World Clinical Settings

EBP Competencies for Practicing Professional RNs

1. Questions clinical practices for the purpose of improving the quality of care.
2. Describes clinical problems using internal evidence.[a]
3. Participates in the formulation of clinical questions using a PICO(T) format.
4. Searches for external evidence[b] to answer focused clinical questions.
5. Participates in critical appraisal of preappraised evidence (such as clinical practice guidelines, evidence-based policies and procedures, and evidence syntheses).
6. Participates in the critical appraisal of published research studies to determine their strength and applicability to clinical practice.
7. Participates in the evaluation and synthesis of a body of evidence gathered to determine its strength and applicability to clinical practice.
8. Collects practice data (e.g., individual patient data, quality-improvement data) systematically as internal evidence for clinical decision-making in the care of individuals, groups, and populations.
9. Integrates evidence gathered from external and internal sources in order to plan evidence-based practice changes.
10. Implements practice changes based on evidence and clinical expertise and patient preferences to improve care processes and patient outcomes.
11. Evaluates outcomes of evidence-based decisions and practice changes for individuals, groups, and populations to determine best practices.
12. Disseminates best practices supported by evidence to improve quality of care and patient outcomes.
13. Participates in strategies to *sustain an evidence-based practice culture.*

(continued)

EXHIBIT 8.1 EBP Competencies for Practicing RNs and APRNs in Real-World Clinical Settings (*continued*)

EBP Competencies for Practicing APRNs

These include all the competencies of registered professional nurses *and the following*:

14. Systematically conducts and exhaustive searches for external evidence[b] to answer clinical questions.

15. Critically appraises relevant preappraised evidence (i.e., clinical guidelines, summaries, synopses, syntheses of relevant external evidence) and primary studies, including evaluation and synthesis.

16. Integrates a body of external evidence from nursing and related fields with internal evidence[a] in making decisions about patient care.

17. Leads transdisciplinary teams in applying synthesized evidence to initiate clinical decisions and practice changes to improve the health of individuals, groups, and populations.

18. Generates internal evidence through outcomes management and EBP implementation projects for the purpose of integrating best practices.

19. Measures processes and outcomes of evidence-based clinical decisions.

20. Formulates evidence-based policies and procedures.

21. Participates in the generation of external evidence with other healthcare professionals.

22. Mentors others in evidence-based decision-making and the EBP process.

23. Implements strategies to sustain an EBP culture.

24. Communicates best evidence to individuals, groups, colleagues, and policy makers.

[a] Evidence is generated internally within a clinical setting, such as patient assessment data, outcomes management, and quality-improvement data.
[b] Evidence is generated from research.

EBP, evidence-based practice; PICO(T); Patient/population, Intervention/area of interest, Comparison, Outcome(s), Time.

Source: Copyright 2013 Melnyk, Gallagher-Ford, & Fineout-Overholt.

---

improvement and not being competent in any of the 24 competencies. Although master's-prepared clinicians reported a higher level of competency across all of the competencies compared to those who were baccalaureate prepared, the only competency that advanced practice nurses reported being competent in was questions clinical practices for the purpose of improving the quality of care (Melnyk, Gallagher-Ford et al., 2018). The EBP competency scores were not significantly different across gender, race/ethnicity, and working in or not working in a Magnet-designated organization. There were strong positive relationships between EBP competency with EBP beliefs and EBP mentoring, moderate positive relationships between EBP competency and EBP knowledge, and a small association between EBP competency and EBP culture. The results of this study indicated that this sample of nurses across the United States believe they need improvement in and do not believe they are yet competent in the 24 EBP competencies.

Another set of EBP competencies, the Core Competencies in Evidence-Based Practice for Health Professionals, were recently developed to standardize and improve EBP education in academic curricula (Albarqouni et al., 2018). In the process of development, the authors first conducted a systematic review of educational studies in which they identified 86 EBP competencies. This systematic review was then followed by a modified Delphi survey study of 234 multidisciplinary health professionals. The final set of 68 competencies were grouped into six domains of EBP, including (a) step 0: introductory, (b) step 1: ask, (c) step 2: acquire, (d) step 3: appraise and interpret, (e) step 4: apply, and (f) step 5: evaluate. The steps were broken down into substeps that included multiple competencies. The level of detail for each competency also was described, including the time that should be dedicated to each competency, including (a) explain, (b) mention, and (c) practice with exercise (Albarqouni et al., 2018). The two sets of research-based competencies had many similarities with the EBP steps. The competencies developed by Melnyk et al. (2014) take EBP one step further than those developed by Albarqouni et al. (2018) and include the addition of a final step (Step #6) to disseminate the outcomes of an EBP change. Dissemination of EBP change projects through presentations and publications is critical for others to learn about what works in implementing evidence-based care (Beckett & Melnyk, 2018).

BARRIERS AND FACILITATORS OF EBP

Multiple barriers inhibit the delivery of evidence-based care, including:

a. Misperceptions that EBP takes too much time

b. Inadequate knowledge and skills in EBP

c. Cultures that perpetuate a philosophy of "that is the way we do it here"

d. Lack of resources and support, including budgetary investment by C-suite executives

e. The teaching of rigorous research in academic clinical programs instead of how best to use research evidence and rapidly translate it into practice

f. Resistance to change

g. Lack of evidence-based policies and procedures

h. Lack of autonomy and power to change practice

i. Inadequate numbers of EBP mentors to work with point-of-care clinicians on implementing evidence-based care

j. Lack of support from leaders and managers (Melnyk et al., 2016; Melnyk, Fineout-Overholt, Gallagher-Ford, & Kaplan, 2012; Squires, Estabrooks, Gustavsson, & Wallen, 2011; Wilson et al., 2015)

A national study of more than 1,000 nurses randomly sampled from the American Nurses Association found that leader/manager resistance is a major barrier to evidence-based care (Melnyk et al., 2012). To better understand the barrier of leader resistance, a national survey with 276 chief nurse executives from 45 states across the United States was conducted. This study sought to describe chief nurse executives' own beliefs and implementation of EBP as well as the amount of their budgets they invested in educating and skilling their clinicians in EBP. Findings indicated that chief nurse executives believed in the importance of and value of EBP. However, their own implementation of EBP was low, with more than 50% of them reporting being uncertain about how to measure outcomes of clinical care delivered in their hospitals (Melnyk et al., 2016). A large percentage of the chief nurses also reported that they did not have a critical mass of nurses in their hospital who were skilled in EBP. The majority of these chief nurses only allocated 0% to 10% of their budgets to build, support, and sustain EBP in their organizations. Although the chief nurses reported that their top two priorities in their role were the quality and safety of care being delivered in their hospitals, they ranked EBP as one of their lowest priorities, which indicated that they did not understand that EBP was the direct path to improving quality and safety in their healthcare systems. Therefore, it was not unexpected that one third of the hospitals from this chief nurse survey did not meet the National Database of Nursing Quality Indicators (NDNQI) metrics and almost one third of the hospitals were above national core performance measure benchmarks, including falls and pressure ulcers (Melnyk et al., 2016).

Even if clinicians and healthcare systems do not consistently implement EBP, third-party payers are providing reimbursement only for healthcare practices that are supported by scientific evidence (i.e., pay for performance). Furthermore, hospitals are now being denied payment for patient complications that develop when evidence-based guidelines or policies are not being followed (Melnyk & Fineout-Overholt, 2019). In addition to pressure from third-party payers, patients and family members are often seeking the latest information posted on websites about treatments for their health conditions. This movement by the public is likely to exert further pressure on healthcare providers to provide the most current and best practices and health-related information.

To overcome the multiple barriers in implementing EBP, there must be a multicomponent strategy in place at all levels. Top administrators and directors/managers must "walk the talk" and invest in educational and skills-building programs for their clinicians as well as create a culture and infrastructure support in which EBP is the norm, that is, the standard of performance and care (Melnyk, 2016b). For clinicians to advance the use of EBP, misconceptions about how to implement practice based on the best available evidence need to be corrected, and knowledge and skills in this area must be enhanced. It also must be recognized that a change to EBP is behavior change for many clinicians who did not learn this approach to decision-making and the necessary skills in their educational programs. These deficits can, however, be addressed thorough intensive EBP continuing-education programs that can increase and sustain EBP beliefs, knowledge, and competence. Facilitators of EBP include:

a. Encouragement and support from managers/leadership/administration who delineate clear expectations for all clinicians to be competent in EBP and who themselves role model decision-making based on best evidence

b. Clearly written research publications

c. Protected time allocated for clinicians to participate in the steps of EBP, including writing PICO(T) questions, searching for and critically appraising evidence, and so on

d. A critical mass of EBP mentors who have knowledge and skills in EBP along with expertise in individual and organizational change strategies

e. Resources to assist with EBP at point of care (e.g., computers dedicated solely to EBP, access to electronic databases, access to librarians who are knowledgeable in EBP)

f. Integration of EBP into health professional curricula

g. Performance evaluations, clinical advancement (ladders), and promotion processes that integrate the EBP competencies

h. Interprofessional teams that engage in evidence-based quality-improvement initiatives

i. Policies and procedures that include best evidence (Melnyk, 2016a; Melnyk & Fineout-Overholt, 2019; Stetler, Ritchie, Rycroft-Malone, & Charns, 2014; ten Ham, Minnie, & van der Walt, 2015)

Federal agencies, healthcare organizations and systems, health insurers, policy makers, and regulatory bodies must advocate for and require the full integration of EBP. In a national EBP forum that involved leaders from numerous organizations and federal agencies, reimbursement for EBP was, overwhelmingly, the top recommendation needed to advance EBP (Melnyk, Gallagher-Ford et al., 2018). Funding agencies also must establish translational research (i.e., how findings from research can best be translated into clinical practice to improve care and patient outcomes) as a high priority.

CALL TO ACTION

Ask to see your healthcare organization's policy and procedure manual. Are the policies backed by current best evidence? If not, seek out the chair/director of your policy/procedure committee to bring this issue to her or his attention.

KEY LEADERSHIP STRATEGIES TO IGNITE AND SUSTAIN EBP IN HEALTHCARE

Leaders must first understand that EBP is the direct pathway to achieve the Quadruple Aim in healthcare and be willing to invest in it knowing that healthcare quality and safety will be enhanced, population health outcomes will improve, healthcare costs will diminish, and clinician job satisfaction will increase as EBP diffuses throughout the organization.

Leaders must gain the EBP knowledge and skills that they expect of their clinicians. As is true of any culture change, if leaders do not consistently role model and implement evidence-based decision-making themselves, clinicians are not likely to follow suit. Leaders must actively seek first followers/early adopters of EBP in order to diffuse EBP across the organization because the majority do not act to elicit change until they observe others who have successfully made the change (Rogers, 2003). Strategic engagement of early adopters of EBP in key roles and places of influence is an essential step for leaders to purposefully undertake to successfully build and sustain a cultural change to evidence-based decision-making and problem-solving across the enterprise.

The leadership team, with involvement and input from all levels of healthcare professionals in the organization, should develop an exciting dream/vision for EBP, which will help drive the mission and goals of the organization. Autocratic dictates without involving all levels of the team are often a prescription for failure. However, when a team of leaders and clinicians working in the grassroots of the healthcare system share a common vision for which everyone has had the opportunity for input, there is greater ownership and investment by the team members to facilitate organizational change. The vision, mission, and goals should include clear language reflecting EBP as a core component of practice and be displayed prominently throughout the healthcare system to serve as a visual reminder to all that EBP is deemed important and is part of the organization's strategic plan.

CALL TO ACTION

What are the vision, mission, and goals of your organization? Are they prominently displayed and communicated?

EBP frameworks and models should guide EBP work and system-wide implementation of EBP. There are multiple EBP models, including the ACE Star Model of Knowledge Transformation, the Advancing Research and Clinical practice through close Collaboration (ARCC©) Model, the Clinical Scholar Model, the Iowa Model of Evidence-Based Practice to Promote Quality Care, the Johns Hopkins Nursing Evidence-Based Practice Model, and the Promoting Action on Research Implementation in Health Services (PARIHS) framework (Dang et al., 2019). Most of these are process models that are intended as a structure to support individual EBP projects/initiatives by following the steps of the EBP process. However, there are two models, the ARCC Model and the PARIHS Model, that guide organizations in the system-wide implementation of EBP. Using one of these models will guide the overarching work that needs to be done across the organization to build and sustain EBP culture and supportive infrastructures.

The original version of the **ARCC Model** was conceptualized by Bernadette Melnyk in 1999 as part of a strategic-planning initiative to unify research and clinical practice in order to advance EBP within an academic medical center for the ultimate purpose of improving healthcare quality and patient outcomes (Melnyk & Fineout-Overholt, 2002). Throughout the past two decades, the ARCC Model has been refined as a result of research conducted to empirically support the components of the model. ARCC includes key strategies for individual and organizational change to best practice implementation and sustainability.

The first step in the ARCC Model is an organizational assessment of culture and readiness for system-wide implementation of EBP as workplace culture can either inhibit or facilitate the advancement of evidence-based care (Figure 8.2). The Organizational Culture and Readiness Scale for System-wide Integration of Evidence-based Practice (OCRSIEP) can assess organizational culture (Fineout-Overholt & Melnyk, 2006). This valid and reliable, 25-item Likert scale identifies organizational characteristics, including strengths and barriers to the implementation of EBP within a healthcare system. The central strategy within the ARCC Model is to develop a critical mass of **EBP mentors,** typically master's-prepared clinicians or those with clinical doctorates who are competent in the EBP process and skilled in overcoming barriers to individual and organizational behavior change. These EBP mentors work with point-of-care clinicians to implement EBP and conduct evidence-based quality-improvement initiatives. Other components of the EBP mentor role as defined in the ARCC Model include (Melnyk & Fineout-Overholt, 2019).

a. Ongoing assessment of an organization's capacity to sustain an EBP culture

b. Building EBP knowledge and skills by conducting interactive group workshops and one-on-one mentoring

c. Stimulating, facilitating, and educating nursing staff toward a culture of EBP, with a focus on overcoming barriers to best practice

  d. Role modeling EBP

  e. Conducting ARCC EBP-enhancing strategies, such as EBP rounds, journal clubs, web pages, newsletters, and fellowship programs

  f. Working with staff to generate internal evidence (i.e., practice-generated) through outcomes management and EBPI/evidence-based quality-improvement projects

  g. Facilitating staff involvement in research to generate external evidence

  h. Using evidence to foster best practice

  i. Collaborating with interdisciplinary professionals to advance and sustain EBP

These EBP mentors also have excellent strategic planning, implementation, and outcomes evaluation skills so that they can document the impact of their role in moving the organization to an EBP culture (Melnyk, 2007). Having a critical mass of EBP mentors in a healthcare system increases clinicians' beliefs about the value of EBP and their ability to implement it, which in turn leads to higher EBP implementation and competency.

Ultimately, consistent implementation of EBP by clinicians throughout a healthcare system leads to achieving the Quadruple Aim in healthcare. Multiple studies have supported the key

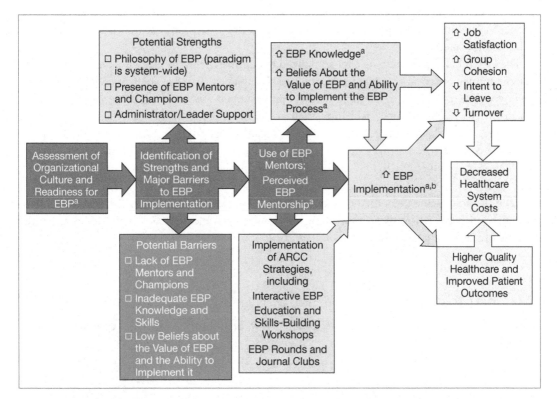

Figure 8.2 The ARCC Model for system-wide implementation and sustainability of EBP.

[a]Scale developed

[b]Based on the EBP paradigm and using the EBP process

ARCC, Advancing Research and Clinical practice through close Collaboration; EBP, evidence-based practice.

Source: Copyright 2017 Bernadette Mazurek Melnyk & Ellen Fineout-Overholt.

role of ARCC EBP mentors as well as the relationships in the ARCC Model, including a higher quality of care, improved population health outcomes, and higher job satisfaction and reduced turnover rates in clinicians working in systems that implement ARCC (Kim et al., 2017; Levin et al., 2011; Melnyk, 2012; Melnyk et al., 2004, 2017; Melnyk & Fineout-Overholt, 2002; Melnyk, Fineout-Overholt, Giggleman, & Cruz, 2010; Melnyk, Fineout-Overholt, & Mays, 2008; Wallen et al., 2010). The ARCC Model has been implemented in numerous hospitals and healthcare systems throughout the United States and the globe by preparing a critical mass of EBP mentors who work directly with point-of-care clinicians to implement and sustain EBP throughout the entire health system.

As a part of implementing the ARCC Model, groups of nurses and other transdisciplinary healthcare providers first attend EBP educational and skilsl-building immersion workshops and then work with clinicians to conduct multiple evidence-based quality-improvement projects to improve outcomes that have been identified as challenging or problematic in the healthcare system (e.g., patient falls, hospital-acquired infections and injuries, rehospitalizations). These EBP immersion programs have prepared over 3,000 nurses and transdisciplinary clinicians across the nation and globe as EBP mentors. Some of the individuals who have attended these immersion programs have entered roles as EBP mentors within their healthcare systems. A 5-day EBP immersion program to prepare EBP mentors is available as an on-site workshop or through an online program offered by the Helene Fuld Health Trust National Institute for Evidence-based Practice in Nursing and Healthcare at The Ohio State University College of Nursing (see https:// fuld.nursing.osu.edu).

The PARIHS framework was conceptualized to capture the many complex factors that influence the implementation of evidence in practice (Dang et al., 2019). The framework has developed over time as a result of ongoing quality-improvement and research projects and contends that in order to achieve successful implementation, one must consider three elements: (a) the nature and type of evidence (e.g., research vs. clinical experience vs. local data), (b) the qualities of the context (i.e., culture), (c) the way the process is facilitated (e.g., doing for others vs. enabling others; Hill et al., 2017; Kitson, Harvey, & McCormack, 1998; Rycroft-Malone et al., 2002, 2004).

Each of these elements is further segmented into subelements and then evaluated on a continuum from high to low with the intent of moving each element to "high" to increase the chances of implementation success (Dang et al., 2019).

CALL TO ACTION

What EBP model is used in your organization? How long has the EBP model been used? Has it improved outcomes?

Once leadership decides upon a system-wide model for EBP implementation, it needs a thorough baseline assessment of the organization in terms of EBP culture and clinician competency so that the outcomes of organizational changes made can be monitored and documented. Many valid and reliable measures of EBP attributes exist in the literature, including the Organizational Readiness ORSCIEP scale, the EBP Beliefs and EBP Implementation Scales (Melnyk & Fineout-Overholt, 2002; Melnyk et al., 2008), the EBP Self-Efficacy Scale (Tucker, Olson, & Frusti, 2009), and the EBP Competency Scale (Gallagher-Ford & Melnyk, 2017).

Now that there is a set of EBP competencies for practicing RNs and APRNs, these competencies should be used in healthcare systems to ensure high-quality and safe care. The vision, mission, and goals of the organization that reflect the importance of EBP should be shared with clinicians in their orientation/onboarding sessions. The EBP competencies should also be integrated at this point. Because clinicians enter healthcare systems with a wide variation in EBP knowledge and skills and attitudes, they should use the EBP Competency Scale to identify areas where they need improvement so that an individualized plan can be developed and implemented.

EBP competence should be assessed in all clinicians. It is quite likely that current employees have not been in school recently and, therefore, have not learned about EBP, so the likelihood of EBP competency deficiencies is high. Thus, current employees should also use the EBP Competency Scale to identify areas where they also need development. Once the EBP needs are identified, workshops and educational skills-building sessions, taught by EBP experts/mentors, should be provided to assist staff in achieving the competencies. Because it is well known that recognition is important to keep people motivated and engaged, ongoing recognition and appreciation programs should be launched to highlight and recognize those clinicians who achieve all of the EBP competencies.

Leaders and managers must create a workplace where EBP can arrive, survive, and thrive. This requires creation and sustainability of two critical, yet discreet attributes: (a) an EBP culture and (b) readiness for EBP. Building an EBP culture, just as with any other culture, is the responsibility of leaders (Gallagher-Ford, Buck, & Melnyk, 2019; Melnyk, Gallagher-Ford, & Fineout-Overholt, 2016). It requires leaders to:

a. Acquire a true understanding of what EBP is and what it is not.

b. Set the vision for an evidence-based enterprise.

c. Integrate EBP into the mission and goals of the organization.

d. Develop a written strategic plan for EBP.

e. Invest adequately in EBP to support the multiple resources and programs that are necessary.

f. Role model EBP in leadership decision-making and practice.

g. Develop a synergistic **evidence-based quality-improvement (QI) process** in the organization.

h. Establish a mechanism to track outcomes and return on investment (ROI) for all EBP initiatives.

i. Build infrastructures that give all clinicians "voice" in the organization.

j. Promote discussion, collaboration, and communication in all teams (Cullen, 2018).

k. Establish clear expectations for evidence-based decision-making across all departments and at all levels of the enterprise.

l. Establish clinical–academic partnerships to support the scholarly requirements of an evidence-based enterprise.

m. Negotiate work conditions to support EBP (protected time for EBP project work).

n. Hardwire evidence into organizational policies and guideline development processes.

o. Develop a specific EBP mentor job description.

p. Conscientiously integrate the EBP competencies throughout the organization.

q. Have courage and the willingness to publicly navigate barriers and resistance to EBP in the early stages.

r. Have persistence in navigating barriers and resistance to EBP over time until EBP becomes the "norm" or default way to practice in the organization.

In addition to creating the culture, leaders must resource the EBP transformation (readiness for EBP). In a recent concept analysis by Schaefer and Welton (2017), EBP readiness was described as similar to military readiness in a model. The four components of EBP readiness Schaefer and Welton describe are:

1. Personnel—EBP readiness requires multiple people with EBP knowledge and skills who are allotted time away from the bedside to conduct EBP activities and who are empowered with the autonomy to change practice.

2. Training—EBP readiness requires purposeful, applicable education and training, beyond nursing school, that is tailored to individual needs.

3. Equipping—EBP readiness requires resources needed to do EBP and effective communication related to resources available and how to access them.

4. Leadership—EBP readiness requires that leaders set the EBP culture, allocate resources, provide support particularly including development and integration of EBP mentors.

This conceptual analysis provides an excellent framework to plan for acquiring the resources that clinicians will need to succeed in delivering evidence-based care. Resources for EBP include:

a. Educational and skills-building programs to learn EBP

b. A critical mass of EBP mentors

c. Protected time for staff to participate in the steps of EBP to bring initiatives to fruition

d. Access to computers and electronic databases for evidence searching; access to dedicated nurse scientists (or other disciplines) who assist clinicians when the body of evidence is inadequate and research is indicated

e. A system to provide continuously current, immediately available, evidence-based policies and procedures to clinicians to underpin best practice every day

There are many tools and resources available to leaders to help them build an environment in which EBP can thrive and the Quadruple Aim can be achieved. The research-based EBP competencies for practicing RNs/clinicians and APRNs/clinicians are an easily accessible and readily applicable resource in any organization. These simple expectations can readily be used to drive the multifaceted integration of EBP, which is essential to the successful transformation of an organization to an evidence-based enterprise. Specific opportunities for use of the EBP competencies include (Melnyk et al., 2016):

a. Integrate the language of the competencies into interview questions for new hires, so candidates are made aware of the expectation for EBP.

b. Ask interview candidates about their level of EBP knowledge and skills.

c. Insert the EBP competencies into job descriptions and performance appraisals for RNs, APRNs, other frontline clinicians as well as managers and leaders.

d. Incorporate the competencies into onboarding/orientation/residency programs to establish EBP expectations from the very beginning of employment.

e. Stratify the competencies into professional advancement programs (also known as *clinical ladders*).

f. Integrate the competencies across shared governance structures to ensure an evidence-based approach to problem-solving/decision-making is hardwired into all councils.

Leaders must make a conscientious and strategic decision to build evidence-based enterprises because EBP is the direct path that will lead to the achievement of the Quadruple Aim in healthcare. Leaders must be prepared for myriad challenges, barriers, and "sacred cows" along the way, but that is what leadership is all about—bringing an organization and its workforce to best performance and outcomes. Only with clear vision, steadfast commitment, a written strategic plan, ongoing measurement of outcomes, and courage and persistence will success be possible. Decades have passed since the Institute of Medicine (now the National Academy of Medicine) called for all healthcare decisions to be evidence-based by 2020; this goal is far from being achieved. The time is now:Leaders must spearhead the EBP revolution to improve care and outcomes for both patients and clinicians.

🔑 KEY TAKEAWAY POINTS

■ EBP achieves the Quadruple Aim in healthcare, which includes enhancing the patient experience, improving population health outcomes, decreasing costs, and improving the work life of clinicians.

■ Clinicians should all become competent in the EBP competencies.

■ Leaders must walk the talk as well as provide the resources and support for their managers and clinicians to become competent in EBP.

■ Implementation of the ARCC Model for system-wide implementation and sustainability of EBP in which the key strategy is developing a critical mass of EBP mentors results in safe, high-quality healthcare and improved population health outcomes.

CASE STUDY

You are the brand-new CEO at a 160-bed rural hospital in the southwestern United States. Upon entering your role at the hospital, you ask your chief nursing officer (Daryl), who has been in his role for 15 years, about the model that he is using to guide EBP and inquire about the number of EBP mentors that are being used to help clinicians implement and sustain EBP. Daryl responds that, to his knowledge, there is no EBP model used at the hospital and he does not have any positions for EBP mentors. The core performance metrics have not been good at this hospital and the CEO believes that accelerating EBP in the organization would help to reduce the organization's high prevalence of ventilator-associated pneumonia, central- line infections, and rehospitalizations.

If you were the CEO, what would your next steps be and why?

Would you consider hiring a different chief nursing officer and why?

REFERENCES

Albarqouni, L., Hoffmann, T., Straus, S., Olsen, N. R., Young, T. Ilic, D., ... Glasziou, P. (2018). Core competencies in evidence-based practice for health professionals: Consensus statement based on a systematic review and Delphi survey. *JAMA Network Open, 1*(2), e18028. doi:10.1001/jamanetworkopen.2018.0281

Beckett, C. D., & Melnyk, B. M. (2018). Evidence-based practice competencies and the new EBP-C credential: Keys to achieving the quadruple aim in healthcare. *Worldviews on Evidence-Based Nursing, 15*(6), 412–413. doi:10.1111/wvn.12335

Berwick, D. M., Nolan, T. W., & Whittington, J. (2008). The Triple Aim: Care, health, and cost. *Health Affairs, 27*(3), 759–769. doi:10.1377/hlthaff.27.3.759

Bodenheimer, T., & Sinsky, C. (2014). From Triple to Quadruple Aim: Care of the patient requires care of the provider. *Annals of Family Medicine, 12*(6) 573–576. doi:10.1370/afm.1713

Cullen, L. (2018). Translating evidence-based practice into reality of daily practice: Leadership solutions for creating a path forward. *Journal of PeriAnesthesia Nursing, 33*(5), 752–756. doi:10.1016/j.jopan.2018.05.009

Dang, D., Melnyk, B. M., Fineout-Overholt, E., Yost, J., Cullen, L., Cvach, M., ... Stevens, K. (2019). Models to guide the implementation and sustainability of evidence-based practice. In B. M. Melnyk & E. Fineout-Overholt (Eds.), *Evidence-based practice in nursing and healthcare. A guide to best practice* (4th ed., pp. 378–427). Philadelphia, PA: Wolters Kluwer.

Dotson, J. A., Roll, J. M., Packer, R. R., Lewis, J. M., McPherson, S., & Howell, D. (2014). Urban and rural utilization of evidence-based practices for substance use and mental health disorders. *Journal of Rural Health, 30*(3), 292–299. doi:10.1111/jrh.12068

Fineout-Overholt, E., & Melnyk, B. M. (2006). *Organizational culture and readiness for systemwide integration of EBP*. Gilbert, AZ: ARCC.

Fridman, M., & Frederickson, K. (2014). Oncology nurses and the experience of participation in an evidence-based practice project. *Oncology Nursing Forum, 41*(4), 382–388. doi:10.1188/14.ONF.382-388

Gallagher-Ford, L., Buck, J. S., & Melnyk, B. M. (2019). Leadership strategies for creating and sustaining evidence-based practice organizations. In B. M. Melnyk & E. Fineout-Overholt (Eds.), *Evidence-based practice in nursing and healthcare. A guide to best practice* (4th ed., pp. 328–343). Philadelphia, PA: Wolters Kluwer.

Gallagher-Ford, L., & Melnyk, B. M. (2017). *The EBP competencies scale for practicing registered professional nurses and advanced practice nurses*. Columbus, OH: The Helene Fuld Health Trust National Institute for Evidence-based Practice in Nursing and Health Care.

GBD 2015 Maternal Mortality Collaborators. (2016). Global, regional, and national levels of maternal mortality, 1990–2015: A systematic analysis for the Global Burden of Disease Study 2015. *Lancet, 388*(10053), 1775–1812. doi:10.1016/S0140-6736(16)31470-2

Hill, J. N., Guihan, M., Hogan, T. P., Smith, B. M., LaVela, S., Weaver, F. M., … Evans, C. T. (2017). Use of the PARIHS framework for retrospective and prospective implementation evaluation. *Worldviews on Evidence-Based Nursing, 14*(2), 99–107. doi:10.1111/wvn.12211

Johnson, J., Louch, G., Dunning, A., Johnson, O., Grange, A., Reynolds, C., … O'Hara, J. (2017). Burnout mediates the association between depression and patient safety perceptions: A cross-sectional study in hospital nurses. *Journal of Advanced Nursing, 73*(7), 1667–1680. doi:10.1111/jan.13251

Kaiser Family Foundation. (2017). OECD health data: Health expenditure and financing: Health expenditure indicators, OECD Health Statistics. Retrieved from https://doi.org/10.1787/health-data-en

Kim, S. C., Ecoff, L., Brown, C. E., Gallo, A. M., Stichler, J. F., & Davidson, J. E. (2017). Benefits of a regional evidence-based practice fellowship program: A test of the ARCC model. *Worldviews on Evidence-Based Nursing, 14*(2), 90–98. doi:10.1111/wvn.12199

Kim, S. C., Stichler, J. F., Ecoff, L., Brown, C. E., Gallo, A. M., & Davidson, J. E. (2016). Predictors of evidence-based practice implementation, job satisfaction, and group cohesion among regional fellowship program participants. *Worldviews on Evidence-Based Nursing, 13*(5), 340–348. doi:10.1111/wvn.12171

Kitson, A., Harvey, G., & McCormack, B. (1998). Enabling the implementation of evidence based practice: A conceptual framework. *Quality in Health Care, 7*(3), 149–158. doi:10.1136/qshc.7.3.149

Levin, R. F., Fineout-Overholt, E., Melnyk, B. M., Barnes, M., & Vetter, M. J. (2011). Fostering evidence-based practice to improve nurse and cost outcomes in a community health setting: A pilot test of the advancing research and clinical practice through close collaboration model. *Nursing Administration Quarterly, 35*(1), 21–33. doi:10.1097/NAQ.0b013e31820320ff

Makary, M. A., & Daniel, M. (2016). Medical error-the third leading cause of death in the US. *BMJ, 3*(353), i2139. doi:10.1136/bmj.i2139

McClellan, M. B., McGinnis, M., Nable, E. G., & Olsen, L. M. (2007). *Evidence-based medicine and the changing nature of health care.* Washington, DC: National Academies Press. doi:10.17226/12041

McGinty, J., & Anderson, G. (2008). Predictors of physician compliance with American Heart Association guidelines for acute myocardial infarction. *Critical Care Nursing Quarterly, 31*(2), 161–172. doi:10.1097/01.CNQ.0000314476.64377.12

Melnyk, B. M. (2007). The evidence-based practice mentor: A promising strategy for implementing and sustaining EBP in healthcare systems [Editorial]. *Worldviews on Evidence-Based Nursing, 4*(3),123–125. doi:10.1111/j.1741-6787.2007.00094.x

Melnyk, B. M. (2012). Achieving a high-reliability organization through implementation of the ARCC model for system-wide sustainability of evidence-based practice. *Nursing Administration Quarterly, 36*(2), 127–135. doi:10.1097/NAQ.0b013e318249fb6a

Melnyk, B. M. (2016a). An urgent call to action for nurse leaders to establish sustainable evidence-based practice cultures and implement evidence-based interventions to improve healthcare quality. *Worldviews on Evidence-Based Nursing, 13*(1), 3–5. doi:10.1111/wvn.12150

Melnyk, B. M. (2016b). Culture eats strategy every time: What works in building and sustaining an evidence-based practice culture in healthcare systems. *Worldviews on Evidence-Based Nursing, 13*(2), 99–101. doi:10.1111/wvn.12161

Melnyk, B. M., Buck, J., & Gallagher-Ford, L. (2015). Transforming quality improvement into evidence-based quality improvement: A key solution to improve healthcare outcomes [Editorial]. *Worldviews on Evidence-Based Nursing, 12*(5), 251–252. doi:10.1111/wvn.12112

Melnyk, B. M., & Fineout-Overholt, E. (2002). Putting research into practice. *Reflections on Nursing Leadership, 28*(2), 22–25.

Melnyk, B. M., & Fineout-Overholt, E. (2019). *Evidence-based practice in nursing & healthcare: A guide to best practice* (4th ed.). Philadelphia, PA: Wolters Kluwer.

Melnyk, B. M., Fineout-Overholt, E., Feinstein, N. F., Li, H., Small, L., Wilcox, L., & Kraus, R. (2004). Nurses' perceived knowledge, beliefs, skills, and needs regarding evidence-based practice: Implications for accelerating the paradigm shift. *Worldviews on Evidence-Based Nursing, 1*(3), 185–193. doi:10.1111/j.1524-475X.2004.04024.x

Melnyk, B. M., Fineout-Overholt, E., Gallagher-Ford, L., & Kaplan, L. (2012). The state of evidence-based practice in US nurses: Critical implications for nurse leaders and educators. *Journal of Nursing Administration, 42*(9), 410–417. doi:10.1097/NNA.0b013e3182664e0a

Melnyk, B. M., Fineout-Overholt, E., Giggleman, M., & Choy, K. (2017). A test of the ARCC model improves implementation of evidence-based practice, healthcare culture, and patient outcomes. *Worldviews on Evidence-Based Nursing, 14*(1), 5–9. doi:10.1111/wvn.12189

Melnyk, B. M., Fineout-Overholt, E., Giggleman, M., & Cruz, R. (2010). Correlates among cognitive beliefs, EBP implementation, organizational culture, cohesion and job satisfaction in evidence-based practice mentors from a community hospital system. *Nursing Outlook, 58*(6), 301–308. doi:10.1016/j.outlook.2010.06.002

Melnyk, B. M., Fineout-Overholt, E., & Mays, M. (2008). The evidence-based practice beliefs and implementation scales: Psychometric properties of two new instruments. *Worldviews on Evidence-Based Nursing, 5*(4), 208–216. doi:10.1111/j.1741-6787.2008.00126.x

Melnyk, B. M., Gallagher-Ford, L., & Fineout-Overholt, L. E. (2016). *Implementing the evidence-based practice (EBP) competencies in healthcare: A practical guide for improving quality, safety, and outcomes*. Indianapolis, IN: Sigma Theta Tau International.

Melnyk, B. M., Gallagher-Ford, L., Long, L. E., & Fineout-Overholt, E. (2014). The establishment of evidence-based practice competencies for practicing registered nurses and advanced practice nurses in real-world clinical settings: Proficiencies to improve healthcare quality, reliability, patient outcomes, and costs. *Worldviews on Evidence-Based Nursing, 11*(1), 5–15. doi:10.1111/wvn.12021

Melnyk, B. M., Gallagher-Ford, L., Thomas, B., Troseth, M., Wyngarden, K., & Szalacha, L. (2016). A study of chief nurse executives indicates low prioritization of evidence-based practice and shortcomings in hospital performance metrics across the United States. *Worldviews on Evidence-Based Nursing, 13*(1), 6–14. doi:10.1111/wvn.12133

Melnyk, B. M., Gallagher-Ford, L., Zellefrow, C., Tucker, S., Thomas, B., Sinnott, L. T., & Tan, A. (2018). The first U.S. study on nurses' evidence-based practice competencies indicates major deficits that threaten healthcare quality, safety, and patient outcomes. *Worldviews on Evidence-Based Nursing, 15*(1), 16–25. doi:10.1111/wvn.12269

Melnyk, B. M., Orsolini, L., Tan, A., Arslanian-Engoren, C., Melkus, G. D., Dunbar-Jacob, J., ... Lewis, L. M. (2018). A national study links nurses' physical and mental health to medical errors and perceived worksite wellness. *Journal of Occupational and Environmental Medicine, 60*(2), 126–131. doi:10.1097/JOM.0000000000001198

Rogers, E. M. (2003). *Diffusion of innovations* (5th ed.). New York, NY: Free Press.

Rycroft-Malone, J., Harvey, G., Kitson, A., McCormack, B., Seers, K., & Titchen, A. (2002). Getting evidence into practice: Ingredients for change. *Nursing Standard 16*(37), 38–43. doi:10.7748/ns2002.05.16.37.38.c3201

Rycroft-Malone, J., Harvey, G., Seers, K., Kitson, A., McCormack, B., & Titchen, A. (2004). An exploration of the factors that influence the implementation of evidence into practice. *Journal of Clinical Nursing, 13*(8), 913–924. doi:10.1111/j.1365-2702.2004.01007.x

Schaefer, J. D., & Welton, J. M. (2018). Evidence-based practice readiness: A concept analysis. *Journal of Nursing Management, 26*(6), 621–629. doi:110:1111/jonm.125999

Shanafelt, T. D., Hasan, O., Dyrbye, L. N., Sinsky, C., Satele, D., Sloan, J., & West, C. P. (2015). Changes in burnout and satisfaction with work-life balance in physicians and the general U.S. working population between 2011 and 2014. *Mayo Clinic Proceedings, 90*(12), 1600–1613. doi:10.1016/j.mayocp.2015.08.023

Shirey, M. R., Hauck, S. L., Embree, J. L., Kinner, T. J., Schaar, G. L., Phillips, L. A., ... McCool, I. A. (2011). Showcasing differences between quality improvement, evidence-based practice, and research. *Journal of Continuing Education in Nursing, 42*(2), 57–68. doi:10.3928/00220124-20100701-01

Squires, J. E., Estabrooks, C. A., Gustavsson, P., & Wallin, L. (2011). Individual determinants of research utilization by nurses: A systematic review update. *Implementation Science, 6*, 1–20. doi:10.1186/1748-5908-6-1

Stetler, C. B., Ritchie, J. A., Rycroft-Malone, J., & Charns, M. P. (2014). Leadership for evidence-based practice: Strategic and functional behaviors for institutionalizing EBP. *Worldviews on Evidence-Based Nursing, 11*(4), 219–226. doi:10.1111/wvn.12044

Tawfik, D. S., Profit, J., Morgenthaler, T. I., Satele, D. V., Sinsky, C. A., Dyrbye, L. N., ... Shanafelt, T. D. (2018). Physician burnout, well-being, and work unit safety grades in relationship to reported medical errors. *Mayo Clinic Proceedings, 93*(11), 1571–1580. doi:10.1016/j.mayocp.2018.05.014

ten Ham, W., Minnie, K., & van der Walt, C. (2015). Integrative review of benefit levers' characteristics for system-wide spread of best healthcare practices. *Journal of Advanced Nursing, 72*(1), 33–49. doi:10.1111/jan.12814

Tucker, S., Olson, M. E., & Frusti, D. K. (2009). Evidence-based practice self-efficacy scale: Preliminary reliability and validity. *Clinical Nurse Specialist, 23*(4), 207–215. doi:10.1177/0193945909342552

Vlada, A. C., Schmit, B., Perry, A., Trevino, J. G., Behrns, K. E., & Hughes, S. J. (2013). Failure to follow evidence-based best practice guidelines in the treatment of severe acute pancreatitis. *HBP Journal, 15*(10), 822–827. doi:10.1111/hpb.12140

Wallen, G. R., Mitchell, S. A., Melnyk, B., Fineout-Overholt, E., Miller-Davis, C., Yates, J., & Hastings, C. (2010). Implementing evidence-based practice: Effectiveness of a structured multifaceted mentorship programme. *Journal of Advanced Nursing, 66*(12), 2761–2771. doi:10.1111/j.1365-2648.2010.05442.x

Wilson, M., Sleutel, M., Newcomb, P., Behan, D., Walsh, J., Wells, J. N., & Baldwin, K. M. (2015). Empowering nurses with evidence-based practice environments: Surveying Magnet pathway to excellence, and non-Magnet facilities in one healthcare system. *Worldviews on Evidence-Based Nursing, 12*(1), 12–21. doi:10.1111/wvn.12077

Healthcare Finance for Leaders

Cheryl L. Hoying, Courtney Campbell-Saxton, and Alma Helpling

"It's good to have money and the things that money can buy, but it's good, too, to check up once in a while and make sure that you haven't lost the things that money can't buy."—George Lorimer

LEARNING OBJECTIVES

- Differentiate between capital and operating budgets and the reason to have both types of resource projections in the budgeting process.

- Determine the external factors affecting the financial viability of healthcare organizations and ways nurse leaders can manage expenditures and increase efficiencies to provide value for the consumer.

- Generate an ideal margin to foster economic stability of an organization.

- Analyze a budget spreadsheet and determine how to identify variances.

INTRODUCTION

We can all relate to money as we use some type of legal tender or script every day. Over the years, money-related phrases and idioms have been embedded in our brains, for example: "Money doesn't grow on trees" (*Cambridge University Press*, 2018), "money can't buy happiness," "no money, no mission" (TeleTracking, n.d.), and "for the love of money is the root of all evil" (King James Bible, n.d.).

We all need financial acumen to function in this world, both in our personal and professional lives. Monetary skills are essential for nurse and healthcare leaders because they are responsible for a large labor force that drives expenses and revenue. For example, chief nursing officers or administrators for patient care are responsible for nursing departments, which often comprise 75% of health system employees (AMN Healthcare, 2017). They are also responsible for many allied health and other departments as well (Advisory Board Company, 2014). In addition, the scope of their responsibility typically involves both inpatient and outpatient services across the continuum of care.

In a recent AMN Healthcare report investigating how nurse leaders spend their time, the respondents indicated that 14% of their time was spent on finances. This major focus on finance attributed to controlling costs, reducing variation, and streamlining processes.The respondents emphasized a greater need to work with tighter margins (AMN Healthcare, 2017).

In turn, healthcare workers need to increase their understanding and impact on resources because they are the ones utilizing supplies and services. Their actions directly affect the financial bottom line. Leaders must educate staff about the finances of their unit or department and the financial performance of their organization to help control costs.

SOURCES OF REVENUE FOR HEALTH SYSTEMS

"The first rule in making money is not to lose it."—Steven Lee

What is *revenue* and what are the sources of revenue? For healthcare organizations, **revenue** represents the estimated amount that will be collected from governmental and commercial payers, as well as from patients themselves, for the hospital or provider services rendered. For most healthcare organizations, revenue is the first line reported in the Statement of Operations in published financial statements because it generally is the most significant source of operational funding. Revenue typically includes estimates of the amount that will be reimbursed for services rendered based upon a guarantor payer. Some examples of payers include Medicare, Medicaid, and commercial organizations, such as Blue Cross/Blue Shield, Aetna, and United Healthcare.

Hospital services can be reimbursed based on a percentage of billed charges or based on an agreed upon contractual rate for a **diagnostic-related group (DRG)** or **Common Procedural Terminology (CPT)** code. Reimbursement can vary for the same procedure or medical service between two different payers. For example, according to a comparison report by America's Health Insurance Plans (2016), "In 2012, 96% of DRGs (48 out of 50) had commercial-to-Medicare payment ratios greater than 1.0, indicating that commercial average payments were overall higher than Medicare average payments for the same DRG (p. 3)." Furthermore, in some cases, the reimbursement difference between commercial payers and Medicare is significant. The same report published that "In 2012, the top 10% of DRGs with the highest ratio of commercial-to-Medicare payments had payment ratios ranging from 1.89 to 5.26, indicating that there were some DRGs where average commercial payments were more than double the average Medicare payments (p. 3)" (America's Health Insurance Plans, 2016). This means that, for the same service, commercial payers may reimburse between 200% and 500% of the amount reimbursed by Medicare. As the population continues to age and become Medicare eligible, and as reimbursement for hospital services becomes increasingly Medicare dependent, reducing the cost of goods and services provided to amounts that approximate Medicare reimbursement will be of paramount importance.

Other sources of revenue for healthcare organizations could include, for example, grants, philanthropic gifts, income from subleasing space in a hospital or office building, and incidental revenue received from the sale of products in a hospital gift shop. A grant is money that is awarded to an individual or an organization by a nonprofit or government entity. Generally, grants fund specific projects, research studies, or initiatives in response to a written proposal or application. Revenue is recorded as the funds are used or spent in accordance with the grant contract. Other revenue typically consists of funds received for other incidental services such as cafeteria food sales or parking fees. In some cases, the activities producing other revenue for nonprofit corporations are considered unrelated business activities and, as a result, are subject to tax.

The health system revenue cycle is every operation that is involved in collecting revenue. "All administrative and clinical functions that contribute to the capture, management, and collection of patient services revenue" (Oregon Health & Science University, n.d.). The revenue cycle includes the entire "life" of a patient account. For example, the revenue cycle includes "front-end" activities such as scheduling, pre-registration, financial counseling, and registration. Front-end revenue-cycle activities also include clearing patients financially for services by verifying insurance eligibility, obtaining necessary insurance authorization, and clearing the services requested for medical necessity. In addition, the revenue cycle includes "middle" functions such as ensuring all clinical documentation is complete and accurate, charges are captured with integrity, and transcription and coding of the medical record are done.

SOURCES OF HEALTH SYSTEM EXPENDITURES

"Beware of little expenses; a small leak will sink a great ship."—Benjamin Franklin

Health systems invest dollars in many different ways. Some expenditures are operational in nature; others constitute capital expenditures. *Operational expenditures* are defined as ongoing costs (excluding expenses related to production) for running a business or organization. Salaries and benefits for nurses and physicians, pharmaceutical supplies and drugs, rent, and utilities are all health system operational expenditures. *Capital expenditures* are finances used on materials to increase productivity or efficiency "spent to acquire or upgrade productive assets (such as buildings, machinery and equipment, vehicles) to increase the capacity or efficiency of a company for more than one accounting period" (Capital expenditure, 2009). Examples of capital assets include land, buildings, and surgical robots. Organizations must ensure the facilities they operate are equipped to handle the required patient care. In addition, labor supply combined with supply and equipment needed to provide care are an institution's top priorities.

As health systems evaluate the ways in which they will invest capital into the operation, there are many things to consider. For example, a health system may determine that there is demand where a certain market need is not being met. In such a situation, the health system may determine it is a wise investment to start a new program or open a new facility depending on the scope of the market need. Like other businesses, health systems must determine how to prioritize their capital resources to utilize them efficiently. They do not have unlimited resources, so choices have to be made. Health system leadership commonly goes through a strategic-planning exercise to determine how resources will be allocated from an investment perspective. In addition to large capital investments, health systems spend dollars as part of the normal course of business. These expenditures are typically referred to as the costs required to operate on a day-to-day basis—or *operating costs*.

Operating costs in a health system can be defined as *direct* or *indirect costs*. *Direct cost* is the cost to run a particular department, including the labor, supply, and service costs for that department. *Indirect costs* are those that are incurred, but may not be directly attributable to a department. An example of **indirect costs** could be the cost of utilities or other support areas that cannot be wholly attributed to a patient department, such as a nursing unit.

Perhaps one of the largest expenditures for many healthcare systems is the investment in human capital, including salaries and benefit costs. Ensuring that salaries and benefits offered to employees are market based is extremely important. Reviewing salary costs for various roles that may be in high demand in a market ensures that the organization is competitive and can attract and retain the needed staff. Lagging on market competitiveness with regard to salary and benefit offerings can lead to reactive compensation practices. An example of this might be an area that lagged in market competitiveness but then offered signing bonuses to ensure the appropriate staffing for patient care. When one organization follows a practice such as this, there is sometimes a ripple effect, creating a bidding war on staff for a given market that also tends to drive the market rate up for a particular supply of labor.

Supply costs in a health system also can be significant expenditures. These can be anything from materials that are directly related to a patient condition (such as surgical supplies), items necessary for patient care in the patient room or clinic (e.g., thermometers, bed pans, gowns), or supplies required in the support areas. In many organizations, patient supply costs can be driven by clinical leader preference. For example, a surgeon may have a preference on the type of stapler that he uses in the operating room.

Health organizations are increasingly aware of the opportunity to review supply expenditures to see whether there is opportunity to reduce costs. One way some organizations have done this is to institute value analysis committees with representation from various disciplines within the hospital. A good framework for a value analysis committee would be to include frontline staff, finance, purchasing, supply chain, and clinical leadership (including providers). These committees can review new supply requests to ensure there is line of sight into any increase in cost or opportunity to evaluate vendors. In addition, they can review opportunities to change a supply that may have cost-savings opportunities.

Health systems also tend to have a large investment in procuring services to run their operation, such as laundry/linen services, cafeteria services, if outsourced, and other services. As healthcare becomes more data driven, many health systems have seen large increases in costs related to information technology infrastructure like the licensing fees related to operating an electronic medical record. Many organizations have processes in place to review the cost for these outside services. A best practice is to ensure that the higher cost services are reviewed on a regular basis and that they are competitively bid for on a schedule, which may vary from yearly to every 3 years or some other time frame.

There are many other ways that health systems spend dollars—for example, some organizations are involved in research designed to improve patient care or outcomes and some are heavily involved in supporting the health and wellness of their communities. Each organization must evaluate how resources are spent to ensure the investments have the desired results.

 CALL TO ACTION

Meet with a financial analyst at a healthcare facility and ask questions about organizational costs. Ask to see some financial statements to learn what the overall expenditures are for the organization.

◆ STRATEGIES THAT BRING THE MOST RETURN ON INVESTMENT

"Money is only a tool. It will take you where you wish, but it will not replace you as the driver."—Ayn Rand

Due to the smaller margin yields that many healthcare organizations face, understanding the return on investment (ROI) related to a potential investment is critical. ROI is a way to evaluate the success or worth of an investment. "ROI measures the gain or loss generated on an investment relative to the amount of money invested. ROI is usually expressed as a percentage and is typically used for personal financial decisions, to compare a company's profitability or to compare the efficiency of different investments" (Investing Answers, n.d.). Essentially, in very broad terms, the organization nets more financial outcomes than the amount invested. An investment could be something as large as opening a new hospital or something smaller such as recruiting a new nurse practitioner. The most commonly used approach to identifying whether there will be a positive ROI is to do a formal business plan, which includes writing a **pro forma financial statement**. A financial projection contains the key assumptions of the investment and the expected outcomes or return. The more explicit and accurate the assumptions are, the more likely that the outcomes or return will be exactly as planned. For example, in the case of recruiting a new nurse practitioner, the following key assumptions could include:

1. Market-demand knowledge: Is the opening for a specialty for which there is known demand? If so, what is the demand? Is it a completely new service line or is it a response to high wait lists because the existing providers are at maximum productivity and cannot absorb any additional patient loads?

2. Volume assumptions: Calculate how many visits/patients the nurse practitioner could see.

3. Revenue assumptions: Use the volume assumption and a charge per patient to determine the patient revenue charges that would be generated.

4. Reimbursement assumptions: Review the payer contracts for the particular service and the patient insurance mix (i.e., 50% commercial insurance, 50% Medicare, etc.) to calculate the actual net cash that could be generated.

5. Expense assumptions: This would include the salary and benefit costs for the provider and any associated support staff (e.g., nurses, office staff). In addition, this would include any supply or services costs necessary for patient visits. Finally, it is important to evaluate whether there are any organizational indirect costs that will be increased as a result of adopting the business plan. This could include support staff (e.g., increases in the revenue cycle office, human resources, marketing) that may not be explicitly related to the proposed plan but for which there would be an increased burden as a result of adding additional staff. Other indirect cost considerations would include overhead type items that would be necessary if adding new clinic space, such as utilities and insurance. Indirect cost assumptions in a business plan are typically some of the most difficult to calculate down to the dollar, but there should be an effort to make a reasonable estimate.

The more accurate the assumptions in a financial analysis, the more likely the operation will experience the intended financial result. Financial summaries can be used for items as large

EXHIBIT 9.1 Example of a Financial Pro Forma

Requesting Department	Department ABC							
Project Name	Project 1							
Capital Purchase / Investment								

Financial Performance Ratio's	
Profitability Index	#DIV/0!
ROI (target ≥ 100% for a positive return)	#DIV/0!
Net Impact on Earnings (w/o deprec exp) / Initial Investment Amt	
5 Year IRR (target > 25%)	0.0%
Payback Period (target < 60% of depreciable life)	0.00
Discounted Payback Period	0.00

CALCULATION OF FINANCIAL IMPACT	Year 0	Year 1	Year 2	Year 3	Year 4	Year 5	Grand Total
Incremental Revenue Generated From Investment:							
Gross Hospital Billings							
Deduction Rate							
Billing Write-offs							
Expected Hospital Billing Receipts							
Physician Billing Receipts							
Other Revenue							
(specify source)							
Total Net Revenue							
Incremental Operating Expense Associated With Investment:							
New Expenses:							
Salaries							
Benefits							
Direct Expense							
Depreciation							
Indirect Expense							
Expenses (Avoided):							
(specify)							
Total Expense Impact							
Net Impact on Earnings							
Net Impact on Earnings for ROI calc. (EBITDA)							
Net Earnings / Total Net Revenue							
Operating Cash Flow (Net Earnings Plus Depreciation)							
Cash outlay by year							
Salvage value (net book value)							
Total Net Cash Flow	-						

EBITDA, Earnings before interest, taxes, depreciation, and amortization; IRR, Internal rate of retur; ROI, Return on investment.

as a new facility and items much smaller such as implementing a new service line. An example financial pro forma, which demonstrates ROI, is provided in Exhibit 9.1.

To evaluate a financial pro forma and determine whether the proposed ROI is accurate, the first step is to understand the assumptions and determine the probability of their accuracy. In some cases, assumptions are very black and white and it is easy to know that the intended financial outcome is assured. In other cases, the assumptions may be high-level estimates based on the available information but without as much certainty. Healthcare leaders need to evaluate financial summaries and the estimated outcomes to determine whether an organization should move forward with a proposed investment. The organization's priorities and financial position are two key factors that influence which business plans receive prioritized investment dollars.

CALL TO ACTION

Ask to be included in the process for requesting funding for a new investment. Learn how the requestor arrives at his or her assumptions and how the or she determines the probability of the intended financial outcome.

▶ HOW THE CURRENT CLIMATE OF HEALTHCARE IMPACTS THE BOTTOM LINE

"Don't tell me what you value, show me your budget and I'll tell you what you value."
—Joe Biden

The United States spends the most in healthcare of any country, accounting for 17.8% of the national gross domestic product (GDP). In 2016, the United States spent $3.3 trillion or $10,348 on healthcare per person (Centers for Medicare & Medicaid Services [CMS], n.d.-b). The "U.S healthcare's world-leading spending is driven by the higher cost of everything from drugs, salaries and administration, not greater utilization, para. 8" (Meyer, 2018). As the healthcare industry continues to face different financial challenges to reimbursement, healthcare leaders are vying to remain financially stable.

Healthcare leaders must be strategic partners with colleagues to provide financial oversight and operational efficiency (Crawford, Omery, & Spicer, 2017). They must be diverse in thought and engage the staff to achieve the organization's mission and vision. In a nurse leadership position, specifically, having a financial liaison embedded into the department is a benefit to both the nursing and the finance departments. It is beneficial for those in nursing to have someone with a background in finance to be able to advise the nurse leader. The partnership, with a finance professional and his or her vast expertise ensures mutual goals and expectations are developed and achieved in the organization. In turn, for the finance partner, that collaboration illuminates the challenges the clinician is faced with in delivering quality care. In addition, the nurse leader must become familiar with furthering his or her comprehension of financial acumen and principles. This can be achieved by attending graduate courses on finance, or reading books or journals on economics.

Many efforts are taking place in healthcare organizations across the country to reduce waste. Leaders often look at labor costs for immediate fixes, because a large portion of dollars can be found there; however, consequences may surface when staff are required to care for an increase in patients/consumers. Dissatisfaction and burnout may occur when staff do not feel they have the time to deliver the care needed for patients (Gooch, 2015). Adjusting staffing to meet consumer need requires great coordination. Flexible staffing resources should be available when the patient need is increased as should opportunities for staff to remain financially whole when the need lessens. Cross-training from inpatient to outpatient areas and having other activities with which staff can engage helps with nurse retention.

There are multiple other aspects to evaluate and consider to decrease costs (Advisory Board Company, 2015). One method is to look at nonlabor activities, such as contracts, by having a group of individuals from the care areas, along with individuals from finance and legal, review contracts on a periodic basis. It is eye-opening to list all the contracts for one department and note the amount of duplication of services for which an organization is paying. In many instances, the individual divisions do not realize others are using similar outside services. Combining contracts can often lead to a better arrangement.

All who work in the organization are responsible for decreasing costs and adding value for the consumer. Therefore, the leader should engage the staff in activities that promote ideas to decrease waste and increase value for the consumer. Although this can be achieved within a specific department, there are multiple benefits to having the staff engaged in organization-wide activities as well. Having interprofessional teams collaborate increases teamwork and highlights the impact on others of the suggestions put forth (Thew, 2016).

Ongoing efforts are deployed to teach and involve those in the organization to improve care and reduce waste. One such method is the Lean methodology. The concept grew out of the Toyota Motor Corporation in the 1950s, created by Toyota's chief of production Taiichi Ohno. The methodology is based on principles from manufacturing and is referred to as the *Toyota Production System*. The model grew from manufacturing to other areas of business, including healthcare, in the 1990s from the result of research by the Massachusetts Institute of Technology (MIT). MIT found it was more effective and efficient than other mass production techniques and coined the term *lean* to differentiate this new approach to production. "The core idea is to maximize customer value while minimizing waste" (Marchwinski & Shook, 2014). It means creating more value for customers using fewer resources. The goal is to provide perfect value to the customer through a process that has no waste from beginning to end (Lean Enterprise Institute, n.d.).

CALL TO ACTION

Collaborate with your coworkers to come up with a process to generate cost-efficiency ideas and evaluate them for implementation. Evaluate their success at specific intervals.

EXTERNAL FACTORS IMPACTING HEALTHCARE FINANCE TODAY AND INTO THE FUTURE

"Price is what you pay. Value is what you get."—Warren Buffet

The CMS has forecasted the following projections for national healthcare expenditures from the years 2017 to 2026:

1. Health spending is expected to grow at an average rate of 5.5% per year for 2017 to 2026 and reach $5.7 trillion by 2026.

2. Health spending is expected to grow faster than the GDP. As a result, the healthcare share of GDP is expected to rise from 17.9% in 2016 to 19.7% by 2026.

3. Economic and demographic factors affecting the growth include changes in projected income growth, increases in prices for medical goods and services, and enrollment shifts from private health insurance to Medicare related to the aging of the population.

4. The trends reflect an aging population. For Medicare, projected enrollment is a factor and for Medicaid, an increase in the share of aged and disabled enrollees is a factor.

5. Primary factors, such as projected GDP growth and employment trends, will contribute to a slight decline in the insured share of the population from 91.1% in 2016 to 89.3% in 2026.

6. By 2026, federal, state, and local governments are projected to sponsor 47% of total national health expenditures, up from 45% in 2016 (CMS, n.d.-a).

These CMS predictions alone are challenging for organizations to remain viable, but these are not the only issues of which an organization should be cognizant. Other factors, such as increased vacancy and turnover of new nurses (Kovner, Brewer, Fatehi, & Jun, 2014) and the baby boomer retirement wave (Kacik, 2018), pose hardships for organizations to maintain a stable workforce and an accurate labor budget.

An additional external force impacting healthcare finance is the redesign of healthcare. Partnering with patients and families is shifting how care is being transformed. Healthcare systems are moving to value rather than volume. Results will continue to focus on quality measures and patient/consumer engagement (Meadows, 2016). To accomplish this, strategies will have to be implemented that go across the healthcare continuum, partnering with community leaders, and moving beyond traditional walls. Focusing on standardizing care to reduce unnecessary variation increases the time required for individualized care. Reaching into the community, utilizing digital care, and promoting wellness will lead to a decrease in hospitalizations (Stempniak, 2015). This opens many opportunities for nurses to work in home care, clinics, and outpatient centers to foster well-being and keep consumers from hospitalization and out of acute care settings.

Considering the increased focus on healthcare costs, why is the cost of care not more transparent to those working in the field and those being served? Often those who are ordering the treatments or procedures and using materials are not aware of their cost. When one does not know a cheaper medication or therapy will suffice, this can lead to increased costs. Organizations need to have the costs of the treatment readily at hand, at the point of care, so that it is translucent to the provider and patient. Calls from consumers seeking information on the cost of care are on the rise. Tools are being developed for cost comparisons of procedures and services (Sinaiko & Rosenthal, 2016). One can easily go to the Internet to compare costs and look at quality and patient satisfaction scores as well. Even when he or she is aware of the costs of the care, it is still confusing for the consumer to realize the true price because there are differences in consumer copays, health insurance, and self-pay methods. Reviewing the quality indicators posted online is perplexing as well for the consumer, as he or she tries to decipher the acuity of those provided services and their long-term outcomes.

 CALL TO ACTION

We often use supplies, treatments, medications, and services without ever knowing the cost of them. Find out the costs of three items used in your workplace. Calculate the utilization and cost of each on a weekly or monthly basis. Share this information with your coworkers.

HOW TO CREATE A MARGIN

"The budget is not just a collection of numbers but an expression of our values and aspirations."—Jacob Lew

For any organization to remain functional, it needs a positive financial bottom line. In healthcare organizations, the excess of revenues over expenses in the statement of operations represents the organization's "bottom line." A positive bottom line or an excess of revenue over expenses needs to be made, not only to pay the staff, but to invest in the future. For both not-for-profit and for-profit organizations, a margin needs to be generated, but the expected amount may be different. For healthcare organizations that have outstanding debt that is rated "A" or above, an operating income (i.e., total operating revenues less operating expenses) of 2.3% or more is typical (Moody's Investor Services, 2018).

Leaders will often hear the acronym EBITDA during the course of a finance meeting. Just like in the medical field, the finance world has its own vocabulary. *EBITDA* stands for earnings before interest, taxes, depreciation, and amortization (EBITDA, n.d.). It is used to analyze and compare profitability and cash generated by operations. The algorithm gives the organization an idea of how it is doing financially and how much cash is on hand before paying debts. EBITDA is calculated as: operating income + depreciation expense + amortization expense. A more literal formula is: EBITDA = net profit + interest + taxes + depreciation + amortization.

An **EBITDA margin** is an assessment of an organization's profitability as a percentage of its total revenue (EBITDA margin, n.d.). It indicates an organization's cash flow. EBITDA is different from the operating margin, which excludes depreciation and amortization. Usually the EBITDA margin is higher than the profit margin.

Although having a positive margin is essential for an organization's longevity, in some circumstances, a business line might generate a loss scenario. Many healthcare organizations might have a few services that are considered important to the mission of the organization and, thus, a certain loss for that service line might be tolerated. Healthcare leaders can ensure that if they have oversight for such a service line, they limit the organizational loss to that which the organization has committed. Losses also can occur as a result of poor business management or an unintended shift in reimbursement due to external factors. For these losses, the leader must partner with others in the organization (e.g., unit management and/or finance staff) to put action plans in place to mitigate losses or turn them around. Organizations must ensure they generate a positive EBIDTA overall. Therefore, it is important to ensure that any service lines for which there is a loss have a plan so that the number of losses does not outweigh those areas with positive cash flow.

CASE STUDY: CONSERVING COSTS, PRESERVING PATIENT VALUE

The medical center has a long history of a strong balance sheet. Because of reimbursement changes at the state and national levels, the organization made the decision to reduce spending in the system by $50 million/year for the next 5 years. In retrospect, this was done at an opportune time to initiate such an endeavor since the process could be implemented over a period of time and presented the opportunity to thoroughly evaluate each initiative versus hastily making budget cuts. Ground rules were established prior to implementation that focused on maintaining the quality of care for patients and preserving human resources at the organization as much as possible.

Each division was asked to participate and was given a designated amount of money to conserve. To ensure transparency and to engage staff in the effort, the Patient Services division utilized their shared governance structure to implement the goal, employing the medical center's Interprofessional Practice Model (2013). The model utilized six councils: Safety, Best Practice, Collaborative Relationships, Comprehensive Coordinated Care, Innovation and Research, and

Professionalism. The Best Practice Council was assigned the task of achieving $1 million in savings. The council consisted of staff from various departments and units, financial business directors, and senior leadership—all of whom drove the process. Ideas were generated from the staff and vetted with the group. The staff were the ones to come up with recommendations because they were the ones closest to the point of care and knew how care could be affected. The $1 million in savings was achieved and quality care was maintained.

In addition, that same year, four groups within the medical center were established to focus on clinical practices, support services, financial services, and physician practices and research. Each group was responsible for a designated amount of savings as well. Employees from various levels in the organization were a part of each of the four teams. Again, ideas were generated from the staff, including physicians, as they were employees of the medical center. The strategies were conceived out of such factors as ease of implementation, patient outcomes, and staff impact. Major savings were generated from this group as well.

Although $50 million in savings was a monumental goal, it was achievable. Staff involvement was integral to the goal's success. The savings achieved could then be passed on to the patients to reduce service charges, used for future capital expenditures, and staff benefits.

KEY TAKEAWAY POINTS

- Nurse and healthcare leaders play an integral part in the financial viability of an organization due to the size of their budgets and impact on care.

- With the healthcare field changing rapidly, healthcare leaders need to find reliable sources to remain current on healthcare economics.

- All staff in an organization have the responsibility to be good stewards of the resources, whether human or material. Leaders need to foster this philosophy.

- Nurse and healthcare leaders need to partner with finance colleagues in the organization to achieve the strategic plan and goals of the organization.

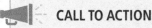

CALL TO ACTION
Learn how to read a budget

"A budget is telling your money where to go instead of wondering where it went."
—Dave Ramsey

Healthcare leaders need to be familiar with the actual financial performance for the areas for which they are responsible. Many organizations have established processes to determine an annual budget as a guideline to analyze whether the actual financial performance is in line with expectations. The budget is based on assumptions regarding volume, revenue, and expense. Typically, there are budget reports for department leaders to review to ensure the actual financial performance is within the parameters established in the budget. Review of the budget report typically includes analysis of actual expenses to budget performance. Other useful data points are the performance compared to the prior year (e.g., Is the department doing better than the prior year even if it is below budget?) and comparison to a volume-adjusted budget. A volume-adjusted budget calculates what the anticipated financial performance would be at a given budget level. For example, if an area budgets 100 patient visits for the month but the actual patient number is 150, the volume-adjusted budget determines what the department would have expected to budget at that higher volume. The patient visit is considered the unit of service by which the department is measured. If the financial performance for the department is trending favorably to the volume-adjusted budget, the department is demonstrating improved efficiency (i.e., it is taking care of more patients at less cost per patient than anticipated). A best practice is to review financial performance on a regular basis and provide explanations for variances and, if necessary, offer mitigation strategies that will enable any gaps in performance to be closed. A sample budget report is shown in Exhibit 9.2.

Key performance metrics can be used to determine whether a department is operating in line with expectations. For example, cost per unit of service is a common key performance metric used in many healthcare organizations. Units of service can vary by department. For example, on an inpatient nursing unit, the unit of service might be the nightly patient census. In an ambulatory clinic setting, it might be the number of visits per day. Other examples of units of service can look at a more granular level, such as procedures per day. Departments should think about the unit of service that most directly correlates with the care being provided. A common measure that is used in many settings is *adjusted patient days*. This unit of measure weighs inpatient and outpatient visits to provide a broader measure of volume for the healthcare organization.

EXHIBIT 9.2 **Example of a Budget Report**

ABC Department Budget Report							
	Actual	Fixed Budget	Prior Year	Var to Bud	Var to PY	Vol Adj Budget	Explanation
Unit of Service	1,000	1,300	1,200	(300)	(200)	1,000	Patient volume lower than anticipated due to significant winter storm
Gross Charges	500,000	750,000	700,000	(250,000)	(200,000)	576,923	Charges per visit lower than anticipated due to change in service mix
Contractual Adj.	(240,000)	(360,000)	(336,000)	120,000	96,000	(276,923)	
Net Revenue	260,000	390,000	364,000	(130,000)	(104,000)	300,000	Net reimbursement trending as expected - payor mix stable but service mix per patient resulting in lower cash collection
Rev per UOS	260	300	303	-40	-43	300	
Reimb %	52%	52%	52%			52%	
Salary	100,000	125,000	112,000	25,000	12,000	96,154	Flexing of staff per patient did not occur resulting in higher salary cost per UOS
Benefit	28,000	35,000	30,240	7,000	(28,000)	26,923	
Supplies	10,000	12,000	10,000	2,000	-	9,231	Supply cost per UOS higher than anticipated due to service mix
Services	5,000	4,000	4,500	(1,000)	(500)	4,000	Unanticipated increase in cost of ABC service paid annually, working with purchasing to renegotiate contract
Total Expense	143,000	176,000	156,740	33,000	13,740	136,308	Cost per UOS unfavorable due to change in patient acuity combined with lack of staff flexing to volume
Exp per UOS	143	135	131	-8	-12	136	
Net Margin	117,000	214,000	207,260	(97,000)	(90,260)	163,692	Mitigation - will monitor flex staffing and determine if opportunity to review charges for increased acuity
Margin per UOS	117	165	173	-48	-56	164	

PY, prior year; UOS, unit of service.

Now that you know what elements to analyze in a budget, you can begin to determine whether your organization is on the right track financially. Review your departmental financial performance compared to its budget. Evaluate whether revenue and costs are in line with volumes. If there is a significant variance, identify opportunities to mitigate.

REFERENCES

The Advisory Board Company. (2014). *Nursing executive center interviews and analysis: 2014 NEC changing CNO role survey—The Advisory Board survey solutions* (Advisory.com 29759C).

The Advisory Board Company. (2015). Nursing executive center. Retrieved from https://www .advisory.com/research/nursing-executive-center/studies/2015/untapped-opportunities -for-saving-millions

America's Health Insurance Plans. (2016, February). National comparison of commercial and Medicare fee-for-service payments to hospitals. Retrieved from https://www.ahip.org/ wp-content/uploads/2016/02/HospitalPriceComparison_2.10.16.pdf

AMN Healthcare. (2017, September 19). Nurse executive summary: Clinical leadership trends & strategies. Retrieved from https://www.amnhealthcare.com/industry-research/survey/ nurse-executive-survey

Cambridge University Press (2018). Money doesn't grow on trees. In *Cambridge advanced learner's dictionary and thesaurus*. Retrieved from https://dictionary.cambridge.org/us/ dictionary/english/money-doesn-t-grow-on-trees

Capital expenditure. (2009). In *Farlex financial dictionary*. Retrieved from https://financial -dictionary.thefreedictionary.com/capital+expenditure

Centers for Medicare & Medicaid Services. (n.d.-a). National health expenditure projections 2018–2027. Retrieved from https://www.cms.gov/Research-Statistics-Data-and-Systems/ Statistics-Trends-and-Reports/NationalHealthExpendData/Downloads/ForecastSummary .pdf

Centers for Medicare & Medicaid Services. (n.d.-b). National health expenditures 2017 highlights. Retrieved from https://www.cms.gov/Research-Statistics-Data-and-Systems/ Statistics-Trends-and-Reports/NationalHealthExpendData/Downloads/highlights.pdf

Cincinnati Children's Hospital Medical Center. (2013). *Interprofessional practice model.* Cincinnati, OH.

Crawford, C., Omery, A., & Spicer, J. (2017). An integrative review of 21st-century roles, responsibilities, characteristics, and competencies of chief nurse executives. *Nursing Administrative Quarterly, 41*(4), 297–309. doi:10.1097/NAQ.0000000000000245

EBITDA. (n.d.). In *Investopia*. Retrieved from https://www.investopedia.com/terms/e/ebitda .asp

EBITDA margin. (n.d.) In *Investopedia*. Retrieved from https://www.investopedia.com/terms/e/ebitda-margin.asp

Gooch, K. (2015, August 13). *5 of the biggest issues nurses face today. Becker's Hospital Review*. Retrieved from https://www.beckershospitalreview.com/human-capital-and-risk/5-of-the-biggest-issues-nurses-face-today.html

Grant. (n.d.). In *Financial glossary*. Retrieved from https://financial-dictionary.thefreedictionary.com/Grant

Investing Answers. (n.d.). Return on investment (ROI). Retrieved from https://investinganswers.com/financial-dictionary/technical-analysis/return-investment-roi-1100

Kacik, A. (2018, May 7). Building the bench: Hospitals and health systems prepare for boomer retirement wave. *Modern Healthcare, 48*(19),12–14.

King James Bible. (n.d.). Timothy 6:10. Retrieved from https://www.kingjamesbibleonline.org/1-Timothy-6-8_6-11/

Kovner, C., Brewer, C., Fatehi, F., & Jun, J. (2014, August 25). What does nurse turnover rate mean and what is the rate? *Policy, Politics, & Nursing Practice, 15*(3/4), 64–71. doi:10.1177/1527154414547953

Lean Enterprise Institute. (n.d.). What is lean? Retrieved from https://www.lean.org/WhatsLean

Marchwinski, C., & Shook, J. (2014). Toyota production system. In *Lean lexicon* (5th ed.). Boston, MA: Lean Enterprise Institute. Retrieved from https://www.lean.org/lexicon/toyota-production-system

Meadows, M. (2016, May). New competencies for system chief nurse executives. *Journal of Nursing Administration, 46*(5), 235–237. doi:10.1097/NNA.0000000000000336

Meyer, H. (2018, April 7). Blame it on the prices. *Modern Healthcare*, 48(15), 20–24.

Moody's Investor Services. (2018, August 28). Appendix 2: Freestanding hospitals, single-state and multi-state healthcare systems, medians by broad rating category, fiscal year 2017. *Sector in-depth: Not-for-profit and public healthcare.*

Oregon Health & Science University. (n.d.). Revenue cycle. Retrieved from https://www.ohsu.edu/xd/about/services/patient-business-services/revenue-cycle

Return on investment (ROI). (n.d.). In *Investing answers*. Retrieved from https://investinganswers.com/financial-dictionary/technical-analysis/return-investment-roi-1100

Sinaiko, A., & Rosenthal, M. (2016, April). Examining a healthcare price transparency tool: Who uses it and how they shop for care. *Health Affairs, 35*(4), 662–670. doi:10.1377/hlthaff.2015.0746

Stempniak, M. (2015, October 7). IHI lays out 10 ways to radically transform health care. *Hospitals & Health Network*. Retrieved from http://www.hhnmag.com/articles/6569-ihi-lays-out-10-ways-to-radically-transform-health-care

TeleTracking. (n.d.). No margin, no mission: Flying nuns and Sister Irene Kraus. Retrieved from https://www.teletracking.com/resources/no-margin-no-mission-flying-nuns-and-sister-irene-kraus

Thew, J. (2016, January). Interprofessional collaboration: The impact on eliminating individual silos and meeting industry goals. *HealthLeaders, 18*(10), 19–22.

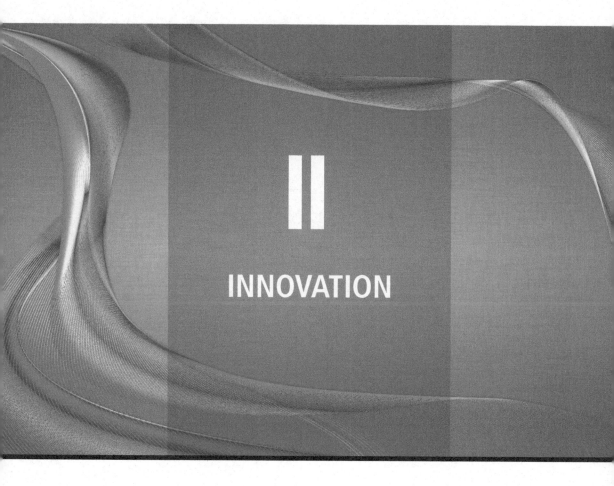

II

INNOVATION

Healthcare Innovation: Bringing the Buzzword to Real-World Healthcare Settings

Nancy M. Albert and Tim Raderstorf

"Innovation does not happen in a straight line; be prepared for bumps in the road; trials and errors."—Nancy M. Albert

LEARNING OBJECTIVES

- Describe how innovation is a core competency of healthcare practice.
- Concretely describe the value of clinical innovations in healthcare settings.
- Explain how innovation influences health transformations.
- Enumerate the key characteristics that promote innovation by healthcare employees.
- Identify foundational structures/systems/processes that drive real-world innovative thinking.
- Summarize principles that facilitate healthcare providers to be innovators.

INTRODUCTION

Buzzwords get their name because they are used, and even overused, in a specific context. *Innovation* is one of many buzzwords used in real-world healthcare settings, as leaders want to believe they support innovation. But do they? What does it mean when a healthcare setting advertises that it is innovative? Are employees innovative? Are systems and processes in place to cultivate innovation? Or, is the buzzword *innovation* used to imply that digital technology, supply and equipment purchases involve start-up products and solutions? Is innovation an event or a foundational element of everyday life? If it is a foundational element, how strong is the foundation? Does the foundation support all employees, or only specific groups, such as physicians or basic scientists? Does the innovation infrastructure allow for variations or does it have customizable features to meet the needs of different work teams?

A second buzzword, *value*, is heavily used in relation to the economics of healthcare, as we are in the age of value for patients. Value for patients can be achieved by innovation. For example, value-enhancing innovations surrounding our knowledge explosion from big data and artificial intelligence can improve patient mortality, morbidity, and quality of life. Innovations that improve patient assessment and prevent unnecessary treatment may decrease cost of care. It is also important that we understand the value of employee-generated innovation in complex, real-world healthcare settings.

But here's the issue. *Innovation* and *value are not* buzzwords in healthcare. They are *core competencies* of healthcare; core competencies that can be overlooked, misinterpreted, or misaligned by healthcare providers and organizations alike. In this chapter, we explore how embedding innovation into your organization will improve outcomes and the overall health of your organization.

THE VALUE OF INNOVATION IN REAL-WORLD HEALTHCARE SETTINGS

Hospitals and health systems are constantly changing to deliver high-quality, safe, client care, and to improve clinical outcomes and the health of their communities. Employee-generated and developed innovations have the capability of enhancing compassionate, evidence-based practices and improving equity of care, quality-of-care delivery, and clinical outcomes. Healthcare workers can articulate and discuss the details of gaps in care and of tools, algorithms, and processes needed to deliver optimal care. Further, when healthcare workers identify client, provider, and hospital system issues that create quality and safety risks and prevent optimization of care delivery, they need to be empowered to communicate and implement innovations. Thus, the obvious *client and community* value of employee-generated and developed innovations are lower cost of care; improved satisfaction; health promotion; and more effective, high-quality clinical care and outcomes. Hospital and health system leaders and providers benefit when hospital-monitored quality and safety performance metrics improve, Centers for Medicare & Medicaid penalties are reduced or eliminated, and hospital reputation improves. Of equal importance, when innovative practices, processes, and systems improve the health of the community, hospital and health systems can expect to see higher utilization of services. Thus, employee-generated and developed innovations are a return on investment (ROI) that can reduce costs of care, create efficiencies and effectiveness paradigms, and ultimately create revenue for hospital and health systems (Figure 10.1; Joseph, Rhodes, & Watson, 2016; Kelly, 2005). You'll learn more about how you can measure the ROI for innovations within your organization in Chapter 16, Negotiating Complex Systems.

The value of employee-generated and developed innovation to real-world healthcare settings does not end with value to clients and communities. The community of healthcare workers that makes up a healthcare system workforce may also derive value from innovations. All leaders should believe that their workforce will benefit from owning their profession/work through innovation. Leaders have an obligation to promote employee-generated innovations as one aspect of investment in their workforce. In essence, when leaders actively promote innovation among

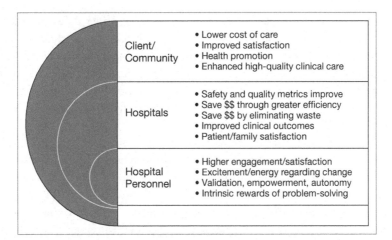

Figure 10.1 The value of innovation in healthcare settings.

their workforce, they are directly supporting the work-related journey of individual employees in their work. Leaders who support work as a journey understand the complexities of work; they understand that work is made up of more than the tasks and events that must be dealt with now or before the shift/workday ends. Leaders who support work as a journey understand that change, flexibility, ideas for improvement and novel innovations, even disruptive innovations, can enhance outcomes for individuals and teams. Leaders must actively listen to employee ideas and innovations and facilitate implementation of innovation-related policies, practices, technology, knowledge, resources, and solutions that lead to professional benefits or that benefit the health of those they serve. When leaders ensure that employees understand that their ideas and innovations are welcomed and encouraged, employees may feel more engaged as an integral member of their healthcare setting and be less likely to seek employment elsewhere. The downstream effect for leaders is that their workforce may be more satisfied with their work life and job roles and be more engaged in meeting the mission and values of the healthcare system, which ultimately affects the health and healthcare of clients.

From a healthcare worker's perspective, a culture of innovation creates value for healthcare settings and, also, personal value. First, there is an excitement that occurs when innovative/ creative ideas are thoughtfully assessed and evaluated (regardless of actual implementation); for example, submitters of innovations may feel validated, empowered, energized, and autonomous. Second, submitters may be engaged in developing new solutions to gaps in care or ongoing issues after they received a positive response from a previous submission of an innovative idea. For some, the challenge of developing a solution may be rewarding in itself as it provides an opportunity to learn more about current evidence that may reshape or stretch thoughts about the original gap in care or problem. For some, the challenge of developing a solution may foster ownership of the problem that may lead to generating hypotheses and conducting research and/or recruiting other healthcare workers to participate in generating solutions. Third, there is value for those who learned that an innovation was developed by a colleague. The noninnovator may also feel empowered to voice innovative ideas and may believe that simply working in an environment that supports innovations is exciting, as it means the noninnovator will benefit from new ideas and solutions. Fourth, when a healthcare setting demonstrates a culture of innovation, inter- and intradisciplinary internal and external collaborations are encouraged and supported. When different disciplines or groups work together toward new solutions, they learn how individual perspectives and interrelationships can alter innovative thinking and spark new ideas. Teamwork is fostered when disparate and like-minded teams converge to solve problems.

Ultimately, the value of innovation to real-world healthcare settings is multidimensional. Many of the effects are cyclic—as the culture of innovation grows and infrastructure and resources are developed to aid growth, innovation is strengthened, thereby reinforcing the original value and creating new value. Most real-world healthcare settings have hierarchical workforces, including multiple levels of leadership. For innovations to hold value within a real-world healthcare setting, at minimum, there must be synergy among workers within a department regarding the value of innovation and also, supportive structures and resources that may be system or department wide (see "Permission to Innovate" and "Engaging Innovators" sections). In addition, each healthcare setting must define *innovation* so that others understand the breadth and depth of the term as it is applied within the healthcare setting.

Call to Action

A commitment to innovation in healthcare includes financial and resource commitments to employee-generated and developed innovations. Explore what resources are provided by your organization to help employee-generated innovations and share that information with your team.

WHAT IS INNOVATION IN REAL-WORLD HEALTHCARE SETTINGS?

There is no one right definition of *innovation* that applies to all healthcare settings; however, there is a difference between seeking to get or be better (incremental improvement) and seeking to do something differently (innovation). In Google Online Dictionary (n.d.), *innovation* was defined as the introduction of "a new idea, device or method" (www.google.com). The Google definition is useful as it helps healthcare workers understand that innovation goes beyond products purchased from companies; for example, it may involve a supply, instrument, or device used in care delivery or a device used in assessment or evaluation of care. Innovation can be the result of knowledge work; for example, it might be an algorithm that is applied as a device or telehealth application or a step-by-step process that is developed into a policy or procedure. One issue with the Google definition is that an innovative or new idea is not the same as an innovation. To be an innovation, there must be concrete implementation of the creative idea that brings ROI (or value) to an individual/group or the healthcare setting. The value can be intrinsic and/or extrinsic and can involve one work area/group or multiple interdisciplinary groups. Thus, we define *innovation* as the implementation of new products, services, or solutions that *create new value*.

There are two key features of innovation in healthcare settings. First, as implied by the definition, there must be novelty. Innovations can be disruptive (first of its kind) or an advancement on something already in use in healthcare (built on the ideas of others). To rephrase, a nondisruptive innovation can be a novelty that has a basis in a currently used product, service, or method. As an example, call lights have been attached to patient beds for years. They promote patient–caregiver voice communication at a distance, but often required a third-party responder to interface with the stationary device located at a nurse's station. An innovation, which was also an improvement to call light patient–caregiver communication, involved implementation of a small wearable communication device that replaced the nursing station stationary device. When worn by nurse caregivers, voice response to patients was instantaneous and the device also allowed for caregiver-to-caregiver voice communication regardless of the caregiver's location, without an interface with the stationary device. The innovation decreased communication time, enhanced patient safety and delivery of high-quality care, and enhanced caregiver colleague communication, to name a few benefits (Fang et al., 2017; Friend, Jennings, Copenhaver, & Levine, 2017) and also led to some new noise concerns (Friend et al., 2017). Since the innovative communication platform was released, improvements have been made, for example, allowing for text communication with a hospital-based cell phone.

In addition to novelty, the second feature of innovation in healthcare is usefulness; essentially, the innovative device or method must be useful to healthcare settings. Usefulness answers why we should care about the innovation. Is there evidence that the problem solved by the innovation is meaningful in terms of changing health, solving inconvenience, improving assessment, altering clinical outcomes, preventing side effects, minimizing health issues, and solving for inefficiency? Usefulness can be defined in many ways, based on the healthcare setting's current status. For example, disposable electrocardiographic lead wires were available for purchase as an alternative to reusable lead wires many years ago. Disposable lead wires may be a very valuable innovation to specific high-volume areas with temporary/short-term use; for example, in a radiology area. In the right environment, disposable electrocardiographic lead wires eliminated the need for cleaning in between cases and were affordable, creating a positive cost:benefit ratio. However, in critical care environments, disposable electrocardiographic lead wires must be durable over time and provide reliable data. The cost per lead wire set is more expensive than short-term-use disposable lead wires and when compared to reusable lead wires, the cost to the healthcare setting might be very high. To meet usefulness criteria, the cost (personnel time and supplies) of cleaning reusable lead wires must outweigh the cost of disposables (which most likely is not the case); thus, the innovation would require other supportive usefulness criteria. If hospital-acquired infection rates decreased significantly after switching to disposable electrocardiographic lead wires, that could be powerful usefulness criteria; however, when research was conducted, disposable lead wires did not reduce hospital-acquired infection rates among critically ill adults (Albert et al., 2014) and the quantity of adenosine triphosphate in relative luminescence units (that correlated with microbial cell counts) was not reduced beyond the first 24 hours of assessment on disposable compared to reusable lead wires among children treated in a pediatric intensive care unit after open heart surgery (Addison et al., 2014).

Differences Between Innovation and Evidence-Based Practice or Continuous Improvement Projects

In real-world healthcare settings, high-quality care can be fostered by (a) innovations, (b) translation of evidence-based practice into clinical care and/or decision-making, and (c) continuous improvement projects aimed at improving processes or outcomes. All three project types use data to guide the approach (evidence-based practices and quality improvement) or to define the problem, issue, or gap (innovation), and all three are useful to healthcare settings, but innovation is uniquely different.

Novelty is the key ingredient that differentiates the three project types. When translating evidence into clinical practice, project leaders may utilize innovative education and/or implementation strategies, but the intervention to be implemented is evidence based, so it is assumed to be based on appraisal of the literature for evidence and it may also involve clinical expertise and client preferences. Continuous improvement strategies are a problem-solving approach to achieve quality improvement. Methodologies can involve Lean, Kaizen, Six Sigma, or others. Healthcare workers may raise ideas during the process, but, based on the nature of the work, the ideas are generally incremental improvements, based on current practice, and not truly novel. If novelty is involved, the novel components of the intervention might need to be vetted for usefulness or other outcomes before used systematically.

 Call to Action—Rapid Prototype/Rapid Conceptualization Exercise

At your next team meeting (or over lunch in the breakroom), ask your team to become engaged in the 15-Minute Rapid Conceptualization Exercise. Here's how to make it happen:

1. Take 3 minutes to discuss the tasks, tools, or barriers that make your job difficult.
   a. List them as quickly as possible. Avoid going down rabbit holes and focus on identification.
2. Take 2 minutes to identify the three most painful tasks, tools, or barriers on your list.
3. Take 1 minute to pick the most painful task, tool, or barrier.
4. Take 6 minutes to conduct a 5 Whys assessment of the problem.
   a. Why is the problem painful?
   b. For whatever answer you come up with, ask "why" of your answer (provide example).
   c. Repeat until you've answered "why" five times.
5. Take 3 minutes to develop a rough solution to the answer of your fifth "why."
6. Assign a team member to speak to your management team/supervisor about your proposed solution within 24 hours.

Note: You will likely not develop a perfect or perhaps even usable solution during this exercise. The purpose is to identify opportunities for improvement in your organization, develop solutions as teams, and take ownership for the processes that need to change to maximize your efficacy as a team.

Leadership Support

Innovation leadership is an important factor in individual innovative behavior; however, it is not just a transformational leadership style used by formal leaders that is important to developing an innovative culture. Self-leadership and individual knowledge sharing are important aspects of innovative leadership as well. In other words, innovation does not just happen; it is created using an infrastructure that includes all levels of healthcare workers (Albert, 2018). The influence of leaders and innovation has not been heavily studied, and most often, reports involve cross-sectional designs involving survey methods. When structured questionnaires were used to assess leadership styles and innovative work behaviors, higher levels of transformational leadership were associated with nurses' psychological empowerment, and psychological empowerment was associated with nurses' intrinsic motivation and knowledge-sharing behavior. It is important to note that both intrinsic motivation and knowledge-sharing behavior are associated with innovative work behavior (Masood & Afsar, 2017). In another report, worksite support was not an important factor in innovation outcomes, but was important to perceived nurse creativity (Tsai, Liou, Hsiao, & Cheng, 2013). Further, in another survey-based research study, the authors learned that both academic and clinical leaders had significant gaps in innovation competencies (White, Pillay, & Huang, 2015); thus, leadership support could be a positive factor in promoting a culture of innovation once leaders understand the value of innovation to their healthcare settings and their roles in creating an innovative culture. Education skills that may assist leaders to be more innovative are provided in Table 10.1.

Skills that apply to leaders (Table 10.1) also apply to healthcare workers who are informal leaders, as self-leadership is an important feature of permission to innovate. In a cross-sectional descriptive study of 347 nurse participants, self-leadership (that included self-observation/positive self-talk, cueing strategies/constructive thinking, self-goal setting, self-rewards/self-determination, and practice) and individual knowledge sharing were important factors in individual innovative behaviors (that included the constructs: opportunity exploration, generativity, formative investigation, championing, and application; Kim & Park, 2015).

TABLE 10.1 **Skills That Promote Innovative Leadership**

Discovery Skills	How to Put Into Practice
Associating	Create connections between problems or issues that are seemingly unrelated to create something new or better; create connections by talking to people across and outside organizational lines; is a cross-pollinator.
Questioning	Voice questions to better understand the current state of work/processes (what, why, how, when) and how current status can be disrupted, changed, or altered.
Observing	Be observant; set aside what is known and preconceived notions to observe with an open mind. Purposely do not judge when observing. Try to see the world as if for the first time; consider everyday experiences and is willing to look beyond the usual places—and also consider a scene before and after people arrive at it; be an anthropologist.
Networking	Use others in his or her sphere to test ideas; consider people with multiple backgrounds and differing perspectives; consider unlikely partners to better allow initial opposition to turn into a positive force; be a collaborator.
Experimenting	Pilot new ideas; enjoys trying new experiences be an experimenter.
Driving	Do not be willing to accept the status quo—move beyond "just doing your job" to circumvent healthcare system bureaucracy and barriers, adapt to changing markets or environments, and be able to overcome failures by having a mind-set toward success; be a hurdler.
Producing	Get people to take chances; build a chemistry to get work done; allow others to take the spotlight; lead when needed; put in the time and energy—long hours, deal with upcoming deadlines, create the best team; lay out the goals and solves problems, including improvising when needed; be a director.
Setting the stage	Consider the setting/environment/workplace; assess space and changes as needed to invite stakeholders to work together; be a set designer.

What to Do If Your Organization Refuses to Innovate?

What happens when your leadership does not provide the tools and resources necessary to innovate? Remember one key fact about your employment: It is conditional upon your decision to work there. If you feel that your ability to innovate is being stifled by your organization, you have three simple choices available to address the issue:

1. Accept that the organization will not change and continue to work in that environment.
2. Follow the steps outlined previously to change your organization. Pay really close attention here. This is a tough one for health professionals.
3. Seek success elsewhere.

Seeking Success Elsewhere

WARNING! CONTRARIAN VIEWPOINT AHEAD

As health professionals, we sometimes forget the value of our skill sets to other organizations. That doesn't just mean other hospitals or clinics. There are multiple opportunities for health professionals to leverage their skills as employees of pharmaceutical companies, medical device distributors, insurance companies, and healthcare software companies to name a few. Healthcare knowledge and clinical expertise are valuable, and there are many pathways to leveraging them to impact the health and wellness of your community.

Real-World Example

As a director in a large academic medical center, Mary was fulfilled by her work. She had the opportunity to interact with patients while serving on teams that tackled some of the largest challenges faced by the organization. Her work was also noticed by others outside of her organization, and she was contacted by a large healthcare information technology (IT) company in her city. After weighing the costs and benefits of staying in her role as a director and following the traditional hospital leadership trajectory, she decided that the opportunity with the IT company would provide her with growth opportunities she couldn't get in her current role. Better yet, it would provide her with a unique perspective, one that could later be leveraged as the executive of major healthcare organizations. She now serves as a director of clinical innovation, and has leveraged her years of hospital and bedside experience to create new value in this new role.

Wait! This chapter is supposed to be about bringing innovation to the bedside, and you are telling me that I should leave my role and go work away from the bedside. If you are thinking this way, you are missing the point. Mary's story is used to illustrate that you have immense power as a nurse, a pharmacist, a respiratory therapist, or in any other type of healthcare role. Do not be afraid to take your own path to innovation to maximize *your impact* on the health of your community at whatever you define to be the "bedside." And if you are constantly running into barriers that prevent you from having impact, seek success elsewhere.

ENGAGING INNOVATORS

Permission to Innovate

Even with a full understanding of the benefits of healthcare innovation, it can be challenging for organizations to put this into practice. Regardless of role, seniority, and profession, the first step to leading innovation is to provide yourself and your colleagues with permission to innovate. Although this concept may seem trivial, think of all the times you heard from your peers something along the lines of "We can't do that, management won't support it." Better yet, how many times have you said those words to one of your colleagues? By providing permission to innovate, teams can develop new value for their organizations without the fear of negative repercussions. When this fear is lifted, dreams become actualized and patients and providers reap the benefits.

Unleashing Creativity

Unleashing creativity is a two-step process that involves both divergent and convergent thinking. *Divergent thinking* refers to a broad search for multiple diverse and novel alternatives to solve a problem, minimize an issue, or move beyond a current state. *Convergent thinking* is a focused and affirmative evaluation of novel ideas generated during divergent thinking. To make creative thinking effective, the divergent process always occurs first, followed by the convergent process. Oftentimes, adults consider their first idea the solution to a healthcare worker's problem. After all, they are highly paid, productive team members who understand the problem to be solved. But, if they force themselves to really follow the steps of divergent and convergent thinking, they will find that novel ideas may emerge that could be much more effective than the first idea presented.

The value of divergent thinking is based on the following principles. First, you must defer judgment about the many diverse alternative ideas raised when trying to respond creatively to a problem. For example, both negative comments ("That will never work, that will cost too much, that takes too much time, the boss will never agree to that, or we did this 10 years ago and it did not work then…") and positive comments ("I love that idea, cool idea, forget the other ideas, let's move this one forward…") can derail the creative process, as responders may be afraid of further criticism after receiving negative feedback or responders may only want to consider ideas related to those that led to praise. Second, make connections to other fields. For example, when addressing patient satisfaction in healthcare, many hospitals looked at theme parks (such as Disney World) to learn how they maintained customer satisfaction. When developing ideas to improve quality and safety in the operating room, many hospitals looked to the airline industry to learn how they continually maintained high quality and safety. Third, go for quantity in generating ideas. It is OK to include things you've already tried, things you've already thought of before but rejected, things that are new to your healthcare system, and things that are new to healthcare. The more ideas, the better! Fourth, seek novelty by encouraging wild or unusual ideas. Finally, incubate. Incubation involves thinking about the problems and developing ah-ha moments. Allow time for incubation as it may not occur at the divergent-thinking session.

Convergent thinking involves a focused and affirmative evaluation of novel ideas. There are only a few rules to the convergent-thinking process. First, be affirmative to keep novelty alive, to keep the goal in mind, to improve ideas, and to incubate. One way to provide feedback is to use the POINT system. P = plusses (what is good about the idea?), O = opportunities (what are the future benefits?), I = issues raised as questions (How might we . . .) to prevent shutting down a potentially viable idea, and NT = new thinking. New thinking creates a focus on exploring the novel ideas that were raised to solve problems/issues. Through the creativity process, the goal is to select the best option and also to make the strange (novel ideas) familiar.

Through the convergent process of unleashing creativity, we must remember that new ways of doing things may be uncomfortable to some people; thus, a creative environment and creative people—for example, those who are flexible, open, and adaptable to new ideas—are needed to support the work. A creative environment may help! Creativity sessions should take place outside of the usual work environment, and may include resources not usually found on a clinical unit. For example, a creativity room may have multiple dry-erase walls (not just boards); comfortable chairs; large pads on which to write ideas; and an assortment of tools, such as putty, colorful paper and markers, sticky notes, rulers, scissors, tape, and glue sticks, pipe cleaners, and other items that allow participants to bring their ideas to life three-dimensionally. A creative environment is one that allows new ideas to be advanced. Leaders must help participants defer judgment when generating and gathering ideas, provide affirmative feedback, take responsibility for creating the right environment, and also maintain balance between divergent and convergent thinking.

Innovation is often a happy "surprise." Once discovered, cultivate it!—Nancy M. Albert

HOW CAN HEALTH PROFESSIONALS DRIVE INNOVATION WITHIN A TYPICAL HOSPITAL SETTING?

Here are a few examples of organizations that have set up programs to turn ideas into actions.

The Innovation Studio—A Success Story of Innovation and Interprofessional Collaboration

Too often in healthcare you hear health providers say something to the tune of "I have this great idea to impact my practice, but I do not know where to begin." At The Ohio State University (OSU) College of Nursing, leaders knew this problem all too well. Students, faculty, and staff struggled with identifying collaborators for projects, lacked the capital to get them off of the ground, and were unaware how to leverage resources in the university to help innovative thinkers mature their innovations.

Through the Office of Innovation and Strategic Partnerships, team leaders conceptualized what a program would look like if it could meet not only the needs of nursing students faculty and staff but also the needs of innovators from all disciplines across the university, including clinical healthcare settings. The team envisioned creating a place where clinicians could meet with colleagues from a variety of backgrounds to identify and discuss the most pressing challenges in healthcare. A place where the healthcare community could speak to an expert to help develop prototypes quickly and at no cost. A place where interprofessional collaboration would be rewarded with capital and other resources. That place became the Innovation Studio. By incorporating healthcare clinicians into the creation of a new healthcare project, the Innovation Studio embraced the core concepts of user-centered design. User-centered design involves a framework that incorporates the user characteristics/experience throughout the design process. You'll explore user-centered design in detail in Chapter 18, Identifying Opportunities to Innovate and Creating Your Niche.

The Innovation Studio is a moveable makerspace/incubator that is filled with 3-D printers, laser cutters, power tools, hand tools, computing hardware, and just about anything else needed to develop a product, service, or solution to improve the health and well-being of the world (Figure 10.2). As everything in the studio is on wheels, the studio is strategically moved to a new high-traffic location every 8 weeks to foster interprofessional collaboration across campus. Teams that meet three simple criteria (1) a team of two or more OSU students, faculty, or staff from (2) two different disciplines or professions who have (3) disclosed their invention to the university (when applicable) are eligible to pitch their health and wellness innovations and request funding.

Here's what the Innovation Studio does differently than any other healthcare makerspace in the world: **They fund everyone.** Each and every team that pitches an idea to the Innovation Studio team is guaranteed to receive at least one round of funding. Once funding is awarded, teams then meet with the Innovation Studio staff to develop actionable milestones that can be accomplished with the funding and resources awarded. Teams are encouraged to complete milestones by the date of the next showcase, so they can again pitch their innovations, demonstrate their progress, and request their next round of funding. Teams remain in a cycle (Figure 10.3) until their innovations are integrated into practice, or the ROI for the project is no longer beneficial.

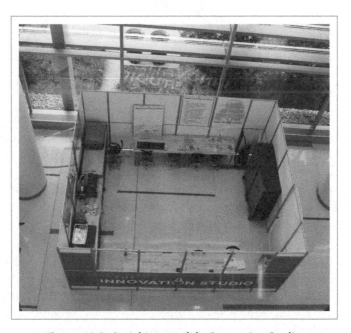

Figure 10.2 Aerial image of the Innovation Studio.

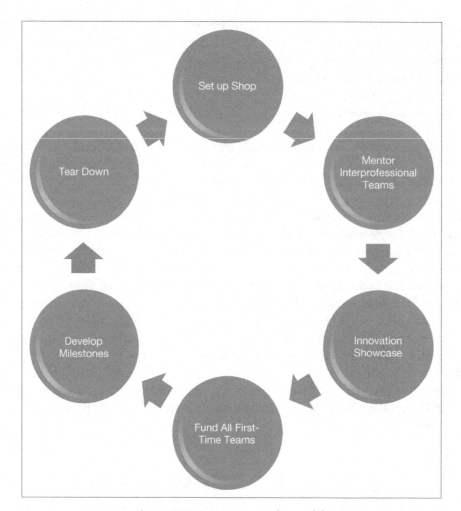

Figure 10.3 Innovation studio model.

Although many projects that have come through the Innovation Studio are physical products, it is important to note that many others are not. Ideas have been pitched about new educational models for psychiatric patients to new productivity software for nurse practitioners. The goal of the Innovation Studio is to improve the culture of interprofessional innovation at the university. To achieve this goal, focus must be placed on the process, not the end product. The organization must not be concerned with the end result, but rather the synergies developed through the convergence of curious clinicians.

Teamwork

Team-building, teamwork, and collaboration are essential elements for launching and leading innovation. An effective team requires selecting people with diverse cultures and heterogeneous traits who will bring depth of creativity to discussion (Davis & Marshall, 2014). In addition, a dynamic, innovative team will embrace shared accountability and networked decision-making, rather than a command-and-control leadership style (Weberg & Werberg, 2014). Interactions within teams are facilitated by innovation leadership characteristics (Table 10.2).

Resources

Multiple levels of resources are needed to bring innovation into real-world healthcare, even if the program is in its inception. Resources must target all levels of stakeholders: leaders, healthcare workers, and even clients and consumers.

Leaders must have at least one go-to person who is responsible for innovation assessment, internal review, and next steps. For example, the go-to person may be responsible for designing, implementing, updating, and maintaining an innovation disclosure form and policies and procedures, and also be the link to outreach personnel (e.g., a patent/intellectual property attorney, venture capitalist, industrial design firm, and licensing representatives who understand the technology and industry involved). Resources that can be extremely helpful to leaders are found in Table 10.3.

Resources are needed to assist healthcare workers to understand that innovation is for all workers, at all levels. Innovation for all will be out of mind if it is out of sight. Innovation must be visible on multiple levels: on the healthcare system intranet, in newsletters, as an element of a nursing professional practice model, in the steps of a professional ladder, and even on a poster board that is located on each unit; thus, resources are needed to initiate, maintain, and update visibility campaigns. Some sites conduct annual "shark tank" events to increase visibility and others may create a moveable Innovation Studio or a more permanent innovations department. A creativity center that stores supplies used in creativity and includes personnel

TABLE 10.2 Innovation Leadership Behaviors That Promote Teamwork

Behavior	Details
Navigation	• Assists with connections to other people to reduce barriers to innovation. • Expands boundaries beyond the current network to unconnected groups to challenge assumptions.
Motivation	• Reads the environment and encourages adaption and change. • Guides others to understand that the vision for the future may be imperfect. • Promotes collaboration to stimulate engagement and instill that there is value in diversity.
Accountability	• Clear-behavior expectations allow the team to move in the same direction, toward the same goal. • Ownership plus a supportive environment stimulates teams to be engaged in the creative process and through their freedom to "work," they will have greater impact.
Tolerance for ambiguity	• Understands that change can be messy; that change is not linear and that change is often complex. • Understands that testing assumptions involves risk taking. • Understands that in complex systems, unpredictability and interdependence are the norm and that every member of the team is a leader and innovator.

TABLE 10.3 **Leadership Resources to Engage Innovation**

Resource	Rationale
Product development fund	• To provide funding for early-stage innovations—allows innovators to validate that the product, service, or technology is efficacious (does what it is supposed to do) and effective (is useful/meets an established outcome)
Law department	• To establish a license agreement • To protect intellectual property by filing a provisional patent application • To assist with spin-off company ventures and regulations
Marketing expert	• To complete a *market analysis* to identify whether market opportunities exist for the product, service, or technology • To complete *active marketing* of the innovation after compiling advantages over the current state of the art and without disclosing proprietary details of the innovation • To show passion for and assist with championing the product, service, or technology; e.g., press releases
Manager	• To ensure progress in innovation development, including writing reviews and reporting • To analyze budgets, operating plans, financing requests, use of funds and regulatory compliance as needed

who can lead creativity sessions is a wonderful resource to have, as it might ignite a spark that will be a future innovation. Resources may be allocated in the form of awards; for example, innovator-team-of-the-year award or information technology, product and service "innovation-of-the-year" awards. Another important resource is funding. Marketing department personnel can develop eye-catching advertisements for funding that engage interdisciplinary innovators to connect and apply for grants or start-up funding.

Ultimately though, the best resources are people who encourage clinical workers to submit innovative ideas that can be cultivated into innovations. Local level leadership (e.g., assistant nurse managers and nurse managers) must be open to recognizing when an innovative idea is voiced and to guiding the innovator to take next steps. Voicing of innovative idea, paired with a reception of support by the idea generator's supervisor is known as the *ideation rate*. Minor, Brook, and Bernoff (2017) concluded that the greatest predictor for a successful innovation program is the "number of ideas approved by management divided by the total number of active users in the system" (p. 2). Essentially, the ideation rate model is based on a combination of idea volume and idea support: the more ideas generated by the individuals most closely associated with the work to be done that receive support from their management team, the more successful the organization.

How the Cleveland Clinic Puts Innovation Into Practice

Enhancing Hand Hygiene

If you work in a healthcare setting and have a clinical role, you know the value of hand hygiene. Healthcare workers, regardless of their roles, are trained in infection control and understand that their hands are the first line of defense. Despite having knowledge about the value of hand hygiene, and despite instructions to wash hands for 15 seconds or clean hands with alcohol-based hand rub, quality-improvement reports from local hospital and healthcare systems often show imperfect hand-hygiene compliance. The chief executive officer at Cleveland Clinic (Cleveland, OH) raised the issue at each town hall meeting and was transparent in sharing our current status and our goal (100% compliance). Further, he encouraged all healthcare leaders and colleagues to hold each other accountable for noncompliance. Hand-hygiene flyers were placed in key patient care areas so that patients also knew the expectations of healthcare providers. The communication plan was effectively disseminated, but junior or lower ranked employees were not comfortable verbalizing the need to perform hand hygiene with more senior or higher level employees. For example, nurses would not publicly tell nurse colleagues or physicians that they failed to perform hand hygiene in front of patients, residents, or other team members during rounding/other patient care activities. There was a perceived sensitivity in calling out someone for missing the expectation and no one wanted patients to lose faith or trust in their care providers.

An infection prevention nurse, Christine Rose, BSN, CIC, at one of our community hospitals raised the need to develop a secret code word that could be used by all practitioners as a real-time reminder to perform hand hygiene. In that way, we could change the culture by discretely communicating the need to perform hand hygiene. Her team assisted in developing the acronym SNAP (*scrub now and prevent*) and bringing the acronym to life (Rose & Siegmund, 2018). For example, someone could snap her fingers as a reminder, or could make vague comments, such as "Do you need to snap?" or "Oh, snap!" to get the right message to the person/people who needed to perform hand hygiene. The innovation also included a marketing plan that used a rice-treat bar that was relabeled, a song (new lyrics to a well-known beat), flyers, and posters. The new acronym was shared at annual patient safety events, used in onboarding and annual education, and the chief executive officer embraced and promoted the concept. In a 2-year period, hand-hygiene compliance improved from 71% to 95% and has remained strong since that time. Ultimately, the innovative idea, once implemented, was extremely useful in promoting hand-hygiene adherence—it changed the culture of transparency and open communication, which were key factors in success.

This case study is an example of an *internal innovation* that was published for external sharing. Hospitals can purchase copyrighted materials developed at the Cleveland Clinic for use in their own setting. Although this innovation is not patentable, it is marketable externally. Features and resources that aided in its success were that it was novel and useful, tool development was provided by the marketing team, and ongoing internal communication was delivered by the chief executive officer and chief nursing officer and communicated downward to all healthcare workers.

Keeping Cool in the Operating Room

An orthopedic operating room nurse, who worked side by side with orthopedic surgeons, watched the surgical team sweat during cases, as the work of orthopedic surgeons can be very physical. The operating room temperature was as low as was allowable, but surgeons were required to wear a leaded apron inbetween their scrubs and a sterile gown, which added to their body temperature. Cooling vests were available in the marketplace, but they had a tether (large corded coil) to a cooling unit and were heavy and uncomfortable to wear. The nurse decided to sew the surgeons a lightweight, disposable vest with strategically placed pockets for ice, to see whether a portable (no tether) lightweight option would be beneficial. The cooling vest was a hit with surgeons and the nurse continued to produce her innovation. When a call was placed for previously implemented innovations, she submitted an entry, which was our first communication about her work. We discussed ice options and other elements of her innovation to enhance the product and completed an invention disclosure form to officially submit her work to Cleveland Clinic Innovations, an office within our system that protects, manages, and commercializes intellectual property. Our Innovations team evaluated the product for marketability, patentability, and commercialization options. The product has been prototyped and licensed for mass production by a company and will be commercially available soon.

This case study is an example of an *external innovation* that represents an improvement on commercially available cooling vests. The improvement was novel as it looked and functioned completely differently than current products, was highly desirable to stakeholders, and was of interest to a company for mass production. The innovator will receive a stake of the proceeds and the product will be available for our surgeons and those around the country. Features and resources that aided in its success were its novelty and usefulness, and support from Cleveland Clinic Innovations.

You'll notice that the Innovation Studio and these case studies from the Cleveland Clinic followed a few key themes to generate success. Innovators identified stakeholders and engaged them from the start. They obtained support from local and global leaders. And they placed the role of reimagining clinical practice in the hands of those who do the work.

🔑 KEY TAKEAWAY POINTS

- Innovation comes from individuals, not bureaucracy; healthcare leaders can harness innovation.

- Creativity and innovative ideas are not the same as innovations. An innovation involves novelty, is useful to the healthcare setting (and is best when it is externally generalizable), and has been concretely implemented.

- Creative healthcare environments have leaders who (a) are dynamic, they provide challenges; (b) provide idea support; (c) take risks; (d) are open to feedback; and (e) are playful/have humor/enjoy the process of novelty.

- Work within teams to create higher impact innovations.

- Problem-solving through ideation is enhanced when we (a) suspend judgment when ideas are raised, (b) strive for quantity of ideas (the more, the better), (c) make connections/interdisciplinary collaborations, (d) seek novelty, and (e) allow for incubation.

■ To create ideas that will lead to innovation, phrase problems as questions; for example: How might we …? What might we …?

■ Take pleasure in looking at healthcare-related problems/issues from multiple perspectives.

REFERENCES

Addison, N., Quatrara, B., Letzkus, L., Strider, D., Rovnyak, V., Syptak, V., & Fuzy, L. (2014). Cleanliness of disposable vs nondisposable electrocardiography lead wires in children. *American Journal of Critical Care, 23*(5), 424–428. doi:10.4037/ajcc2014601

Albert, N. M. (2018). Operationalizing a nursing innovation center within a health care system. *Nursing Administration Quarterly, 42*(1), 43–53. doi:10.1097/NAQ.0000000000000266

Albert, N. M., Slifcak, E., Roach, J. D., Bena, J. F., Horvath, G., Wilson, S., … Murray, T. (2014). Infection rates in intensive care units by electrocardiographic lead wire type: Disposable vs reusable. *American Journal of Critical Care, 23*(6), 460–467. doi:10.4037/ajcc2014362

Davis, P. D., & Marshall, D. R. (2014). Teamwork. An essential for leading and launching innovation. *Nursing Administration Quarterly, 38*(3), 221–229. doi:10.1097/NAQ.0000000000000046

Fang, D. Z., Patil, T., Belitskaya-Levy, I., Yeung, M., Posley, K., & Allaudeen, N. (2017). Use of a hands free, instantaneous, closed-loop communication device improves perception of communication and workflow integration in an academic teaching hospital: A pilot study. *Journal of Medical Systems, 42*(1), 4. doi:10.1007/s10916-017-0864-7

Friend, T. H., Jennings, S. J., Copenhaver, M. S., & Levine, W. C. (2017). Implementation of the Vocera communication system in a quaternary perioperative environment. *Journal of Medical Systems, 41*(1), 6. doi:10.1007/s10916-016-0652-9

Google's Online Dictionary. (n.d). Innovation. Retrieved from https://www.google.com/search?q=definition+of+innovation&ie=&oe

Joseph, M. L., Rhodes, A., & Watson, C. A. (2016). Preparing nurse leaders to innovate: Iowa's Innovation Seminar. *Journal of Nursing Education, 55*(2), 113–117. doi:10.3928/01484834-20160114-11

Kelly, T. (2005). *The ten faces of innovation.* New York, NY: Doubleday.

Kim, S. J., & Park, M. (2015). Leadership, knowledge sharing, and creativity: The key factors in nurses' innovative behaviors. *Journal of Nursing Administration, 45*(12), 615–623. doi:10.1097/NNA.0000000000000274

Masood, M., & Afsar, B. (2017). Transformational leadership and innovative work behavior among nursing staff. *Nursing Inquiry, 24*(4), e12188. doi:10.1111/nin.12188

Minor, D., Brook, P., & Bernoff, J. (2017). *Data from 3.5 million employees shows how innovation really works*. Boston, MA: Harvard Business School.

Rose, C., & Siegmund, L. A. (2018). SNAP: A hand hygiene campaign that improves compliance and fosters a just culture. *Prevention Strategist, 11*(3), 73–76.

Tsai, H., Liou, S., Hsiao, Y., & Cheng, C. (2013). The relationship of individual characteristics, perceived worksite support and perceived creativity to clinical nurses' innovative outcome. *Journal of Clinical Nursing, 22*(17–18), 2648–2657.

Weberg, D., & Weberg, K. (2014). Seven behaviors to advance teamwork: Findings from a study of innovation leadership in a simulation center. *Nursing Administration Quarterly, 38*(3), 230–237. doi:10.1097/NAQ.0000000000000041

White, K. R., Pillay, R., & Huang, X. (2016). Nurse leaders and the innovation competence gap. *Nursing Outlook, 64*(3), 255–261. doi:10.1016/j.outlook.2015.12.007

Emerging Trends in Healthcare Innovation

Bonnie Clipper and Tami H. Wyatt

"Innovation distinguishes between a leader and a follower." —Steve Jobs

LEARNING OBJECTIVES

- Examine three categories of innovation in healthcare and provide examples.
- Describe the impact that emerging innovations have on nursing practice and patient care outcomes.
- Describe strategies by organizational leaders to support the successful adoption and implementation of emerging technologies.

INTRODUCTION

Innovation and the development of new technologies are occurring at a rapid rate: everything from treatment technologies, diagnostic tools, how we educate our clinicians, and even where or how our care is performed is affected. According to *The Economist* (2017), there are currently three distinct groups *working on* innovations in healthcare. These include "traditional innovators," such as pharmaceutical companies, hospitals, and long-standing medical technology players, such as Medtronic, Philips, GE Healthcare, and Siemens; the "incumbent players," such as insurers and pharmacy-benefit managers (PBMs); and finally a group considered disruptive within the healthcare innovation space, known as *insurgents* (Figure 11.1). This group often grabs the headlines: Google, Apple, Amazon, and thousands of start-ups or often unknown innovation companies that create apps, predictive tools, new diagnostic systems, and new devices (*The Economist,* 2017). The emerging trends in innovation that will occur over the next several years will be staggering, including everything from the rapid adoption of artificial intelligence (AI) in healthcare, to virtual or augmented reality (AR) and wearables for both patients and clinicians. In this chapter, you will discover the most common innovation categories in healthcare,

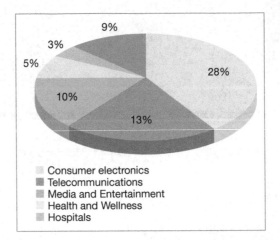

Figure 11.1 Most innovative industries. Consumer electronics (28%), telecommunications (13%), and media and entertainment (10%) rank highest for industries that are the most innovative. Pharmaceutical and biotech (9%), health and wellness (5%), and hospitals (3%) rank significantly lower.

Source: Data from Walker, T. (2017, June 15). Four key trends in healthcare innovation. Retrieved http://managedhealthcare executive.modernmedicine.com/managed-healthcare-executive/news/three-key-trends-healthcare-innovation

the impact of innovation and technologies on healthcare and patient outcomes, and strategies to promote successful adoption of emerging technologies.

There are three broad categories of innovations that impact healthcare—innovations associated with purchasing and using healthcare, innovations in health technology, and innovations in our healthcare-related business models (Herzlinger, 2006). Innovations in buying and using healthcare often strive to offer cost-effective, efficient, more easily navigated models of care delivery, patient (or consumer) experiences, and payment models. Whereas innovations in health technology often capture the greatest attention and involve new treatment therapies, drugs, diagnostic methods and devices that enhance care outcomes, and reduce costs of care. This category potentially connects to desired clinical outcomes more directly (Herzlinger, 2006). Innovations in healthcare business models create new paradigms and tools to reduce time spent by consumers scheduling care, traveling to and from care, methods of delivering care, more convenient locations offering specific care (i.e., urgent care) or prevention-based services (Herzlinger, 2006).

 CALL TO ACTION

Within the next few weeks, introduce yourself to your organization's chief innovation officer, either in person or through email. Share your interest in learning about emerging trends in innovation.

 EMERGING INNOVATIONS IN BUYING AND USING HEALTHCARE

Buying and using healthcare will continue to evolve into an even more consumer-based approach to health insurance, reimbursement, or payment models. This allows consumers (not-yet patients) and patients (currently receiving care) to gain control over their care options if/when they become patients. This model will become customized for different and varied personal spending levels with a heavier shift to a personalized service model. Health insurance plans are rapidly changing to become more specific and offer menu-based options (i.e., a la carte) for each individual user, while remaining economically sustainable.

Buying and using healthcare as a type of innovation also includes the overall healthcare experience and is now known as the *user experience (UX)* or *patient experience (PX)*. A UX with acute care is publicly reported through specific and intentional questions within the Hospital-Consumer Assessment of Healthcare Providers and Systems (2018). These results are related to successful consumer recruitment and retention. There is no shortage of opportunity within healthcare to make the patient and his or her support system the center of the "healthcare universe." Often in healthcare, the "institutions" and providers become consumed in processes and communication systems that silo organizations and prevent the optimal PX from occurring.

One potential area ripe for innovation is the process used to streamline and simplify selection and utilization of health insurance. Emerging innovations in UX about purchasing health insurance are likely to include AI that "overlays" health insurance options and customer service processes to more quickly model the best type of insurance for individual consumers. This experience will continue to improve over time to be nonobtrusive, even more "human-like," and will provide faster and more accurate insurance coverage selection to individuals or families. By incorporating AI for more accurate and quicker insurance interactions with individuals, the number of human service representatives may eventually be reduced. Health insurance coverage will likely become more focused on goals of individuals and families. In turn, insurance companies will examine ways to reduce costs because the more selective individual plans will be costly. One way to reduce labor costs will be through use of AI that can provide consultation and answers about health insurance coverage, premiums, and annual enrollments during "life changes."

The PX is a necessary element of innovation to improve the overall healthcare journey and advance innovation work. The provision of care is more often about existing systems and caregivers than the patients and their support systems. For example, hours of operation for surgical or procedural events are frequently scheduled around provider and staff preferences rather than patient interests. Navigators, whether human, AI, or virtual assistants, may improve timely access to care, determine the appropriate setting of care, eliminate expensive duplication of diagnostics, improve communication among the care team, and more holistically manage a patient's course of prevention or treatment. This, too, may improve the PX within a healthcare system, which is currently often cumbersome and fragmented with duplicitous testing.

Adoption of innovation, specifically technology, will pick up speed as care shifts from sick care to wellness and prevention. Insurance companies that provide employers with annual screening events, including blood work, vital signs screening, biometrics, such as mass index (BMI) screening, and even tobacco use and alcohol consumption histories, have already embraced this shift. They are looking to determine who is at risk and how lifestyle interventions and behavior changes can be introduced sooner in a consumer's life to avoid serious and expensive patient care, courses of treatment, or hospitalization later. Healthcare is transitioning into an era with annual screenings becoming mandatory for provision of insurance services. At some point, these will likely become family or "coveree" based to ensure baseline data on all individuals who are covered by insurance programs.

Some insurance providers track nutrition and fitness data that impact premiums through fitness tracking devices that synchronize activity with database repositories. One example is through a current insurer-based employee wellness program that offers a financial incentive for members to increase their activity though use of a fitness tracker (Fitbit). Eligible employees and their spouses can earn $3 to $4 per day, which is deposited quarterly into their personal health spending account, allowing members to earn nearly $1,500 per member per year for their health spending accounts. In this example, the amount of the incremental daily payments increases based on the number of steps tracked through the fitness tracking device (United Healthcare, n. d.).

The roles of healthcare providers are also undergoing innovations. Some of the fastest growing roles are those of coordinator and navigator. These professionals need to access and synthesize data to develop care maps for patients. Care will eventually be managed for volumes of patients in a seamless and cost-effective manner based on a constant stream of information and options. Healthcare systems will direct patients to the most cost-efficient and appropriate level of care, including outpatient services and even care in a patient's home. Training programs for navigators are growing exponentially to prepare these professionals for 21st-century healthcare. Care coordinators and navigators will use tools that apply big-data analytics and predictive analytics to target at-risk populations to improve patient outcomes and reduce overall costs.

Some innovations in the area of purchasing and using healthcare may not include high-tech solutions but may leverage existing innovations. Ride sharing has emerged to provide on-demand transportation services to and from care appointments because the cost of a ride is cheaper than missing appointments, which may yield expensive inpatient stays.

> *"Without change there is no innovation, creativity, or incentive for improvement. Those who initiate change will have a better opportunity to manage the change that is inevitable."*—William Pollard.

EMERGING TRENDS IN HEALTHCARE TECHNOLOGY INNOVATIONS

The emerging and innovative trends in the areas of treatment therapies, pharmaceuticals, and diagnostic tools are among the most well known in healthcare. However, adoption of these technologies must be affordable and based on evidence. Some of the more exciting and prevalent emerging technologic trends are discussed in the next section.

Telehealth

Telehealth, also known as *telemedicine, virtual care,* or *connected care*, has existed for nearly 20 years and within the last 10 years has gained momentum and interest. Telehealth as an emerging innovation in healthcare typically consists of a camera, smartphone, or monitor with sound and two-way connection, so the practitioner can visualize, hear, and communicate with either a patient or another care provider. Based on current IHS Markit projections, over 5 million telehealth consultations will occur per year by 2020 (*The Economist*, 2017). With a surge in telehealth services may come significant costs for high-quality audio and visual equipment, specific broadband-compliant cabling, and even practitioner coverage. There are also expensive add-ons that positively impact care management as well, such as electronic stetho-scopes and optical scopes, which improve the overall efficacy of patient treatment. However, costs associated with acquisition of telehealth technology are dropping annually. In some cases, healthcare services can be offered through smartphones with Internet connectivity. Ideally, tele-health improves access to healthcare at a significantly reduced cost.

Telehealth commonly allows patients in rural or outlying locations to receive high-quality specialty care that may not otherwise be available. Specialty care services such as cardiology, neurology, neurosurgery, psychiatry, and even maternal services, are specialties that leverage this technology. Telehealth or virtual care may be delivered by a variety of members of the care team, including physicians, advance practice providers, nurses, or psychologists, who are spe-cifically trained in telehealth. The number of telehealth certified nurses, physicians, and coordi-nators is growing as the specialty grows and evolves. There are several companies, even large hospital systems, that provide telehealth services to smaller hospitals, long-term care facilities, and rural based emergency rooms where the number of visits does not offset the expense of providing onsite specialty care services or call coverage.

With telehealth, only those patients who need to be seen in person have clinic visits, reduc-ing costs. One very successful example of this is the current "text only" telehealth program managed by Kaiser Permanente (KP) in Colorado. An emergency department physician talks with between 100 and 200 patients a day through the "Chat with a Doctor" program. The chat consultation identifies and treats conditions such as urinary tract infections, sinus infections, or the flu without requiring an emergency room visit. During the online "chats," physicians are able to diagnose and prescribe medications for more than two-third of the patients thus keeping patients out of the emergency departments and the "chat" is documented in their KP patient medical record. The quality metrics associated with this program indicate patient satisfaction is high, mostly due to the convenience of being "seen" by a healthcare professional and treated for their condition without having to leave their homes to visit a medical provider's office and wait to be treated. The prescriptions are sent electronically to the pharmacy and can even be delivered to the patient. Over the past 10 years, much work has been done to change the coding for patient telehealth visits to allow for payment of such services. This change has contributed to the interest and provision of telehealth as a care modality simply because more providers can bill, and now get paid, for these services. As innovation tends to follow money, expect wide adoption of telehealth as efficiencies develop.

mHealth

mHealth or mobile health refers to mobile medical applications (apps) that can be used on a va-riety of mobile or portable devices, including mobile phones (i.e., smartphones), tablets, or com-puters. It is the fastest growing area of emerging innovations within healthcare. These mobile medical apps "are software programs that run on smartphones and other mobile communication devices. They can also have accessories that attach to a smartphone or other mobile communi-cation devices, or a combination of accessories and software" (Food and Drug Administration [FDA], 2015). When the mobile application offers a diagnosis or care consultation, the FDA considers the application a medical device, and therefore, is regulated as such (FDA, 2015).

mHealth is increasing at a rapid rate, in part, because smartphones share education, can di-agnose breath sounds, monitor electrocardiograms, make appointments, pay medical bills, and many other things. In 2016, there were 259,000 mHealth apps available globally, which were produced by more than 59,000 mHealth app publishers. This trend continues at an exponential rate and has created opportunity within a new industry with explosive growth. mHealth app growth rate was projected to hit $26B by the end of 2017 and exceed $102B by 2022 (Medium, 2017). The majority of mHealth apps are intended to help health consumers with education, preventative services, surveillance, treatment support, and chronic disease management. Clinical trials that evaluate the effectiveness of smartphone apps are moving quickly to appropriately determine if smartphone apps are, in fact, effective for patient use.

The proliferation of mobile health-related apps has triggered the FDA to develop a position statement on mobile health apps (FDA, 2015, para. 14) as follows:

> For many mobile apps that meet the regulatory definition of a 'device' but pose minimal risk to patients and consumers, the FDA will exercise enforcement discretions and will not expect manufacturers to submit premarket review applications or to register and list their apps with the FDA. This includes mobile medical apps that:
>
> - Help patients/users self-manage their disease or condition without providing specific treatment suggestions;
> - Provide patients with simple tools to organize and track their health information;
> - Provide easy access to information related to health conditions or treatments;
> - Help patients document, show or communicate potential medical conditions to health care providers;
> - Automate simple tasks for health care providers; or
> - Enable patients or providers to interact with Personal Health Records (PHR) or Electronic Health Record (EHR) systems.

mHealth, through the explosion of apps, will provide the connections between large, less nimble electronic health records (EHRs) and the variety of new tools and wearables that are booming in the marketplace. Apps will continue to offer healthcare providers information that is gathered through a variety of inputs or wearables. Nurturing the development of third-party apps will become an increasingly critical component as confidence in the data strengthens. The ability to integrate app-gathered data into an EHR system makes the EHR limitless (Mandl, Mandel, & Kohane, 2015). mHealth apps are even being used for epidemic outbreak tracking (Search Health IT, 2018).

One of the fastest growing areas of mHealth is a combination of mHealth and telehealth called the "virtual health assistant." Companies such as Sensely (Sensely Virtual Assistant, 2018) or MDLIVE (2018) offer daily check-in for consumers, as well as chatbots, symptom screening, urgent care, and assessment of any feelings of illness or even mood swings to help consumers maintain optimal health and well-being. The chatbots query patients and gather answers to simple questions. Data from the questions are imported into algorithms that screen patients to determine those who need urgent care or those who can be treated with virtual care.

mHealth adds cost-effective convenience since these devices can be accessed at any time or place by the user due to their portable nature. Through virtual visits and mHealth apps, patients can remain in their own homes, saving them from a trip to a clinic visit or urgent care visit. They can still access a nurse practitioner or physician to evaluate breath sounds, analyze a cardiac rhythm, or evaluate a blood glucose monitoring trend. Additionally, mHealth for surveillance and monitoring can access more accurate patient information, which allows reliability in the health data shared with clinicians and could improve outcomes through more accurate and efficient monitoring and reporting.

Augmented Reality/Virtual Reality

AR is a version of reality that is supplemented or enhanced and created through the use of technology. Typically, technology layers digital information, such as measuring grids, locators, or map coordinates, or even characters over a "real time" screenshot or live-view, that is viewed through a monitor, smartphone, or camera (Merriam-Webster Dictionary, n.d.-b). Pokémon Go is a popular AR game played on smartphones, where generated images appear as if they are truly in the present-time real world.

Virtual reality (VR) is an artificial environment that can be experienced via sensory stimuli (sights and sounds) through a computer influenced directly through an individual's actions (Merriam-Webster Dictionary, n.d.-c). VR cancels out the real world and features complete immersion through specific VR devices such as a VR headset or glasses (The Franklin Institute, 2018, para. 2). While there is often confusion between VR and AR, the two are very different. Simply put, while AR allows users to see the real world and projects digital information into an existing environment, VR eliminates all real experiences offering an entirely simulated world (The Medical Futurist, 2017, para. 2).

Mixed reality (MR) is the combination of AR and VR. MR is very new and the use of cases and outcomes of combining the elements of both AR and VR to allow digital objects and real-world images to interact has not yet been studied in healthcare. The technology necessary for MR is just now hitting the market (The Franklin Institute, 2018, para. 3). It is estimated that in 2017, AR and VR in the healthcare market was valued at $769M and is projected to reach nearly $5B by 2023 (Business Wire, 2018). The benefits of AR/VR in healthcare are exponential and continue to exceed expectations, while the pricing, availability, and benefits to healthcare from MR are yet to be seen.

CALL TO ACTION

In the next month conduct, seek out an opportunity to engage with a virtual or augmented reality product.

Gaming

Game theory is rapidly advancing into healthcare as disruptive treatment and education tool. Generally, gaming in healthcare is through a computer or mobile app-based game to improve a condition, help caregivers monitor their own performance in delivering care, or advance education, whether to clinicians or patients. One example is Ubisoft, the parent corporation of *Dig Rush,* a game to help correct amblyopia or "lazy eye" in children (Lee, 2017). While early results are promising, there are no data that indicate how effective the treatment modality is for long-term results.

Gaming also educates healthcare providers, as with the case of Pediatric Sim (Lee, 2017). It teaches nurses and physicians about several different pediatric emergency care situations such as anaphylaxis, bronchiolitis, diabetic ketoacidosis, respiratory failure, seizure, septic shock, and supraventricular tachycardia, and assesses an individual's performance during the "playing of the game" (para. 10). Gaming, whether for training or treatment, is one of the fastest areas of growth in healthcare consumer and health provider education.

> *"Artificial intelligence will not replace physicians. However, physicians who use artificial intelligence will replace those who don't."*—Bertalan Meskó

Artificial Intelligence

AI simulates behavior and allows the computer to imitate intelligent human behavior (Merriam-Webster Dictionary, n.d.-a). "AI is not intended to replace or replicate human capabilities, but rather to enhance them" (High, 2018, para. 5). The barriers mitigating the advance of AI are similar to those of mHealth: cost, the lack of buy-in from physicians and healthcare executives, as well as the difficulty with interoperability of existing health IT systems (AHIMA, 2017). The use of AI is among the biggest opportunity in health information management (HIM), clinical decision support, hospital/physician workflow, population health, security, and revenue cycle as a way to improve outcomes, treatment options and costs (AHIMA, 2017). In the near future, AI will help clinicians "think" better by supplementing their human thought processes with millions of data points and evidence instead of only the number of studies that have been reviewed and retained by the clinician.

> *"Machine learning will dramatically improve the ability of health professionals to establish a prognosis, Machine learning will displace much of the work of radiologists and anatomical pathologists, Machine learning will improve diagnostic accuracy."*—Matt Asay

Machine learning (ML) is an algorithmic technique used for decades but new to healthcare. In an overly simplified explanation, ML recognizes patterns or predicts trends in data by exposing examples of patterns to ML. "A series of numbers that is associated with something significant, and if that pattern has previously repeated itself, you can teach ML algorithms to recognize that pattern and then use it to predict whether that same significant outcome is going to happen again" (High, 2018, para 7). ML is coupled with AI to build complex algorithms that guide clinical decisions.

Deep learning (DL) is a more recent innovation under the broader umbrella of ML algorithms and uses an algorithmic technique modeled after the neural structures in human brains "DL uses artificial neural networks to dramatically increase the number of dimensions of data it can work with – including unstructured images and sounds" (High, 2018, para 9). DL, most commonly used in engineering, holds great promise when coupled AI and ML to solve complicated healthcare problems. DL is an approach being used for art and music and facial recognition.

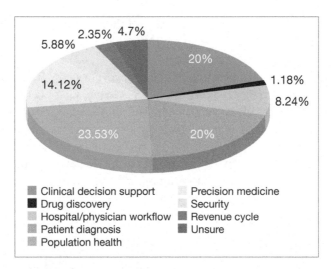

Figure 11.2 AI's greatest initial impact in healthcare.
Source: Data from Sullivan, T. (2017). Half of hospitals to adopt artificial intelligence within 5 years. *Healthcare IT News.* Retrieved from http://www.healthcareitnews.com/news/half-hospitals-adopt-artificial-intelligence-within-5-years

   The impact of AI, whether through ML or DL, will likely revolutionize or eliminate some existing roles within healthcare such as monitor technicians, due to advancing technology that will replace human learning and skills with those of computer models (Figure 11.2).

"The model of medicine can be improved upon by innovative and disruptive technologies."—Bertalan Meskó

Wearables

Wearable computing or "wearables" have existed since 1966, when a computer that predicted roulette was developed. This "wearable" was approximately the size of a package of index cards and contained a computer and four push buttons. To collect data, the "recorder" used the four buttons to indicate the speed of the roulette wheel, the computer then sent radio frequency tones to a roulette player's hearing aid (Lukowicz, 2008). The use of such a system may not be of high value in a general sense and only of importance to a select group of people, but it demonstrates two main properties that define "wearables" (Lukowicz, 2008). These two properties include, first, "the use of electronic assistance in a situation where the use of conventional computers is not feasible," including that it is "unobtrusive and discreet" and can be worn under or as a piece of clothing, hence the term "wearable computing" (Lukowicz, 2008, p. 95). Secondly, the "functionality of the system is related to sensing and analyzing events in the user's environment rather than conventional data processing" (Lukowicz, 2008, p. 95).

   Wearables for patients include devices such as skin tone colored, adherent patches for glucose control, specialized contact lenses, or even smart bandages. These devices continuously monitor and give feedback to improve symptom control or disease management. It is expected that wearables will continue to evolve into even smaller and more discrete systems. There are currently systems, under development, for clinical staff that contacts a patient or calls for help by simply touching the sleeve of a shirt or gown. Once these products meet FDA requirements, they will proliferate.

Google Glass was introduced several years ago. It incorporated AR into a wearable device as it offers a head-up, hands-free (HUHF) experience. Google Glass is the first use of "smart glasses" and is considered by many to be a "wearable"; however, it spans both categories as it is wearable with an AR interface. Google Glass is a way to access smartphone technology, take photos/videos for documentation, and provide Internet searches with verbal, hands-free commands (Tsukayama, 2014). Many other smart glasses technologies are being tested at this time. The next generation of smart glasses will be more discrete, compact, and offer more robust features.

3D Printing

3D printing uses a specifically designed printer to "print" an object using plastic, ceramics, or liquid metal layer by layer. Some 3D printers spray a heated, semiliquid material that hardens as objects are created by the movement of the printer head. The printer's head moves in multiple directions to create the outline of each layer within the object until it is completely printed (Hsu, 2013).

The benefits of 3D printing in healthcare are not fully realized. The Imperial College London has developed a 3D-printing technique that uses 3D printing along with cryogenics to print soft tissues and replicate solid organs (Tan, Parisi, DiSilvo, Dini, & Forte, 2017). This process uses solid-based carbon dioxide to quickly cool down the hydrogel "ink" as it is printed. Thawed printed "tissue" is as soft as human tissue and can support its own weight (para. 11). These printed structures support a new framework where a patient's own tissues, or donor tissues, could regenerate without rejection, thus allowing healthcare teams to print portions of organs or potentially entire organs as replacements when existing organs fail due to disease or injury without the concern of rejection. The capacity to print human tissue has great implications in making transplantation safer by reducing the risk of rejection and possibly even eliminating the need for the myriad of antirejection medications, which eliminates harmful side effects and the exorbitant costs. In the future, advances in this technology may even eliminate the need for transplants altogether.

"There is no innovation and creativity without failure. Period."—Brene Brown

Robotics

There are currently three types of robots in healthcare—the service robot, the clinical/care robot, and the concierge/customer service robot. While the intuitive surgical robotic device (Intuitive, n. d.) has been used in the surgical suite for several years, clinical care robots similar to the surgical robot will gain momentum in healthcare facilities. Clinical robots offer care in a more accurate and precise manner than their human counterparts. The surgical robot eliminates any miniscule hand tremor for precision surgical procedures, thus reducing recovery time and pain for patients. Clinical robots may also provide care in settings where there is not an adequate supply of properly trained clinical providers, such as a battlefield or remote locations.

Service robots will work alongside nurses and other members of the care team to deliver and transport medications, food and supplies to and from patient care areas and patient rooms, thus freeing up caregivers to focus on the important activities that require human interaction, critical thinking, and empathy. Concierge/customer service robots are frequently utilized in Japan for wayfinding, registration, check-in, and food ordering. This type of robot will increase in health-care settings worldwide and will streamline and simplify functions such as scheduling, registration, bill payment, and even education. The services by robots are consistent, eliminating the variation that comes with human interaction and their use allows personnel to be deployed to the highest priority area necessary.

The DNA nanobot is a combination of a robot and a drug delivery device that delivers drugs and they are programmed to fold up microscopically. These tiny robots are deployed into the body searching for their preprogrammed target at which point they open and deliver their medication with pinpoint precision (Buhr, 2018, para. 4). Early testing on cancer-bearing mice and pigs has been successful, thus paving the way for testing on humans. Delivery of medications to specific targets such as tumors could eliminate chemotherapeutic agents improving the overall care to the patient by providing equal efficacy without toxic side effects.

Predictive Analytics

Predictive analytics melds statistics and data, primarily regression analysis, and assumption-based modeling of past behavior to predict future performance and outcomes (Davenport, 2014). This emerging innovation is coupled with AI, especially ML. The ability to use the past as the predictor of the future is compelling (see Figure 11.3). This technology can predict patient outcomes, especially those with negative outcomes, before a human can detect the downward trajectory. Earlier detection of outcomes may result in healthcare providers reacting more quickly and changing the plan of care before the patient experiences the negative or untoward event.

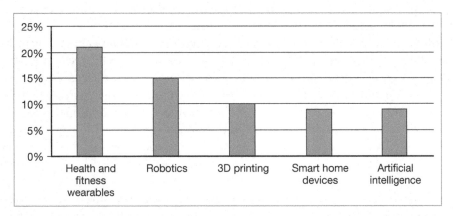

Figure 11.3 Top five technologies predicted to have the biggest impact on people's health in the next 5 years.

Source: Data from Walker, T. (2017, June 15). *Four key trends in healthcare innovation*. Retrieved from http://managedhealth-careexecutive.modernmedicine.com/managed-healthcare-executive/news/three-key-trends-healthcare-innovation

> **CALL TO ACTION**
>
> In the next month, conduct an environmental scan within your own organization to learn which emerging innovations have been adopted within the past year and how they have benefitted your organization.

EMERGING TRENDS IN BUSINESS MODEL INNOVATIONS

Healthcare business models are rapidly evolving and include innovations that further horizontal or vertical integration. New scheduling models and even mHealth (mobile health) apps can reduce the time it takes to see a practitioner or the time it takes waiting once a patient has arrived at their appointment destination. With AI and telehealth, some visits can be avoided altogether and treated instead using virtual care models.

The shift to retail care is another emerging trend with many innovations occurring in this space. Convenience to meet consumer and patient demand is only one of the areas open to innovation. Convenience will be defined by patients and consumers to include access to services including location and the time services are offered. The rise of real-time, demand models of care that incorporated technology to allow provision of care either in person or delivered virtually will grow.

Retail models of care delivery are on the cusp of growth. Current retail models include CVS Minute Clinics, Walgreens Healthcare Clinics, Walmart Care Clinics, and a variety of other urgent care centers, to name a few. These are typically fee-for-service models and are generally for profit organizations or companies offering easy access.

Care will continue to shift to the most cost-effective location for the services. In turn, patients will evaluate episodes of illness with a different lens that includes the cost, convenience, and "downtime" to them and their support systems. In a few short years, it will become commonplace that less expensive and complex procedures will take place in lower cost facilities while more complex, expensive procedures will remain in high-cost settings.

The volume to value shift is a model with consumers demanding value predicated on six themes (Hillary, Justin, Bharat, & Jitendra, 2016). Healthcare should become more patient or consumer focused instead of the current focus on care provider needs. Additionally, the measure of clinical and quality of life outcomes will be discussed with patients. For example, is a hip replacement in an elderly patient with dementia with minimal mobility a success? The answer to this question may be answered differently by the surviving partner tasked paying medical bills and the daily care than it is by surgeons performing the surgery. Such questions will drive many discussions between family members, healthcare administrators, and providers.

Other business model innovations include the migration away from fee-for-service and adoption of more bundled payments for disease management, wellness, and prevention. Price transparency will be the norm. Consumers will demand to know the costs associated with treatments prior to making decisions. Innovations around pricing models will become more apparent as demand-based pricing models are available. Surge pricing may even be trialed as it relates to procedures in demand at specific times of the year.

Ongoing health system integration, both vertical and horizontal, will become more important encompassing the entire continuum of care including urgent/emergent care, acute and long-term acute care, inpatient and outpatient rehabilitation, post-acute care and outpatient/ambulatory care. While many of these shifts are occurring, more co-location of services such as locating primary care services in stores, libraries, or health clubs fostering patient convenience will be the norm. Technologies will facilitate and simplify scheduling appointments and services, and speed up the reporting of lab results and findings. Apps and services to provide patients immediate access to their own health information will make the process of using patient-selected practitioners even easier.

One of the most promising innovation models for healthcare is the growing number of nurse-owned clinics providing primary care to underserved populations. Studies consistently show that primary care nurse practitioners are more likely to provide services to vulnerable populations compared to their physician counterparts (Buerhaus, 2018). Unfortunately, in many states, health policies preclude a nurse's ability to own a clinic because of scope of practice regulations that limit practice autonomy. Those individuals living in states with regulations that restrict a nurse practitioner's scope of practice had significantly less access to primary care (Buerhaus, 2018). Only 23 states allow nurse practitioner practice autonomy (see Table 11.1). The demand to provide care to vulnerable populations continues to grow along with the support for full practice authority and autonomy for advanced practice nurses. If your state is not a full practice authority state, consider how you might influence full practice authority in your own state.

Nurse-owned clinics are innovative in several ways: Nurse-run clinics are more likely to provide services to vulnerable populations and the cost of care to Medicare beneficiaries is less costly than services provided by physicians. Yet, in numerous survey reports, advanced practice nurses provided higher quality care when compared with their physician counterparts but these claims have been challenged in other reports (McCleery, Christensen, Peterson, Humphrey, & Helfand, 2014).

Innovations around quality and access to care will continue at an increasing pace. Technology will grow at an unprecedented rate allowing care delivery in a more accurate and precise manner than ever before. This will improve outcomes and reduce aspects of patient care that have untoward and negative impacts such as the pain and suffering that certain treatments cause in an effort to cure or treat the initial disease. While innovations and technologies race to the marketplace, healthcare advocates must consider the impact that such innovations bring to ethical and cost considerations. While companies will profit, healthcare recipients will potentially experience advancements in quality and convenience.

TABLE 11.1 **States That Support Nurse Practitioner Autonomy**

Alaska	Hawaii	Maryland	Nevada	Oklahoma	Vermont
Arizona	Idaho	Minnesota	New Hampshire	Oregon	Washington
Colorado	Iowa	Montana	New Mexico	Rhode Island	Wyoming
Connecticut	Maine	Nebraska	North Dakota	South Dakota	

Source: From American Association of Nurse Practitioners. (2018). *State practice environment.* Retrieved from https://www.aanp.org/advocacy/state/state-practice-environment

> **CALL TO ACTION**
>
> Identify an emerging innovation relevant to your area of practice and identify ways to learn more about the goals and objectives of adopting such an innovation.

KEY TAKEAWAY POINTS

- Innovations will continue at a rapid pace and revolve around the buying and using of healthcare, innovations in health technology and healthcare-related business models.

- Consumers and patients will demand convenience and simplicity.

- Data portability and sharing will revolve around patient and consumer needs.

- Virtual care, connected health and convenience apps will explode in growth and utility.

- Patients will navigate care using advanced technologies based on costs, outcomes, and perceived value.

REFERENCES

American Association of Nurse Practitioners. (2018). *State practice environment*. Retrieved from https://www.aanp.org/advocacy/state/state-practice-environment

Artificial intelligence use in healthcare growing fast. (2017). *Journal of AHIMA, 88*(6), 76.

Buerhaus, P. (2018). *Nurse practitioners: A solution to America's primary care crisis*. Washington, DC: American Enterprise Institute. Retrieved from https://dokumentix.com/queue/nurse-practitioners.html

Buhr, S. (2018). New DNA nanorobots successfully target and kill off cancerous tumors. *Tech Crunch*. Retrieved from https://techcrunch.com/2018/02/12/new-dna-nanorobots-successfully-targeted-and-killed-off-cancerous-tumors/?utm_content=buffer5f4d3&utm_medium=social&utm_source=linkedin.com&utm_campaign=buffer

Business Wire. (2018). *Global healthcare augmented and virtual reality market 2017-2023: Growing need to reduce the healthcare costs—Researchandmarkets .com*. Retrieved from https://www.businesswire.com/news/home/20180201005633/en/Global-Healthcare-Augmented-Virtual-Reality-Market-2017-2023

Davenport, T. H. (2014). A predictive analytics primer. *Harvard Business Review*. Retrieved from https://hbr.org/2014/09/a-predictive-analytics-primer

The Economist. (2017). *A digital revolution in healthcare is speeding up*. Retrieved from https://www.economist.com/business/2017/03/02/a-digital-revolution-in-health-care-is-speeding-up

Food and Drug Administration. (2015). *Mobile medical applications*. Retrieved from https://www.fda.gov/MedicalDevices/DigitalHealth/MobileMedicalApplications/default.htm#a

The Franklin Institute. (2018). *What's the difference between AR, VR, and MR*. Retrieved from https://www.fi.edu/difference-between-ar-vr-and-mr

Herzlinger, R. (2006, May). Why innovation in healthcare is so hard. *Harvard Business Review*. Retrieved from https://hbr.org/2006/05/why-innovation-in-health-care-is-so-hard.

High, R. (2018). 3 AI terms all business professionals need to understand. *Venture Beat*. Retrieved from https://venturebeat.com/2018/02/24/3-ai-terms-all-business-professionals-need-to-understand/amp/?__twitter_impression=true

Hillary, W., Justin, G., Bharat, M., & Jitendra, M. (2016). Value based healthcare. *Advances in Management, 9*(1), 1–8.

Hospital Consumer Assessment of Healthcare Providers and Systems. (2018). Retrieved from http://www.hcahpsonline.org/

Hsu, J. (2013). *3D printing: What a 3D printer is and how it works*. Retrieved from https://www.livescience.com/34551-3d-printing.html

Intuitive. (n. d.). *DaVinci by Intuitive*. Retrieved from https://www.intuitive.com/en-us/products-and-services/da-vinci

Lee, B. Y. (2017). Virtual reality is a growing reality in health care. *Forbes*. Retrieved from https://www.forbes.com/sites/brucelee/2017/08/28/virtual-reality-vr-is-a-growing-reality-in-health-care/#76bc3bd44838

Lukowicz, P. (2008). Wearable computing and artificial intelligence for healthcare applications. *Artificial Intelligence in Medicine, 42*(2), 95–98. doi:10.1016/j.artmed.2007.12.002

Mandl, K. D., Mandel, J. C., & Kohane, I. S. (2015). Driving innovation in health systems through an apps-based information. *Cell Systems, 1*, 8–13. doi:10.1016/j.cels.2015.05.001

McCleery, E., Christensen, V., Peterson, K., Humphrey, L., & Helfand, M. (2014). Evidence brief: The quality of care provided by advanced practice nurses. In *VA evidence-based synthesis program evidence briefs*. Washington, DC: Department of Veteran Affairs.

MDLIVE. (2018). Retrieved from https://www.mdlive.com/

The Medical Futurist. (2017). *The top 9 augmented reality companies in healthcare*. Retrieved from http://medicalfuturist.com/top-9-augmented-reality-companies-healthcare/

Medium. (2017). *Healthcare mobile app development and mHealth apps in 2017*. Retrieved from https://medium.com/@Adoriasoft_Com/healthcare-mobile-app-development-and-mhealth-apps-in-2017-eb307d4cad36

Merriam-Webster Dictionary. (n.d.-a). *Artificial intelligence*. Retrieved from https://www.merriam-webster.com/dictionary/artificial%20intelligence

Merriam-Webster Dictionary. (n.d.-b). *Augmented reality*. Retrieved from https://www.merriam-webster.com/dictionary/augmented%20reality?utm_campaign=sd&utm_medium=serp&utm_source=jsonld

Merriam-Webster Dictionary. (n.d.-c). *Virtual reality*. Retrieved from https://www.merriam-webster.com/dictionary/virtual%20reality

Search Health IT. (2018). *mHealth (mobile health)*. Retrieved from http://searchhealthit.techtarget.com/definition/mHealth

Sensely Virtual Assistant. (2018). Retrieved from http://www.sensely.com/

Sullivan, T. (2017). Half of hospitals to adopt artificial intelligence within 5 years. *Healthcare IT News.* Retrieved from http://www.healthcareitnews.com/news/half-hospitals-adopt-artificial-intelligence-within-5-years

Tan, Z., Parisi, C., DiSilvo, L., Dini, D., & Forte, A. E. (2017, November 24). Cryogenic 3D printing of super soft hydrogels. *Scientific Reports, 7,* 16293. doi:10.1038/s41598-017-16668-9. Retrieved from https://www.nature.com/articles/s41598-017-16668-9

Tsukayama, H. (2014, February 27). Everything you need to know about Google glass. *The Washington Post.* Retrieved from https://www.washingtonpost.com/news/the-switch/wp/2014/02/27/everything-you-need-to-know-about-google-glass/?noredirect=on

United Healthcare. (n. d.). UnitedHealthcare Motion. Retrieved from https://www.uhc.com/employer/programs-tools/unitedhealthcare-motion

Walker, T. (2017, June 15). *Four key trends in healthcare innovation.* Retrieved from http://managedhealthcareexecutive.modernmedicine.com/managed-healthcare-executive/news/three-key-trends-healthcare-innovation

Patient-Centered Innovation

Adrienne Boissy

"We can do no great things—only small things with great love."
—Mother Teresa

INTRODUCTION

Patient experience emerged as a mere concept decades ago. As originally described, patient experience was articulated as patient-centered care, wherein the patient preferences and values were considered as a core part of treatment. The 2001 publication *Crossing the Quality Chasm* from the Institute of Medicine (IOM) highlighted patient-centered care as a core component in high-quality care (IOM, 2001). The remaining components addressed multiple failures of the current system and called for action to make healthcare safe, effective, efficient, timely, and equitable. *Patient centeredness* was defined as "providing care that is respectful of and responsive to individual patient preferences, needs, and values, and ensuring that patient values guide all clinical decisions." Over the past several decades, healthcare has made substantial strides forward to deliver on this promise. Yet, there is more work to be done.

Six years before the IOM report, the Agency for Healthcare Research and Quality (AHRQ) launched the first Consumer Assessment of Healthcare Providers and Systems (CAHPS) program to better understand the experience of patients. For hospitals that receive Medicare payment, there was a pay-for-reporting incentive, which has evolved into increasing dollars at risk through a pay-for-performance model. This program meant to capture patient experience with standardized surveys and to find ways to disseminate the results for comparison. The surveys vary by setting and include data on topics that are determined to be most important to the patient, including access, communication, discharge, timeliness, and environment. Results of these surveys are publicly posted on the Centers for Medicare & Medicaid Services (CMS) website, although they lag behind by about 2 years. Thus, one of the greatest challenges for hospitals is how to capture the patient experience in a more timely fashion.

Patients often write about their experiences—either as compliments or complaints. Most hospitals have a process to manage this input, which is also regulated by the government. CMS requires that any written complaint about care become what is called a *grievance*. Once a grievance is submitted, CMS mandates that hospitals respond to the patient in writing within 7 days. An example of topics mentioned in grievances from a large healthcare system is provided in Figure 12.1.

The patient voice is captured in healthcare today, whether in patient satisfaction surveys, complaints and grievances, or something else. Each of these methods has its advantages and disadvantages, but organizations need to commit to hearing the patient voice so it may be reflected in practice. A significant disadvantage of these surveys, especially the Hospital Consumer Assessment of Healthcare Providers and Systems (HCAHPS) and CAHPS Clinician & Group Survey (CGCAHPS), is the delay associated with the feedback, which can be up to 6 weeks. In the future, these must evolve to shorter, mobile-deployed, and in-the-moment captures of experience.

All of this feedback is left to hospitals to manage. Many organizations have made it a priority to positively impact the patient experience and have a dedicated chief experience officer (CXO), often a nurse or physician, whose job it is to oversee customer and clinician satisfaction. Originally created by Dr. Toby Cosgrove, former CEO of the Cleveland Clinic, the CXO role was elevated to the C-suite, largely because Dr. Cosgrove recognized that patient experience efforts would not thrive unless the CXO had C-suite visibility. Since then, the role has become quite popular and exists today in close to 60% of all U.S. hospitals. Personnel support and organizational charts are variable.

As an example, the Office of Patient Experience at the Cleveland Clinic includes a focus on human-centered design (HCD), best practices, volunteers, spiritual care, bioethics, complaints

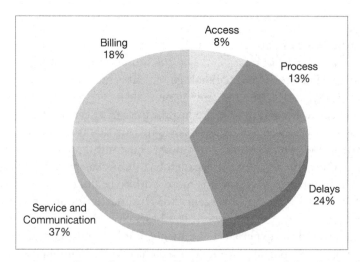

Figure 12.1 Patient dissatisfiers from multiple data sources and the Cleveland Clinic.

and grievances, end of life, research, service excellence, shared medical appointments, clinician communication, and data intelligence. This structure is not the norm, and often practices have one person or a small team responsible for improving patient experience.

Although classic thinking associates the CXO role with driving performance on HCAHPS or CGCAHPS surveys, the future is broader. As the role of the consumer grows in all other industries and new models of delivering health emerge, healthcare is taking notice. The experience of clinical care is only one piece of a patient's journey—attention to his or her emotional and spiritual well-being is an entirely different effort. To that end, many offices of patient experience include spiritual care, volunteers, patient advocates, and service excellence of one kind or another in their considerations of patient experience. Regardless of how it is structured, many, but not all, hospitals and practices deem patient experience a strategic imperative.

PATIENT-CENTERED INNOVATION

To actually capture the experience of our patients and act on it, we must be able to monitor experience in real time. In airline industries, shopping, and retail, the lessons for capturing experience in the moment, recovering service immediately, and pushing for convenience are obvious. A 1990 *Harvard Business Review* article beautifully identified the service recovery paradox—businesses that effectively recover service are multiple times more likely to retain that "customer" than those that don't (Hart, 1990). The ability to capture an experience and then address it is crucial to top-notch service organizations. Yet, most of healthcare doesn't use real-time experience data nor respond in real time. In fact, on the HCAHPS survey, there actually is a question about whether or not the patient wants to be contacted about his or her experience. Yet few hospitals operationalize how to manage this communication.

Learning about the experience of the patient is only half the battle. If you open a channel for patients to communicate with you in real time as a healthcare organization, this fundamentally changes the expectations of the patients. They will expect a responsive system that addresses concerns as soon as we hear of them. Not meeting this expectation runs the risk of disengaging the patient altogether, thereby fracturing trust. In other words, if patients tell us they are waiting too long in a waiting room or the wrong sandwich is on the food tray, we have to be able to reliably recover service in real time. This, in-moment data about the experience of patients—and our response to it—is ripe for innovation.

Not many organizations have effectively mastered operationalized empathy for the patient—building it into processes and systems. Most continue to focus on known evidence-based best practices such as nurse hourly rounding, nurse manager rounds, and a bedside shift report. In addition, communication skills training, scripting, use of the whiteboard for a daily plan of care, sitting at the bedside have all been emphasized. The challenge lies within sustainability of these efforts as the requests of our nurses, APRNs, and physicians grow. Too often the time spent with the patient in meaningful dialogue and connection is the first moment to fall of the priority list.

In the Emergency Services Institute at the Cleveland Clinic, a simple idea was born. Within a patient experience steering committee meeting, a discussion on patient experience improvement in the emergency room (ER) generated many suggestions and ideas. Ultimately, it was decided that the Clinic's greatest opportunity existed in simply letting patients know that the ER caregivers cared about them via a phone call made a day or two after discharge. Maybe not revolutionary or innovative, nevertheless, the effort was absolutely transformative. The ER

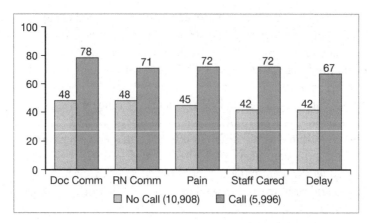

Figure 12.2 Press Ganey score of percentile ranks of EDt overall).

developed a work flow such that every single patient discharged received a follow-up phone call made by one of the caregivers (physician, nurse, medical assistant, etc.). The discharge list of patients was publicly posted and caregivers signed up to call with an expectation that each caregiver would call five patients. Many signed up for more and actively sought out the patients they had cared for specifically. In the first quarter of 2018, the ER caregivers called over 70,000 patients. When the data were divided by patients who received a phone call versus those who didn't, the results were stunning (Figure 12.2).

 CALL TO ACTION

One of the greatest challenges to enhancing the patient experience is sustainability. While everyone is focused and enthusiasm is high, significant improvements can be made. As time goes on, efforts are more difficult to maintain. What methods are effective to sustain improvements and hold people accountable?

Remarkably, this innovation doesn't require any new resources for technology or people, but it has a dramatic impact on the patients, leading to significant improvement in HCAHPS performance across all domains (Figure 12.3). Patients reported that they actually felt cared for as people, not simply as the problem they presented with, and, if their own caregiver called them, the impact was even greater. In fact, multiple comments captured on the patient satisfaction surveys highlighted how surprised and touched patients were to feel individually cared for because of a single phone call. Sometimes the greatest innovations are simple ones, and the power of exceeding expectations with an unexpected gesture is worth noting.

"One phone call, that's all it took." —Pierce Brosnan

Another great example of clinical innovation in experience of patients led by nursing colleagues comes from Intermountain. Partners in Healing® is a program created by frontline Intermountain Healthcare cardiovascular nurses in 2010 to enhance postoperative patient care.

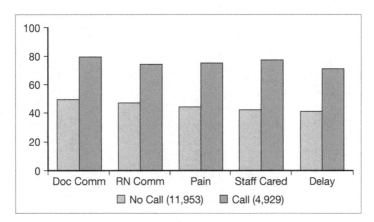

Figure 12.3 The Hospital Consumer Assessment of Healthcare Providers and Systems domain performance based on emergency room discharge phone calls.

These nurses, in collaboration with nurse leaders, sought to improve discharge preparation, consistency of care at home, and the patient and family experience. Michelle Van De Graaff, RN, developed the program based on her experiences in the Peace Corps. Because physicians were rare and nurses often unavailable, Michelle observed families providing the vast majority of care for patients in hospitals in the Republic of Kiribati. She also noticed the patients were calm and the discharge process went smoothly. Based on this premise, the Partners in Healing program was created to formally invite the patients and their family members into the care team.

This voluntary program is also simple. If a patient agrees, nurses invite families to participate, and the Partners are given a badge to wear when they want to function as a Partner in Healing. When the family member needs a break, he or she simply removes the badge. Nurses teach family members certain skills they can perform for their loved one while in the hospital, including incentive spirometer use, measuring intake and output, and supporting activity-related goals. While still closely connected to nurses who can answer their questions, learning these skills fosters empowerment and confidence in performing these tasks when their loved one transitions from hospital to home.

In 2016 to 2017, the program was piloted in multiple nursing departments across various service lines and in both rural and urban geographies within Intermountain Healthcare. Educational materials, tracking systems, and a clear communication structure for nursing leaders, frontline nurses, patients, and their designated caregiver or family member were created. Expansion of the program leveraged high potential, engaged frontline nurses who had participated in and completed Intermountain's Discover Leadership for Nursing course as peer-to-peer champions of the Partners in Healing program.

Bringing these exemplary frontline nurses together in a half-day learning session, focused on team building, learning, and role playing, improved their chances of being successful, effective champions. Taking on the role of champion with responsibilities beyond their own nursing unit was scary, challenging, and rewarding, providing valuable experience in project management and influential leadership.

Comprehensive documentation, including paper-based tracking of data collected for 8 years, facilitated a retrospective review showing a 65% reduction in readmission rates for patients

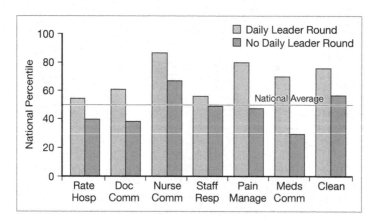

Figure 12.4 Impact of daily leader round on the Hospital Consumer Assessment of Healthcare Providers and Systems scored at the Cleveland Clinic.

whose families participated in the Partners in Healing program (Van De Graaff et al., 2018). In addition, over 90% of participants stated the program improved their transition from being cared for in the hospital to being cared for at home.

At the Cleveland Clinic, one regional hospital consistently scored at or above the 90th percentile of all the HCAHPS domains. The organization applied the success of this hospital as a case study and implemented best practices at other regional hospitals. The process involved interviewing the leadership team and observing operations at the high-performing hospital. In addition to common best practices, the hospital enhanced monthly enterprise leadership rounding by assigning leaders specific units to visit on a weekly basis.

Leaders were engaged in a pilot period wherein we measured the impact of novel rounding methods and asked for their continued commitment of support if effective. The daily leader rounding process included (a) individual leaders receiving their assignments; (b) rounding on the patients; (c) sharing any pertinent information with the nurse manager before leaving the unit and completing an online, customizable questionnaire; and (d) trending the data, including follow-up action taken and sharing this with units. The questions on the questionnaire are used as the process metrics that are being tracked and then compared to the HCAHPS survey, which is the outcome metric. The positive impact of daily leader rounding on HCAHPS is shown in Figure 12.4.

CLINICIAN EXPERIENCE

Another area ripe for innovation with respect to the experience of patients that also follows caregiver experience has to do with efficiency—54% of physicians in the United States fulfill criteria for burnout, including measures of emotional exhaustion, depersonalization, and lack of fulfillment (Shanafelt et al., 2015). For nurses, the numbers are similar (Vahey, Aiken, Sloane, Clarke, & Vargas, 2004).

Reduction of autonomy in practice, the sheer volume of information and data, demands on time, and lack of meaning in work all contribute to the moral distress associated with wanting to care for human beings but feeling locked in a system that makes it difficult to do just that.

Multiple studies have demonstrated the impact of burnout on patient safety, medical comorbidities, suicide, patient satisfaction, and likelihood to leave the profession (Panagioti et al., 2018; Windover et al., 2018). Although conceptually it is believed that clinicians who are burned out deliver worse experiences to patients, this is less clear in the data.

Multiple innovations focus on reducing burnout. One of the most common issues plaguing healthcare is the tremendous requirement for documentation on all caregivers. Nurses at the bedside are often pushing mobile workstations in front of them, and unfortunately, in between themselves and the patients. Reducing the waste and redundancy in nursing workflows is paramount to combatting burnout. Physicians are spending hours after work completing their documentation for all the patients they may have seen in the clinic (Sinsky et al., 2016). Feedback to the government as to how to reduce this burden is one piece of the puzzle, but innovation is necessary to reduce the clerical burden on people who actually want to provide exceptional care. Scribes are being increasingly used in outpatient settings to enable documentation and fulfillment of these documentation requirements. These can work in person or virtually, even through glasses worn by the clinician. Preliminary reports suggest scribes can save clinicians time and are welcomed by patients (Yan et al., 2016). Traditional scribes involve having a third party in the room, which at times can generate discomfort either for the clinician or for the patient when discussing sensitive issues. Virtual scribes, however, remove the physical presence of a third person and allow the scribe to participate either through the use of technology or simply the intercom. The benefits should also be balanced with the notion that we have introduced a third party into the intimate space between the patient and their doctor.

Mircrophones have been used in the inpatient setting to improve communication with patients. Rather than answering the phone or dialing a number, the voice-activated technology allows the nurse to continue doing what he or she was doing and can simply touch the speaker itself to engage in conversation or make a connection. Conversations through these microphones are easily heard by the patient at whose bedside the nurse may be working.

Newly designed hospital rooms will be fully wired. The room will know when the patient is out of bed and when the patient is supposed to be asking for assistance. The room will turn the lights on in the morning to keep the patient oriented to day and night. This connectivity will identify not only safety hazards for patients but also direct patient education, empower patients to order meals, review a plan of care, and additional services. Bedside tablets, like those used at the University of Iowa and Ohio State University, will allow using the room to become a true interactive experience. Too often, the patient in the bed spends a significant amount of his or her time waiting to hear from the medical team about each and every day and the actual schedule of these items often remains amorphous. In the very near future, digital and connected hospital rooms will notify nurses when a patient is up and out of the bed immediately, will use in-room voice-activated technology, and allow virtual visits to distant family as well as clinical consultations. Beyond even that, the patient room will anticipate needs, fully integrate clinical monitoring, and literally "sense" the patient. A fully connected room will allow the patient to manage more of his or her own environment rather than needing the nurse or another caregiver, thereby giving back the gift of time.

Another great innovation example is how clinicians round in the hospital. Teams often huddle in the morning and then round on patients by walking to each room, which often takes up several hours. Technology has emerged wherein the physicians or APRNs can stream into the patient TV platform, or connect via a mobile virtual-rounding interface, and visit the patient from the comfort of his or her home or office (saving time). In addition, nurse-manager rounding is quickly moving from paper rounds, which are later manually entered into a database, to rounds performed with a mobile device. Multiple mobile-rounding platforms exist and can capture not only compliance with safety requirements but also track trends and issues over time. Issues identified on rounds are automatically routed to the appropriate party and resolved without a single phone call.

CALL TO ACTION

In your own field, reflect on a typical day. The workflows, the steps you take, the time you spend in different tasks. Select one that would substantially benefit from becoming more efficient. What would be the impact on the caregiver and the patient?

COMMUNICATION

Communication is the most common procedure performed in healthcare. Decades of literature associate effective communication with enhanced trust, loyalty, stronger relationships, and reduced malpractice suits (Levinson, 1994; Moore, Adler, & Robertson, 2000). Although all of these have value, at a more basic level, communication is key to healthcare. Keeping patients well is a worthy and appropriate focus of population health efforts. In many other areas of healthcare, patients are living with chronic diseases and coming into hospitals with acute illness. To care for them, we are asking them to undergo procedures that might hurt, surgeries that might have complications, and medications they might not fully understand. These requests are substantial—physically and emotionally. Our ability to communicate engenders trust and aligns the treatment with patient values.

When communication comments are broken down in patient satisfaction surveys, patients continue to highlight basic respect as well as need for empathy in communication. Lack of coordination is a recurring problem identified by patients, showing gaps in transfer of care across settings, inconsistent quarterbacking of care, and multiple care teams using multiple care plans. Patients can identify their preferences in tools like customer relationship management systems—systems used in nearly every industry outside healthcare to create a 360° view of the customer. Innovation will capture patient preferences, respect these through customized automation, and limit the number of interruptions for any given patient.

As for interpersonal communication, change has already arrived. Mobile phone users are beginning to text more than they talk on the phone, so effective engagement of many future patients will be about text and voice recognition. The few well-known models of effective communication (Frankel & Stein, 1999; Windover et al., 2016) will need to be adapted to these new settings, including virtual visits. In addition, how we teach effective communication must shift to a digital mode as well through nano-coaching and e-learning modules. All the while keeping in mind the most effective means of connecting with another human is still through effective use of empathy.

DIGITAL TOOLS AND WHAT THEY MEAN FOR PATIENT ENGAGEMENT

Digital tools that empower the patient and send messages at any time have exploded on the healthcare landscape. However, clinicians remain somewhat confused about the differences between *patient experience* and *patient engagement*. Making the distinction is important, so we are all speaking the same language about which we are referring to, hoping to improve, and what tools we will use to get us there. Table 12.1 highlights the similarities and differences between patient experience and patient engagement (Boissy, 2018).

Mercy Healthcare System designed healthcare without walls by investing in remote monitoring as a means of caring for their patients outside of the hospital and clinic. The $54 million Virtual Care Center offers multiple programs, including remote monitoring for ICU care, stroke, sitter care, and clinical alarms. Although this may seem like an innovation simply in healthcare, imagine a better patient experience than one wherein you don't have to go to the hospital at all? Yet these experiences still need to be designed well. Uncoordinated touches that bother the patient about things that are not important to them, but rather to us, will prevent patients from taking advantage of all these tools have to offer.

Ochsner Health System embraced similar digital solutions years ago and also created the O-bar, a literal bar where patients could come to learn about apps and devices to support management of their health. The O-bar distills the hundreds of apps available to a given patient to the ones that might be right for that patient. By integrating with the Apple Watch,

TABLE 12.1 Patient Engagement Versus Patient Experience

	Patient Engagement	Patient Experience
Goals	1. Drive better health and outcomes 2. Empower patients and loved ones to be active in their own care 3. Reduce costs	1. Drive better health and outcomes 2. Exceed expectations 3. Reduce suffering 4. Brand differentiation
Stakeholders	Patient, others are likely	Patient, others are likely
Context	Patient's own health	All encompassing (access, communication, food, etc.)
Patient involvement (behaviors and ownership)	Required	Not required (though in an ideal experience, patients are partners and codesigners)
Time	Transactional or longitudinal	Transactional or longitudinal
Use of health self-management tools/services	Yes	No
Validated measurement	Patient Activation Measure, Patient-Reported Outcomes Measurement Information System, Patient Health Engagement Scale	Hospital Consumer Assessment of Healthcare Providers and Systems, CAHPS Clinician & Group Survey, etc.

CAHPS, Consumer Assessment of Healthcare Providers and Systems.

Ochsner created a hypertension monitoring program wherein 71% of patients achieved target blood pressure control in 90 days compared to 41% of those engaged through the usual means (Milani, Lavie, Bober, Milani, & Ventura, 2017). These tools can also remind patients to take their medications and maintain physical activity goals well beyond counseling in the doctor's office, all of which more effectively engage the patient in hos or her own health management.

Digital engagement tools have flooded into the healthcare ecosystem, and can meet needs involving navigation, longitudinal relationship building, and improved patient activation. Because there are so many tools in the marketplace, there is potential for this approach to become fragmented. Considerations for the future of the work include the ability for a healthcare professional to review significant data elements, evolving artificial intelligence to understand the data and its meaning, and cohesive designs of a digital experience that extends across the continuum of care.

BILLING AND PAYMENT

Engaging our patients through digital tools is about both the clinical and nonclinical parts of a patient journey. Think for a minute about the banking industry. Years ago, you would receive a check in the mail, you would sign it, drive over to the bank or the automated teller machine (ATM) and make the deposit into your accounts. The total time spent between the moment the check was issued and your deposit was 10 to 14 days if not more. Today, a check can be automatically deposited in your account directly or, if the check arrives at your home, you can snap a picture and complete the transaction through an app on your phone. Now let's consider what happens in healthcare.

A patient arrives for an outpatient appointment, pays a co-pay depending on what his insurance requires and has his visit—labs and an MRI of the brain are ordered. The MRI of the brain has to undergo a preauthorization process, which can take several days and, if denied, the physician has to call to appeal this decision. There are no expectations set prior to the appointment about what it will cost or what insurance covers. Can you imagine if you went shopping at the grocery store and the first time you saw a price tag or understood what you were paying for was at the register? Makes no sense, and therefore, is ripe for disruption.

To add more complexity, most people don't pay their bill the first time they get it. Why, you ask? Because not only do they believe the bill is inaccurate, but that if they wait long enough, insurance will pay it. When the Cleveland Clinic interviewed patients in their homes about the bill, the reasons why they didn't pay their bill varied. Some were actually struggling financially, whereas others were skeptical about the bill itself. One perplexed patient stated: "I didn't know it was going to be that much! They should have warned me!" And patients are right, transparency of costs of care is a major factor in decision-making and innovation has arrived in real-time verification of insurance, personalized payment plans, and mobile payment options.

CLINICIAN-CENTERED INNOVATION

Perhaps the most innovative thing we can do in a digital world is to continue to find and promote meaning for the frontline caregiver. There isn't a single solution for this problem. Organizations, schools, and businesses are working to engage a more distracted workforce. Yet we know that having meaning in your work can protect against burnout, so find ways to foster meaning. Just as we seek to personalize care for patients, we need personalized care for the frontline. Not all wellness programs or art classes work for all caregivers. Some find meaning by spending time with family, others do yoga, and others golf. Traditional methods of in-person classes and all-day retreats may also need to incorporate new methods, including digital platforms with smaller bites of learning, to reach caregivers where they are. Today, it is unlikely that one organization can produce individualized wellness for each caregiver, but it certainly is aspirational. A digital experience of the future also needs to enhance the lives of the people providing the care and experiences for our patients.

To make the lives of our caregivers and patients easier, new methods to drive efficiency and design new systems and processes have evolved. Efficiency is largely driven by continuous improvement, exemplified by philosophies like LEAN. Continuous improvement uses a cycle of plan, do, check, act to drive incremental improvements, and often involves those doing the work to eliminate waste in their environment and to optimize processes. Other improvement methods include the more recently popular AGILE, which originated in the software industry as a new way to manage project development. AGILE focuses on face-to-face transparency with the user and development of products in short sprints, with the idea that they won't be perfect but will be constantly iterated.

When it comes to experience or service design, a third method of innovation and improvement, human-centered design (HCD), is commonly used. HCD has similarities to the other methods previously described, mainly the involvement of multiple stakeholders, exploration of the needs of the end user, and inclusion of those who will be impacted by the service. All methods are used in a variety of industries, with HCD often used in service design to drive ideation and products based on what the end user sees, does, feels, and says—and ultimately on what the end user values. HCD uses a consistent process: empathize, define, ideate, prototype, and test. It is also important to recognize that these methods can complement each other and often overlap, rather than existing as separate entities.

Kaiser Permanente has blended methodologies into a process they called *CoDesign*, which has resulted in better engagement of staff when they participate in the program. Furthermore, substantial improvement was made to operations, including transport time, communication of radiology costs, and dementia care. To be specific, score for patients' likelihood to recommend Kaiser Permanente increased over fourfold when a new process about communicating radiology costs based on processes was implemented (Kachirskaia, Mate, & Neuwirth, 2018). Another great example of HCD in innovation is the Helix Centre in the United Kingdom. They developed the Amber care plan, wherein a chatbot walks patients through articulating their advance care plans—their wishes, goals, emergency contacts—from the comfort of their own home. Risk calculators are being developed in other organizations wherein patient wishes and preferences are indentified and a healthcare power of attorney (HC-POA) is designated, and these wishes are made transparent in the electronic health record (EHR). Designing a better end of life, and more appropriate, a better experience of living at the end of life, should also be considered part of the patient experience. All too often, this is left to palliative care specialists. Although nearly all patients want to die at home, a staggering small percentage actually do. HCD can change all of that if we take time to listen.

Jonathan Bartels, a palliative care liaison and prior ER trauma nurse at the University of Virginia Medical Center, noted in his practice that after resuscitation efforts, often the clinicians would turn from the deceased body and walk away. Inspired by witnessing a chaplain stop a team to lead a prayer, Jonathan had an idea—an idea that required no additional resources or an app to bring to fruition. What ultimately evolved was a movement called *The Pause*, wherein the caregiving team and ideally the family gather together to *literally* pause and verbally recognize the efforts of the care team and to honor the life of the patient after he or she dies. As a caregiver doing the work of caring for patients, he saw the pain in their experience and took the opportunity to change a life. As a result, he has touched innumerable lives around the globe as hospitals adapted this approach. The beauty of this innovation was its humanity—pausing to reflect on the privilege we have to care for human beings, the despair we feel when we lose someone we care for, and inviting all those impacted by the loss to come together in a moment.

CONCLUSIONS

Jonathan Bartels's innovative gesture serves as a reminder to patients and caregivers alike. Just because technology has exploded and many devices show promise, we must remember that at its core, healthcare is still a remarkably human endeavor. Wearables and remote monitoring are absolutely going to make healthcare and management of one's own health easier and more convenient—as it should. These devices and their use need human guidance and processing. Just because you can check your heart rate every 2 minutes doesn't mean you should. Just because we care for you, doesn't mean your data are ours to use as we wish. Just because facial recognition exists doesn't mean we should use it without patient consent. We will likely to change nearly every touch point we have with patients by embracing digital tools. Yet the most powerful tool we have—*and this will not change*—is our language. Through our spoken words and physical touch, we can engage, we can inspire, and we can connect as only humans can.

✦ KEY TAKEAWAY POINTS

- Simple well-organized ideas can have a big impact on patient experience, as measured in surveys and operations.

- The digitally connected room will change the way we care for patients by empowering them to manage their environment, schedule, and data.

- Better financial journeys in healthcare will provide greater transparency on costs and insurance coverage at the point of service.

- Human-centered design helps industries, including healthcare, deeply understand the values and behaviors of end users.

- A major goal of any patient experience improvement effort will move us from transactional care to care across a lifetime, including end of life.

REFERENCES

Boissy, A. R. (2017). Patient engagement versus patient experience. Retrieved from https://catalyst.nejm.org/patient-engagement-vs-patient-experience

Frankel, R. M., & Stein, T. (1999). Getting the most out of the clinical encounter: The four habits model. *The Permanente Journal, 3*(3). doi:10.7812/TPP/99-020

Hart, C. W., Heskett, J. L., & Sasser, W. E. (1990). The profitable art of service recovery. *Harvard Business Review*. Retrieved from https://hbr.org/1990/07/the-profitable-art-of-service-recovery

Institute of Medicine (2001). *Crossing the quality chasm: A new health system for the 21th century*. Washington, DC: National Academies Press.

Kachirskaia, I., Mate, K. S., & Neuwirth, E., (2018, June 28) Human-centered design and performance improvement: Better together. *Catalyst*. Retrieved from https://catalyst.nejm.org/hcd-human-centered-design-performance-improvement/

Levinson, W. (1994). Physician–patient communication: A key to malpractice prevention. *Journal of the American Medical Association,272*(20), 1619–1620. doi:10.1001/jama.1994.03520200075039

Milani, R. V., Lavie, C. J., Bober, R. M., Milani, A. R., & Ventura, H. O. (2017). Improving hypertension control and patient engagement using digital tools. *American Journal of Medicine, 130*(1), 14–20. doi:10.1016/j.amjmed.2016.07.029

Moore, P. J., Adler, N. E., & Robertson, P. A. (2000). Medical malpractice: The effect of doctor-patient relations on medical patient perceptions and malpractice intentions. *Western Journal of Medicine, 173*(4), 244–250. doi:10.1136/ewjm.173.4.244

Panagioti, M., Geraghty, K., Johnson, J., Zhou, A., Panagopoulou, E., Chew-Graham, C., . . . Esmail, A. (2018). Association between physician burnout and patient safety, professionalism, and patient satisfaction: A systematic review and meta-analysis. *JAMA Internal Medicine, 187*(10), 1317–1330. doi:10.1001/jamainternmed.2018.3713

Shanafelt, T. D., Hasan, O., Dyrbye, L. N., Sinsky, C., Satele, D., Sloan, J., & West, C. P. (2015). Changes in burnout and satisfaction with work–life balance in physicians and the general US working population between 2011 and 2014. *Mayo Clinic Proceedings, 90*(12), 1600–1613. doi:10.1016/j.mayocp.2015.08.023

Sinsky, C., Colligan, L., Li, L., Prgomet, M., Reynolds, S., Goeders, L., . . . Blike, G. (2016). Allocation of physician time in ambulatory practice: A time and motion study in 4 specialties. *Annals of Internal Medicine, 165*(11), 753–760. doi:10.7326/M16-0961

Vahey, D. C., Aiken, L. H., Sloane, D., Clarke, S. P., & Vargas, D. (2004). Nurse burnout and patient satisfaction. *Medical Care, 42*(2 Suppl.), II57–II66. doi:10.1097/01.mlr.0000109126.50398.5a

Van De Graaff, M., Beesley, S. J., Butler, J., Benuzillo, J., Poll, J. B., Oniki, T., . . . Brown, S. M. (2018). Partners in healing: Postsurgical outcomes after family involvement in nursing care. *Chest, 153*(2), 572–574. doi:10.1016/j.chest.2017.09.046

Windover, A. K., Boissy, A., Gilligan, T., Merlino, J., Velez, V. J., & Rice, T. W. (2016). The REDE model of healthcare communication: Optimizing relationship as a therapeutic agent. *Journal of Patient Experience, 1*(1), 8–13. doi:10.1177/237437431400100103

Windover, A. K., Martinez, K., Mercer, M. B., Neuendorf, K., Boissy, A., & Rothberg, M. B. (2018). Correlates and outcomes of physician burnout within a large academic medical center. *JAMA Internal Medicine, 178*(6), 856–858. doi:10.1001/jamainternmed.2018.0019

Yan, C., Rose, S., Rothberg, M. B., Mercer, M. B., Goodman, K., & Misra-Hebert, A. D. (2016). Physician, scribe, and patient perspectives on clinical scribes in primary care. *Journal of General Internal Medicine, 31*(9), 990–995. doi:10.1007/s11606-016-3719-x

Positive Deviance: Advancing Innovation to Transform Healthcare

Kathy Malloch and Tim Porter-O'Grady

"Do not go where the path may lead, go instead where there is no path and leave a trail."—Ralph Waldo Emerson

LEARNING OBJECTIVES

- Describe the origins and value of positive deviance (PD) as a precursor to innovation.
- Understand the principles underpinning PD to enhance the role of the contemporary leader.
- Explain the interpretation of PD in at least two practical applications.

INTRODUCTION

Often, positive deviance (PD) is viewed as negative and counterproductive. However, a closer look at PD reveals strong links to innovation. In this chapter, we present the origins of PD, the principles underpinning PD, the discipline of PD, the relationship of PD to innovation, and scenarios in which PD occurs.

"Whatever you can do or dream you can, begin it. Boldness has genius, power, and magic in it. Begin it now."

THE ORIGINS OF POSITIVE DEVIANCE

Have you ever noticed some people whose sometimes weird and unusual behavior does not fit the norm, yet produces positive results for them? They often seem "in their own world," but find unusual solutions to problems and have creative approaches to difficult problems. These are society's deviants, also known as *hurdlers*, or individuals who continually challenge

> **Box 13.1   Positive Deviance Descriptions**
>
> - *Positive deviance (PD)* is defined as an act that is outside of the norm, but that may actually be heroic rather than negative (Tuhus-Dubrow, 2009).
> - Involves behavior that over-conforms to social expectations—over-exercising; over-dieting.
> - PD takes the opposite approach to traditional design and problem-solving; traditional design is primarily prescriptive based on consultants or content experts telling communities what they should or should not be doing to achieve a specific outcome.
> - PD places the community at the center of the problem-solving process, with the belief that the best solution can be found within the community members themselves; it is about cocreation, designing interventions *within* communities rather than *for* communities.
> - PD involves behavior that is outside the norm but with no intention to harm.
>
> *Source:* Tuhus-Dubrow, R. (2009, November 29). The power of positive deviants: A promising new tactic for changing communities from the inside. *Boston Globe.* Retrieved from http://archive.boston.com/bostonglobe/ideas/articles/2009/11/29/the_power_of_positive_deviants

assumptions and find ways to overcome obstacles (Kelly, 2005). They seem to have an unusual supply of internal resources available to solve unusual problems using creative strategies even though they have no more apparent talents or resources than their peers.

This unusual set of circumstances was first noticed formally in the 1970s when social researchers studying community resources in areas noted for their higher levels of poverty found some unusual circumstances related to the nutritional status of children. Although most of the children in the researched region of poverty had generally low levels of nourishment, there were some poor families whose children actually had higher levels of nourishment even though their financial situation was no different. These poor families who had especially well-nourished children found a way inside of their circumstances to make sure that their children were adequately nourished. It is in these circumstances that the social scientists identified these individuals as positive deviants (Box 13.1).

THE PRINCIPLES UNDERPINNING POSITIVE DEVIANCE

Several principles emerged with the suggestion that there were consistent terms of understanding that related specifically to the phenomenon identified as PD:

1. Communities and teams already have solutions located within their own members for solving problems and addressing issues. The relational dynamics and expertise necessary for doing so was already present. One could consider this "thinking *inside* the box."

2. Resources, processes, and organization around issues or problems are sufficiently present inside communities and teams. Often, although the resources are present, content experts in the organization are not involved in the initial development of solutions, thus limiting the applicability of the solution.

3. Communities and teams have a collective wisdom that is sufficiently distributed among members (not necessarily present in leadership), adequate to address concerns. Using the

discipline/process of PD draws upon this collective intelligence as a source for relevant problem-solving. The believed adequate and appropriate solution is discarded or worked around by the content experts.

4. An organized and disciplined PD approach engages the community or team members to collectively discern and obtain viable solutions because either the behaviors and practices are already present or potentially present in a way that aligns well when accurately addressing the issue or concern. Rather than continuing to perform work that is not effective, positive deviants modify the work processes knowing that the deviant processes are more effective. Positive deviants focus on getting work done in the safest and most effective manner.

5. PD reflects the saying: "it is wiser to act your way into a new way of thinking than think your way into new way of acting." In PD, it is easier to change behavior by acting on it or practicing a new behavior than to have deep knowledge about it. This orientation to action, challenging, impacting, or changing behavior, and subsequently, ways of thinking, is a cornerstone to successful use of the discipline of PD. Most positive deviants prefer not to over-discuss or over-examine potential processes for improvement; rather they move quickly to action as the appropriate way to get work done.

THE DISCIPLINE OF POSITIVE DEVIANCE

Over the years, a wide variety of approaches have been used to implement the principles of PD in a manner that was both useful and sustainable. Two social scientists, Jerry and Monique Stermin, developed a discipline and subsequent mechanism for formalizing processes associated with PD in a way that was useful and highly effective. Working with Save the Children in Vietnam in the 1990s, Jerry and Monique developed a process for addressing a population of malnourished children using the community's own resources to address strategies that would address the nutritional circumstances of these children. Dramatic results in applying the principles and processes associated with PD reinforced their understanding of the validity and relevance of the PD process they developed. Using the community's own resources, the PD approach harnesses the cultural resources of the community or team by helping them seek the already present but unique and uncommon behavior shown in small community cohorts, that when aggregated and generally adopted from these small points of practice toward community patterns of behavior, predicted achievable positive and sustainable outcomes. The Stermins quantified this process and structured it into a useful problem-solving approach (Dorsey, 2017). Similarly, in practice applications of new policies and protocols developed from published research, there is a mismatch or gap in application to local settings. These gaps make it difficult or nearly impossible for individuals to implement the protocols not designed for their setting. Thus, a positive deviant recognizes the mismatch and determines a different way to achieve the desired goals.

 CALL TO ACTION

As a leader, create an infomercial for your team informing members of the principle, values, and benefits of positive deviance.

The components of the Stermins' process that were generated from their experience and applications are:

- An invitation to change
- Defining the problem
- Determining the presence of PD individuals or groups
- Discovering uncommon practices or behaviors
- Program design
- Monitoring and evaluation
- Scaling up

Since this initial work by the Stermins, many social science scholars, business leaders, and community organizations have taken the process of PD, generated data supporting its characteristics and attributes, and implemented a wide variety of projects and processes that validate its utility and veracity. Businesses, not-for-profit organizations, and community services have used the associated processes of PD to make a sustainable difference. A brief understanding of each of the elements of the process can help translate PD utility and application in an almost unlimited variety of circumstances. Harnessing the dynamics of PD provides leaders an opportunity to operate inside existing resources and to charge the talent already present inside the organization to think differently about problems and challenges and to find solutions within their own work culture to master work challenges and changes. This approach recognizes the value and significance of innovation-based practice as well as the nature of an appreciative approach to problem-solving. Further, using an appreciative approach toward PD, individuals are valued for their willingness to solve problems in meaningful and effective ways. Applying this systemic and organized approach to solutions moves the locus of control for decisions and actions to participants and teams at the point of service, empowering them to find and use already present insights and resources (Singhal, Buscell, & Lindberg, 2014).

STEP 1: AN INVITATION TO CHANGE

The first step is helping the community realize that a problem or issue exists in the group. To implement effective PD, leadership should understand the community within the context of its own lived experience and its culture. In healthcare, as service providers, healthcare systems are organizations that know precious little about the character and culture of the community within which they find themselves. Because of the historic "late-stage engagement" model of healthcare delivery in which treatment intervention drives care, there has been little impetus for healthcare facilities to deeply explore the critical elements and character of the communities within which they reside.

To combat this lack of awareness, read the local newspaper and note the priority of issues that continually appear as news. Often, these persistent challenges are fertile ground for PD and ultimately, innovation. The first stage of addressing any issue is to obtain a sense of how the community perceives the issue. Any substantive response to healthcare concerns or other problems will depend on the accuracy and veracity that underpin existing personal and community problems. Once that identification occurs, the pockets of PD are more likely to counter the prevailing concerns or issues or provide small exemplars to thrive in the face of such issues and can emerge and be observed.

Part of this invitation to change is reflected in leaders' capacity to mindfully listen to the community as it tells the story. Reading and observing the community yields only limited results, and the leader's insights or biases may not truly exemplify the underlying dynamics informing or affecting any given issue. Opportunities to converse and connect with community members provide both formal and informal mechanisms to share concerns in a way that reveals common insights, views, perspectives, and experiences. Use community forums, political and social structures, churches, and other collective forums for a broad-based, accurate description of the community perceptions about specific priorities and concerns. It is generally through this dialogue that common themes emerge, and priorities are revealed in a way that is useful to leaders as they attempt to identify the breadth and depth of issues and the related root-cause elements. This becomes the birth of an appreciative approach in which PD can result in an improved process and outcome.

STEP 2: DEFINING THE PROBLEM

Following these identified processes, leadership should not only help the community gather information leading to specific insights but also help the community own and investment in the emerging priorities that best represent legitimate concerns. The community must be part of this process and, of course, feel ownership for the problems or issues it has defined. Here, a crisp and clear articulation of the issue provides health and community leadership the best opportunity to look for the positive deviants that offer unusual strategies to sustain their positive response to concerns that otherwise negatively impact the community.

Evidence-based approaches to problem definition and clarity provide the rigor that ensures the accuracy and veracity of the concern identified. The usefulness and use of tools for helping the community in its assessment are as important as the assessment itself. Through both human dynamics and evidence-based methods, the community's assessment of the specifics of an issue yield accurate and legitimate results. Understanding the community's perceptions and insights about the issue alongside more rigorous methodological and statistical processes gives leaders some sense of the diversity, dichotomy, and/or synergy and integration of the issue and the community perspective. The capacity to identify and pursue community-positive deviants whose personal success related to the issue runs counter to prevailing community concerns will depend on how narrow and clear the substance of the issue is from the broader community perspective (Parkin, 2010). Positive deviants focus on the desired end point rather than spend time on the current processes that lead to the desired outcome. Too often, individuals and communities get stuck in the current processes and view them as untouchable, eliminating the opportunity for PD.

Leadership in this more unusual approach to community problem-solving helps the community understand its differences in the value of a PD approach. Long experience of individuals and communities suggests to them that it is at this point that a broad-based problem-solving process is undertaken by the community to collectively "solve their problem." However, in the PD approach, the community-based identification of a problem leads to a second level of identification of those going through the same issues but who have positively resolved them on an individual or family level. The work of PD becomes the opportunity to eliminate this discordance between current and deviant practices.

STEPS 3 AND 4: IDENTIFYING POSITIVELY DEVIANT INDIVIDUALS, GROUPS, AND PRACTICES IN THE COMMUNITY

Positive deviants are usually highly engaged, interactive, and relationally based individuals. They are often reflective and capable of objectively analyzing issues and circumstances using goal-oriented approaches to solve problems. They tend to be creative and innovative, independent and unbound by routine and structural or organizational limitations. These people are positive and diligent and not easily dissuaded from their own frequently self-created processes and solutions. They often can be heard saying "we tried that before" or "that has worked in the past" and are not limited by approval or disapproval of their actions. They repeatedly ask, "Why is this occurring"?

The positive deviant is unconstrained by other's behaviors or approaches. He or she seeks approaches to problem resolution that are immediately practical, applicable, and useful. She or he easily surrenders attachment to current practices when they no longer work and transforms them within a changing context to again be more relevant and useful. His or her energy keeps him or her from a "ritual and routine" trap that allows the PD individual to experiment freely with new approaches and processes. These patterns of behavior seem to be deeply embedded in the positive deviant's DNA (Singhal, Buscell, & Lindberg, 2010). Positive deviants are seldom deliberately trying to create chaos or conflict; the goal is how to achieve a better process and outcome and eliminate ineffective processes.

Leaders and researchers can easily seek out these individuals who are unconstrained by the community's immobility on an important issue or priority. They are usually found because they are anomalous to other members of the community and seem to be demonstrating positive practices or outcomes while the community as a whole is suffering from a general lack of solution and/or sustainability.

When discovered, leaders study the action approach of the positive deviant for both process effectiveness and positive outcome or impact. Objectively examine the PD approach to determine its efficacy in process, resource use, specificity, effectiveness, and sustainability (generalizability). Leadership and researchers should conduct a study of the positive deviant as a person

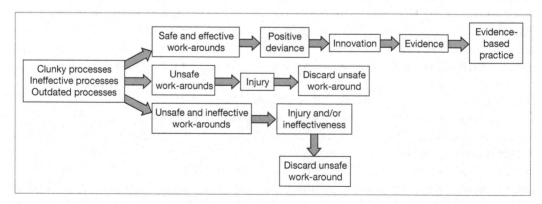

Figure 13.1 Exploring the relationships among work-arounds, positive deviance, and evidence-based practice.

and his or her specific characteristics that can be transferred or learned and the practices that can become an ongoing part of the work structure of organizations, systems, or communities. Once these practices have been determined, examined, and formalized, they become the basis for generalizing to the community as a whole and for providing creative and innovative solutions to the community's issue or problem. PD has transformed a clunky ineffective process into a safe and effective work-around that can likely lead to a formalized innovation. The innovation is examined and tested from an evidentiary position and becomes positioned to advance to evidence-based practice (Figure 13.1).

STEP 5: PROGRAM DESIGN

At this stage, leaders formalize the creative and unique approaches discovered from working with a community's positive deviants. They must clearly identify the generalizability of the positive deviant's particular approach to ensure that it addresses the larger issue and offers a viable solution. The community-based program design and initiative should identify replicable behaviors, processes, and best practices that adequately and sustainably provide a solution to the issue. It is here that the evidence of "acting into a new way of thinking" becomes apparent, as solutions not previously conceived by the entire community form the basis for community action going forward. Because evidence-based data generation and strategies follow a rigorous vetting before being applied to the community at large, the veracity of the approach and its predictability for success is more positively predictable. Community members are encouraged to undertake the unique but tested approach and offer their support when questions and reactions emerge. Community members are encouraged in their effort through the participation in small tests of change and in the evidence of viability and positive impact.

STEPS 6 AND 7: MONITORING, EVALUATION, AND SCALING UP

Evaluation and monitoring are related, but separate processes. Evaluation looks specifically at systematically and objectively examining the effectiveness, efficacy, and impact of particular actions on a defined goal. It looks at the workability and viability of specific actions on the point of impact, whereas monitoring looks at the impact of change over the long term. Monitoring is more consistent and is focused on the long-term effectiveness and efficacy of a particular process considering previous expectations or goals. Both practices are important to assess the viability and generalization of the application of a particular PD and its long-term sustainability.

During the monitoring process, data are gathered regularly at specific junctures in the process to determine their effectiveness and to track the long-term progress over the life of the process. The evaluation looks more specifically at the positive deviant approach considering the expectations and goals of a specific change. The point is to see whether the application of the unique approach is demonstrably more effective, has the desired impact, and produces the expected positive results or positive results beyond those anticipated. Also, continually addressed is an examination of the PD approach itself so that its dynamics and mechanisms can be more objectively evaluated to determine how they affect management decision-making, organizational learning, and best work practices.

CALL TO ACTION

Pushing harder: Identify at least one positive deviant practice in your organization that is allowed in one area and not in others. What are the opportunities to scale the positive deviant practice to benefit other areas in the organization?

Scaling Up

In the case that small tests of change or components of the change process undertaken in parts of the community demonstrate success, leaders must decide appropriate mechanisms and processes to "scale up" the implementation of the PD plan in a way that addresses the entire community. Scaling up requires attention to resources and energy generated by the community to ensure a sustainable level of impact at a larger level of measure. Efforts undertaken in smaller units may be successful because they are judicious and economical regarding resource use and human dynamics. Yet, when applied to the whole community, the scaling up of resource use, human dynamics, and other opportunity and work costs may be considerably different and the risk more broadly expanded.

Scaling up reflects the community's commitment to broad-based action. Leadership, once the community affirms the viability of a specific deviant practice, must get community commitment and engagement. They need to translate the preferred practice in a way that is amenable to the larger group. It is here where scaling up demands continuous broad-based monitoring and support, giving the community the information, tools, system support, and broad-based encouragement to make significant changes in behaviors and practices in a way that affects the community at large. When small components of the community resist changes, leaders must generate opportunities for highly successful community cohorts to mentor and model their successful management of the change process in a way that encourages those in the community who are less successful.

Scaling might generate evidence that suggests shifts, adjustments, or alterations in the methodology or mechanisms of the deviant changes applied to the whole community. Larger aggregates of data production and analysis can reveal significant opportunities for adjusting past practices and behaviors. Leaders may need to make shifts at critical points in the implementation process. Evidence-based practice demands that when the evidence indicates the emergence of a best practice or a need for a practice change based on a reduction in value, it is possible to change the work and methodologies quickly and seamlessly as a way of doing business. Habits, rituals, and routines may mitigate against these incremental but necessary changes either in various pockets of the community or across the entire community. Built into the processes, scaling up is this implementation and application of an evidence-driven response and incorporating it into new practices and processes. Although the discipline and practice of PD certainly has structure and form, leadership, communication, relationship, and high levels of interaction in the community are highly critical competencies necessary to support and advance commitment, engagement, problem-solving, and advancing viable and sustainable solutions (Benjamin & Buscell, 2017).

CALL TO ACTION

In a group of four to five individuals, select three current policies in your unit or department. Analyze each policy and identify potential positive deviant behaviors as a result of these policies. Are there changes that could be made to update the policies that would improve patient quality or safety? Employee quality or safety? Organizational quality or safety? Develop a plan to propose, gain support, and institute changes to benefit patients, employees, or the organization.

KEY TAKEAWAY POINTS

■ Not all noncompliant behavior is negative; there is value in PD.

■ If the deviance is harmful, then stop!

■ Learn to formally identify PD based on principles and share this phenomenon with others—sooner rather than later!

CASE STUDIES

In this section, relatively straight forward examples of PD are presented to illustrate the activities of PD and the thinking of positive deviants. In the first case study, new pathways in a community park are considered as the PD. Behaviors based on a PD approach to change guide the work of positive deviants rather than the traditional approach to change (for more information, go to https://theachiever2011.wordpress.com/2011/09/16/scout-for-your-secret-change-agents).

CASE STUDY 13.1. **An Alternate Pathway**

Think about your local community and the beautiful parks and landscaping that have been planted to beautify the environment and make recreation accessible. An individual in a hurry comes along and moves off the sidewalk to the grass to get around another person and to move faster to his or her destination. More and more individuals see the pathway through the grass as a better option than the paved sidewalk. Eventually, the pathway through the grass becomes the main travel route and the sidewalk is seldom used (Figure 13.2).

An Invitation to Change

In an informal manner, the invitation to change was the availability of another option to get to one's goal: the grass area near the sidewalk. The availability of an alternate pathway or option is an important consideration in this process. The absence of a ready alternative would require new and different thinking to achieve the goal of decreased time for walking such as using a bicycle or a similar implement.

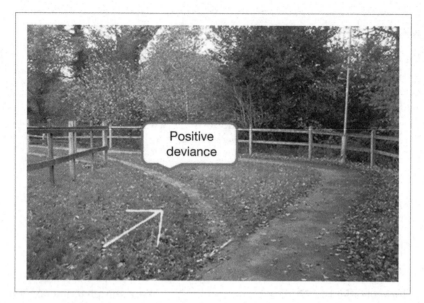

Figure 13.2 Shorter pathways as positive deviance.
Source: Copyright Jonathan Billinger. Retrieved from https://www.geograph.org.uk/photo/6020249

Defining the Problem and Recognizing Positive Deviants

The definition of the problem also occurred informally; namely, individuals wanted to get to destinations more quickly and in a direct manner. These positive deviants continued walking on the new pathway and others followed, knowing the positive outcome.

One reaction to the deviance could be to post signs requesting individuals to stay on the pathway and to block the alternate pathway with ropes and barriers. Be sure this is counterproductive in most situations when a great opportunity lies on the other side of the ropes. Individuals jump the barriers and continue to use the deviant pathway.

CALL TO ACTION

Break a rule today: If you could break one rule today, what would it be? What are the benefits of this broken rule to healthcare or patients?

Designing the Program and Scaling Up

As the community recognizes this alternative pathway, not only at this location but also at many other locations around the community, individuals come together to design a new program for creating walking paths. When new areas are built, sidewalks are not built until the common pathways are created by the users. Then, the sidewalks are created where individuals walk most often. PD now becomes the norm for creating pathways in the community. This practice is scaled up across the community and even throughout the state and nation. This approach and analysis can be applied in numerous situations.

CASE STUDY 13.2. **Healthcare Practices**

> *"Only those who will risk going too far can possibly find out how far one can go."*
> —T. S. Eliot

Consider the work of nursing in which policies require routine vital signs are taken at a specified time, medications given at specific times, or reports submitted in a specified format. In many situations, vital signs are not taken at the specified time because a patient is sleeping, bathing, or involved in another activity. The patient obviously has a blood pressure and is not in any distress. Or, a daily medication scheduled to be given at 8 a.m. is not given until nearly 10 a.m., for similar reasons. No harm to the patient, but the patient could complete tasks—taking a shower and undergoing physical therapy. In fact, the outcome is better than if the patient was required to stop or delay the shower until after medication time or a physical therapy treatment.

Consider, too, the daily reports submitted for inventory accounting. It is known that the reports are not used or reviewed until Monday of each week, yet the daily requirement remains while work requirements continue to increase. It is important to note that positive deviants seldom avoid the deviant practice when there is the probability that the risk is minimal, and the outcomes will be better. The positive deviant recognizes there is always a risk in not following established protocol; however, he or she is able to assess the degree of risk and potential benefit and chooses the benefit when appropriate. In all three situations, PD has occurred.

Although many individuals may have been shifting their practices to these changes, it is not until the community of individuals recognizes and embraces the changes and positive outcomes that the community at large embraces the PD. Scaling up to the system occurs. Policies and practices are considered and strategies to shift policies and practices are then developed to reflect what the community of individuals already knew was a better practice. They had figured it out "inside the box."

In these situations, the invitation to change emerged from the need to either be timelier, allow patients to complete therapies, to continue sleeping, or in the case of the report not used daily, to provide more timely care instead of spending time on a report that would not be missed or used. Often times, the invitations to change occur in subtle ways and positive deviants find themselves asking questions like, why is this necessary, is there a better alternative, and what will happen if I change practice?

The problem, in most cases, is the potential failure to meet patient needs safely in a timely manner. The prescribed precision of taking vital signs at a certain time or delivering medications at a specific time is the problem in these situations. Failure to provide the services at exactly the precise time seldom negatively impacts patient wellness and safety. There is latitude in the time for service that is rarely defined in policy; latitude that a positive deviant is able to determine especially when other events are occurring that would increase the overall benefit to the patient.

An Invitation to Change

The invitation is subtle and emerges from patient needs for care and timeliness. Also, the need is for sleep when an assessment of vital signs is involved.

Defining the Problem

The problem is a policy or practice that lacks sufficient evidence and latitude to provide the best patient care.

Determining the Presence of PD Individuals or Groups

As previously noted, these practice deviations most likely occur quite often in the healthcare community but are seldom acknowledged for fear of punishment for failure to follow established policies. Recognizing the practices and gathering positive deviants in the community to build a case for change is a critical step in changing practices in a formal manner. Interestingly, these kinds of situations are less likely to occur when the individuals involved in the specific practices are included in the design of policies and guidelines. Positive deviants tend to provide the best care when there are guidelines rather than specific policies. For example, medications are provided in a consistent and safe manner rather than medications are given at 10 a.m. Similarly, vital signs are monitored once in 24 hours, unless there is a change in patient comfort or mental status.

Program Design

Designing community policies begins with gathering the individuals who have achieved better results with PD for review of appropriateness of current policies to be sure there are minimal obstructions to providing the safest and most efficient care. Although not labeled as an exercise in PD, the Institute for Healthcare Improvement (IHI) recently sponsored a "Break a Rule for Better Care" in which healthcare workers were challenged to identify "If you could break or change one rule in service of a better care experience for patient or staff, what would it be and why?" More than 240 organizations from 21 countries participated in the IHI global "Breaking the Rules for Better Care" in 2018. This exercise provided guidelines to identify those practices that might be habits rather than policies, individuals in the community with better ideas, and the community receiving care to support a much-needed approach to supporting PD and positive deviants.

Monitoring and Evaluation

Discussion with the healthcare community and individuals providing care should occur on a regular basis. The IHI model provides a great starting point to support this work.

Scaling Up

Expanding the new practices as well as the entire process of supporting PD can move from a small unit to large systems. Further embedding this work in a quality-management program could strengthen the value of this work.

CONCLUSIONS

The work of innovation begins with many sources and is an important knowledge base for all healthcare workers. In this chapter, the nature of PD was presented as an important behavior that can lead to multiple innovations when evaluated and framed as positive acts. As with any innovation, a disciplined approach is necessary for success and recognition by the larger community.

"You must do the thing you think you cannot do." —Eleanor Roosevelt

REFERENCES

Benjamin, S., & Buscell, P. (2017). *Unexpected guests: Solve tough problems with adaptive positive deviance.* Washington, DC: Plexus Institute.

Dorsey, D. (2017). *Positive deviant.* Fast Company. Retrieved from https://www.fastcompany .com/about-us

Gary, J. (2012). *The use of positive deviance to deliver patient-centered care* (Paper 28). Retrieved from http://hdl.handle.net/10950/77

Institute for Healthcare Improvement. (2018). Breaking the rules for better care. Retrieved from http://www.ihi.org/Engage/collaboratives/LeadershipAlliance/Pages/Breaking-the-Rules .aspx

Kelly, T., & Littman, J. (2005). *Ten faces of innovation.* New York, NY: Doubleday.

Parkin, S. (2010). *The positive deviant: Sustainability leadership in a perverse world.* London, England: Earthscan.

Singhal, A., Buscell, P., & Lindberg, C. (2010). *Inviting everyone: Healing healthcare through positive deviance.* Washington, DC: Plexus Presse.

Singhal, A., Buscell, P., & Lindberg, C. (2014). *Inspiring change in saving lives: They positive deviance way.* Washington, DC: Plexus Institute.

Tuhus-Dubrow, R. (2009, November 29). The power of positive deviants: A promising new tactic for changing communities from the inside. *Boston Globe.* Retrieved from http://archive .boston.com/bostonglobe/ideas/articles/2009/11/29/the_power_of_positive_deviants/

Measuring Innovation and Determining Return on Investment

Deborah Mills-Scofield, Sidney Kushner, Stefanie Lyn Kaufman, and Eli MacLaren

"What matters in the new economy is not return on investment, but return on imagination." —Gary Hamel

LEARNING OBJECTIVES

- Understand the complexity of measuring innovation.

- Develop a method to measure innovation within your organization.

- Examine three unique organizations and how they measure their own innovation return on investment.

INTRODUCTION

The debate on how to measure innovation never ceases, regardless of industry or sector. Most organizations use the same metrics they use for more mature and traditional businesses. That can work, but it usually doesn't. As you think about how to get the return on investment (ROI) you want or need from innovation, start thinking differently—change your mind-set, innovate how you measure!

Start by thinking about innovation as not just doing new cool stuff. Let's think about innovation as a form of risk management—risk mitigation, elimination, and, if things don't go as well, risk rescue. In today's world, if you don't innovate, you die. Just look at one of the economic measures of success—the S&P 500. In the 1950s, the average life span of an S&P 500 company was 60 years; today it is under 20 (Credit Suisse, 2017).

Iconic names have dropped off the S&P 500: Sears, Lehman Brothers, Dell, to name a few. GE, which had been on the Dow Jones Industrial Average since 1907, was delisted in June 2018, and the list goes on (e.g., AT&T, General Motors, Hewlett-Packard, etc.). These are companies that, among other things, didn't innovate well. They may have been inventive, but innovating—when you successfully bring inventions that meet real customer needs to the market—is a lot harder and more rare.

🔲 INNOVATION AS INSURANCE

Because innovation is a form of risk management, it's also a type of insurance that protects an organization from dying, being severely, or permanently injured, or obsolete. Innovation has both a positive and negative aspect of insurance. The positive is that if you innovate, you are protecting your organization from someone else cannibalizing your business or becoming irrelevant. By innovating, you are continually looking at how to add more meaningful, real value to your product or service based on the real and pressing needs of your customers. The negative can also be viewed positively. If you innovate and it doesn't work (assuming you didn't totally swing and miss), then maybe that innovation isn't as big a threat as you thought. Innovation initiatives are valuable, even if they don't (all) pan out and even if you don't use all of them. You've still learned a lot about what will and what won't work, and as important, the reason why.

All said, an organization needs to measure innovation, though not necessarily by using the same metrics as more mature, traditional businesses. Finding and using the right metrics is critical and requires time, discussion, and reflection on impact and consequences. What you measure drives behavior, so this needs to be approached carefully and thoughtfully. While in the end you want to measure ROI in some way, it is usually calculated based on many underlying assumptions and measures, not just ROI over some specified time period. Think about why you're measuring—innovation—is it just "ROI"? What do you want to accomplish—communication? Performance? Learning (hint: Big yes!)? Also, make sure your metrics match the degree of innovation you're doing (e.g., incremental, somewhat disruptive, really disruptive). The range of possible things to measure is vast—such as diversity of teams, funding, resource quality, training, R&D (research and development) turnover, investments, percentage of growth coming from innovations, learning, and so on. So, when you're thinking about ROI, think about what metrics you will use, the time frame during which you will use them, and the decisions you'll be making based on those metrics to determine an acceptable ROI. It's not as straightforward as revenue and/or profit over x years.

Metrics are a way to measure performance and mitigate risk. There are a few types of risk: technical, market, execution, and financial. Technical risk occurs whether what you're "making" will work or not—for example, do molecules bend the way you want them to? Speed is key here—**time to market!** Market risk is the risk of product/service acceptance and adoption. Doing extensive bottom-up research and ethnographic studies to understand customers' real needs (not what you want them to need) is critical. Scale matters a lot here, especially if you are addressing the customers' needs really well—and that's **time to volume.** Execution risk is the risk of being able to pull it all off—from the start of creating the product/service through to commercialization, launch, market penetration, and service. Execution has a profound impact on financial risk, also called *putting good money after bad.* Leaders may think "If we just have $x more, it'll work, we can get the right suppliers, we can get the right stores to sell it, we can, we can, we can." This type of thinking can be a slippery slope, which is why you need watchful, honest, unbiased eyes.

One way to determine the right metrics is to think of the traditional factory as a model (Figure 14.1): raw materials come in, they get processed, put into the market, and voilà—results.

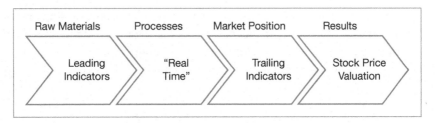

Figure 14.1 The factory model.

RAW MATERIALS: LEADING INDICATORS

A critical lesson in identifying metrics is that you need leading indicators—metrics that tell you when things could be going wrong (or right) before they do. Most metrics trail (or lag)—they become clear after the fact. Lagging indicators can lead to surprises; leading indicators can give more insight earlier in the process. However, leading indicators are usually harder to think of. Also, one person's leading indicator is another person's trailing indicator depending where you are in the factory model. Leading indicators measure:

• Tangibles—Capital and time spent/dedicated to innovation (research and development [R&D] as a percentage of sales), dedicated talent, software, physical infrastructure, equipment, space, quality of tools, resources, skills, research partnerships, number and value of ideas being proposed, and so on

• Intangibles—Talent, external networks, engagement, culture, knowledge, training, brand, reputation, learning and knowledge growth (depth and breadth), and so forth

• Innovation structure—Open innovation networks, venture capital (VC) model, separate group, team diversity, and so on

• Innovation strategy and portfolio management—a mix of incremental, quasidisruptive, disruptive, degree of separation from core strategies, and so on.

PROCESSES: REAL-TIME INDICATORS

Okay, you've got the raw materials, the ingredients needed for innovation. How well do you process what you have? These are your real-time indicators (or near-real time) because you can see how well things are going as you're going! These indicators include how fast and how well you identify required resources and the combination and coordination of those, effectiveness and efficiency of your ideation and vetting process, speed and performance of your processes as intended, implementation execution, time and cost reduction in new product/service/process development over time, actual versus planned cycle times, new patents, and so forth.

MARKET POSITION: TRAILING INDICATORS

These are the "easy" ones. These include metrics like intellectual property and/or licensing, success of new product launches, sales or revenue and profit (overall, per product/service, per employee, per customer, per market, etc.), market share, market creation, market adoption, sales/

profits from each type of innovation in your innovation portfolio, cost of infrastructure versus revenue, new customer acquisition, existing customers trading up, customer loyalty, and so on. Also, though few companies do this, the cost of not innovating (which may show up more next, in results) is a critical metric, and at times hard to calculate.

 ## RESULTS: "STOCK PRICE" AND VALUATIONS

For most organizations, public or private, this is where the rubber meets the road. If your innovations result in increased revenue, profitability (project, product/service, customer), life-cycle value, and so forth, it's a win. Your stock goes up (literally and figuratively). Perhaps your innovations let you charge more (extract more value), or you gain customers. Maybe your existing customers buy more and buy up, or you launch more and more products/services and your launch effectiveness and efficiency improves and the time from idea to your customer's hand decreases. All of these raise the value of your enterprise, and make it easier to attract, retain, and develop top talent, get investment, and continue to meet or exceed customers' needs. These are the indicators that increase value and continue to increase value the better you get at doing them—the most important of which is delighting your customers.

Using metrics like those mentioned previously enable you to collect the data to figure out what ROI is best for your organization and your products and services. Don't just assume you have to use the traditional ones—and in some (many) cases, you may have to make a strong case why the traditional ones are not appropriate. You don't judge the capabilities of a child the same way you do an adult. Be cautious. Too many people assume that the cost of innovation outweighs the benefit—that the status quo prevails. It doesn't (just ask GE today.). Remember, innovation is insurance. Keep an eye out for how the competition, the market, and customers are changing and innovating.

And then there's the wonderful term, *sunk costs*. Well, they're sunk. Gone. Not getting them back—and not worth sending an expedition crew to raise them up to the surface. The desire to leverage sunk costs could result in leveraging something that is or has become irrelevant or obsolete. And remember those young kids innovating in the garage? They don't have any sunk costs!

 ## SO HOW DOES ALL OF THIS GET PUT INTO PRACTICE?

As you read the following three stories of innovation's impact on family health and well-being in Texas, on mental health support and healing, and on children with cancer and their families, you will see how sometimes innovation doesn't have to be complicated, highly technical, or require years spent in a lab before reaching the patients. Sometimes, many times, innovation's healing power is seen through people—normal human beings. You'll also see that a key metric is not just ROI where I = investment, but ROI where I = impact. That's the kind that matters most. And that's what the following three stories will show.

> *"Not everything that can be counted counts, and not everything that counts can be counted."* —Albert Einstein

How the Business Innovation Factory Measures Innovation

By Eli MacLaren, Chief Market Maker at Business Innovation Factory

For 14 years, the Business Innovation Factory (BIF) has been working with leaders in healthcare to make transformational change safer and easier to manage. Our point of view is that innovation exists on a spectrum. On the one hand, there is the well-established science behind incremental improvements. On the other hand, there is the exploratory practice of transformational innovation. Both are important in an innovation portfolio, but both need to be structured differently. Here's why.

Incremental innovation is inherently about improving what is, which can be measured by organizational efficiency. Transformational innovation is a generative act and is ultimately a practice of exploration. The leading cause of death for transformational exploration is when innovation leaders are asked to defend the ROI of exploratory efforts. It is incumbent upon innovation leaders to both structure transformational activities to demonstrate early wins, create new measures and metrics for accountability, and share their learnings early and often to bring others along for the journey. The case study that follows describes how BIF worked with the Children's Health System of Texas (Children's Health), as their innovation team to do just that.

Background

Children's Health, like other medical centers across the country, was seeing an uptake in visits to the ED for nonemergent issues that could be served better and less expensively through primary care. Increasingly, the visitors to the ED were no-pay or Medicaid patients, causing strain on the hospital's financial model. The CEO wondered whether there was a better way to serve this population; he brought in BIF as a consulting partner to help structure this exploration for success. In the 5 years that BIF worked with Children's Health, we created a foundation for innovation that led to incremental and transformational practices while prototyping concepts and new business models. This process led to the commercialization of a well-being-based business model. The core practices that led the organization to success are listed in the following text.

Create a Connected Adjacent

Innovation initiatives are often structured separately from the core operations in an effort to ensure the integrity of the exploration. This has the negative side effect of creating an "us and them" mentality among core operations and innovation leaders. Often described as *skunk works*, these separate initiatives can be perceived as a space where the "cool kids" get to be creative, and raises organizational issues that inhibit new opportunities for change.

To avert this challenge, Children's Health created a "connected adjacent." Although separate from core operations, the innovation space and its core activities were connected back to the core, such that:

- Learnings and "next practices" could be easily communicated to the core staff to improve the way the existing model currently works.

- The innovation team was accessible to the core staff to provide training and to troubleshoot emerging challenges.

- Core staff came along on the innovation exploration, often cocreating solutions based on emerging insights, to create an environment in which change was done "by us" rather than "to us."

The cornerstone of this "connected adjacent" was a piece of foundational research. Taking a human-centered approach, the innovation team sought to understand how families in the greater Dallas area experienced "their health," how they experienced "healthcare," and how they experience accessing the materials, resources, and information to engage in "healthy behaviors." The key insights emerging from this foundation were as follows:

- Children grow up in a system, and that system is the family (broadly defined)—a pediatric health system seeking to serve children needs to do so within the family unit.
- Health does not have an immediate and tangible ROI for children or families (like the output of being a first-generation college-goer), and to engage people in their health requires making health tangible.
- Families desire an overall sense of well-being—as defined as confidence in the right information, a sense of belonging, social support, and personal power (individual agency) in their decisions and behaviors.

From this, the innovation team extracted a series of "jobs to be done"—problems that patients needed solved (Table 14.1).

These insights and jobs to be done served to improve the existing model, and to explore new family well-being business models. But before the team could do that, the innovation team needed to measure and prove that they could have a positive impact on well-being. This required new metrics.

Establish New Metrics

The first new metrics were defined as the Family Well-Being Quotient and measured whether the team could improve family well-being (and if so, why and how). It defined a set of behaviors under each element of wellness, creating a well-defined and illustrative spectrum across each

TABLE 14.1 **Jobs to Be Done**

Element of Wellness	Need	Job to Be Done
Sense of self	Spiritual	Self-awareness: I want to see my potential reflected back to me.
System of support	Social	Supporting relationships: I want to belong and contribute to a community that reflects my values and beliefs.
Personal power	Emotional	Agency: I want opportunities for responsibility, reciprocated trust, and interdependence.
Connected knowledge	Functional	Interpretation: I want to spark my curiosity to explore, translate, make meaning, and choose wisely.
Balanced outlook	Functional	Resourcefulness: I want a stronger ability to understand, seek, and secure the resources I need.

behavior. The spectrum was then translated into a numeric score, and an algorithm was created that tracked changes across each behavior; the algorithm also analyzed the relationships between the factors to understand independent and dependent variables.

The data were collected through self-assessments—completed by individual participants, and survey assessments and qualitative interviews done by the innovation team. The results were then cross-analyzed to define a common assessment for each individual and for each family, an assessment that blended the multiple data sources and added a nuanced context to each of the data sources.

The data were collected in three different increments—before the first round of prototyping to establish a baseline, in the midst of the prototyping, and at the close of each prototype. Two different prototypes were created through the program: (a) What's Cookin' Dallas and (b) Your Best You. Participants went through the same cycle for each prototype.

The data, described in Figure 14.2, show the changes in the youth's sense of well-being, as well as changes in the individual elements of wellness before their engagement in the prototypes and after their engagement. It also shows the changes in the family's overall sense of well-being before and after engagement in the prototypes. Further, we break the data by element of well-being to demonstrate the specific shifts that occurred for youth and families. For example, in assessing people's sense of agency, the shift is specific from the degree to which people feel that they are dependent on others or other forces to improve their health and well-being or the degree to which they have autonomy and independence to achieve positive changes (Figures 14.2–14.7).

The second new metrics came later—after the innovation team was able to demonstrate that the prototypes could change people's sense of well-being. Based on the evidence, the leadership team made a decision to explore a family well-being business model. In this second phase of prototyping, the innovation team prototyped the entire business model, and the evidence

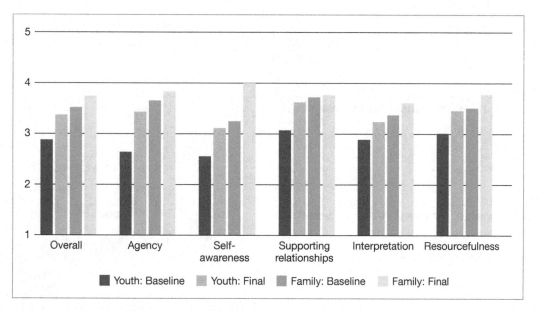

Figure 14.2 Well-being prototype. Elements of wellness.

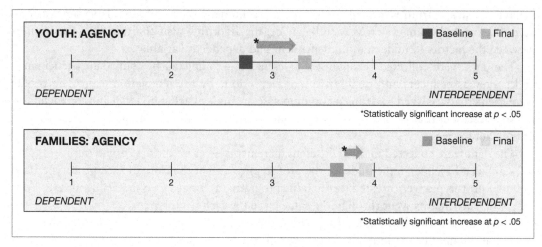

Figure 14.3 Agency.

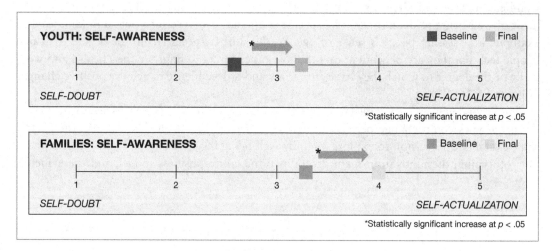

Figure 14.4 Self-awareness.

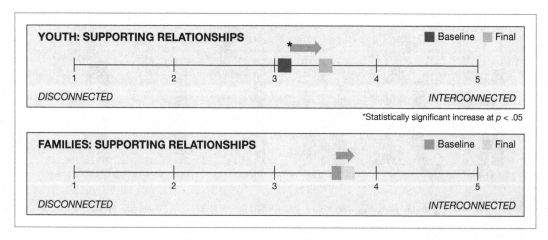

Figure 14.5 Supporting relationships.

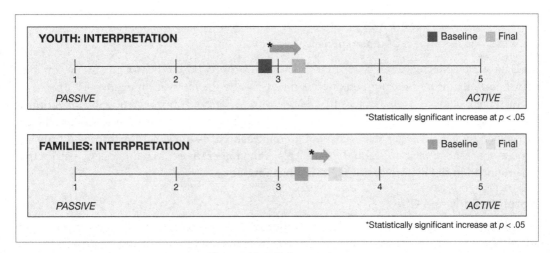

Figure 14.6 Interpretation.

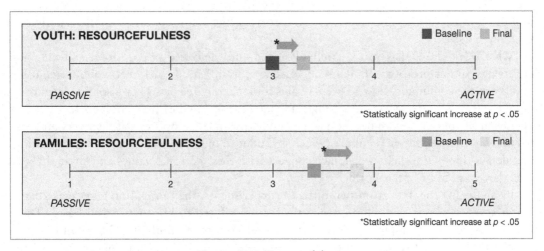

Figure 14.7 Resourcefulness.

required to commercialize was based on the quality of the experience. To do so, we needed to know the answers to these questions:

- Could we create a compelling experience that engaged individuals in their personal and family well-being?
- Could we deliver on that experience by combining capabilities in new and different ways?
- Did this experience improve well-being?
- What impact did improving well-being have on signaling health data outcomes, for example, compliance with diabetes control?

To measure the answers to these questions, we developed a model derived from a traditional Kirkpatrick Model with four tiers of learning:

- Do people enjoy the experience?
- Did they learn from the experience?

- Did they change behaviors as a result of that experience?
- What was the impact of that experience?

Data were collected weekly during the 12-week prototype, both through surveys by individual participants and through qualitative interviews by the innovation team.

Incremental innovation is measured based on efficiency. Transformational innovation is about exploration, and therefore cannot be measured based on what is known and/or efficiencies gained by what is. That said, it cannot go unmeasured, as the lack of metrics will translate into an open-ended lack of accountability. This is the imperative for creating new metrics that are grounded in the hypotheses of the experimentation.

Prototype Early and Often

To reduce the risk of transformational innovation, the innovation team had to measure impact and ROI from different angles. This helps the team understand the differences between correlation and causation in the experiments. To this end, prototyping early and often was core to success. The first two prototypes, described in the following text, tested different approaches to improving family well-being. They were, in theory, testing a concept and hypothesis and not a solution in itself.

What's Cookin' Dallas was a family-designed and -delivered pop-up food and nutrition experience. In this prototype, families operated a "pop-up" food truck that would teach other families in the community how to prepare and cook healthy recipes. They also organized community trips to supermarkets—teaching individuals and families how to shop for low-cost healthy meal options. You're Best You was a family-designed "camp" for self-discovery and contribution. It married hip-hop culture (which is grounded in self-reflection and self-exploration) and design thinking to help individuals connect with their personal values and strengths, and who they want to be in the world.

By analyzing the data from two different experiments, the innovation team was able to better assess the how and what of relevant factors related to improving well-being. These prototypes provided ample evidence that we could improve family well-being and how to do it. Key learnings became next practices for the community health team and became the basis for the next prototype. The next prototype moved beyond point solutions, to test the entire desirability, feasibility, and viability of a new family well-being-centered business model.

Many organizations have "bolted on" well-being efforts to their existing business model under the hypothesis that improving health would improve well-being. The Children's Health prototype put well-being at the core, testing the inverted hypothesis that if we improved well-being, we would improve health. This model assumed that we had to address the social determinants of health, and recognized that Children's Health did not have the necessary capabilities to do this. However, they could deliver value by creating an integrator function. To this end, Children's Health contracted with social service agencies to address the social determinants of health, paying a portion of the premium dollar in exchange for their services. At the time, Children's Health had developed a new insurance capability, and was enrolling patients. This gave them flexibility to play with the premium dollar in new ways.

The prototype tested (a) whether the value proposition resonated strongly with customers, (b) whether Children's Health could successfully contract with social service agencies for an individual versus a population, and (c) what impact the program had on health outcomes (as assessed by signaling, not confirming data).

Develop a Storytelling Practice

The underlying practice that enabled this exploration is storytelling. Storytelling took a variety of forms:

- The innovation team digitally captured emerging insights and turned them into patient "testimonies" that helped leaders and core staff shift their lens, witnessing the healthcare experience through the stories and voices of patients.
- It turned key insights into animated graphics that engendered empathy and the ability to relate to their patients' experiences—while suspending judgment.
- It created digital opportunity spaces that helped staff understand possibilities in a future-facing, exciting (nonthreatening way).
- It translated stories into meaningful data such that staff and leaders were prepared to make a case for further exploration in an evidence-based culture.

This practice both engendered buy-in and attracted the necessary resources (both financial and political) that enabled the work to grow and thrive.

Conclusions

After this exploration, the Family Well-Being Quotient was taken to scale through the population health division of Children's Health. Children's Health used an agile methodology to help the staff incorporate next practices and effectively redefine and rewire their existing capabilities to deliver value to patients in new ways. The connected approach to innovation created an inclusive environment in which staff sought to support and explore with the innovation team rather than be threatened by it. Building a storytelling practice helped the organization as a whole to shift its lens, get excited by new and emerging insights, and participate in the journey, versus observing it. New metrics held the integrity of transformational innovation, while also helping the core staff understand what they could do immediately to better serve patients. Prototyping early and often provided meaningful data that engendered continued support and resourcing.

Every good innovation portfolio requires a mix of strategy that improves how the model currently works and leads to transformational opportunities. It also requires a culture of inclusion and transparency—the product of working out loud and sharing compelling stories. The challenge is not that transformational innovation is scary or riskier than incremental innovation. The opportunity is to catalyze a class of leaders who have the skills, tools, and mind-sets to structure transformation successfully.

 CALL TO ACTION

Don't rely on existing metrics; create your own indicators to assess exploratory innovation. Test hypotheses and not just potential solutions. Consider how learnings can improve the way the existing model works *and* acts as a springboard into new models.

HOW PROJECT LETS MEASURES INNOVATION

By Stefanie Lyn Kaufman, Founder of Project LETS

What Is the Problem?

During my freshman year at Brown University, I scotch-taped part of my leg back together after a severe self-harm episode to prevent being forced on medical leave and losing my place in academia. I wasn't alone. Many peers were afraid to use university mental health resources because they didn't know what the explicit policies were for issues like self-harm, suicidal ideation, psychosis, and eating disorders. Ambiguous policies—and stories about students who experienced forced hospitalization, constant surveillance, and mandated leaves from school—made students hesitant to disclose their concerns to the administration or university mental health centers. Oftentimes, students who did try to seek help were unable to see a therapist because on-campus centers were booked for months at a time, and off-campus providers were too expensive. Other friends did not find traditional forms of mental healthcare to be especially culturally relevant to them, and struggled to connect with therapists who did not understand critical parts of their identities.

These policies institute fear and take power and autonomy away from students. On top of these institutional power imbalances and issues, rates of mental illness among college students are at a record high (National Alliance on Mental Illness, 2012). Individuals with mental illness face societal stigma, discrimination, and oppression—which is known as *ableism*—and many barriers exist within the current model of mental healthcare that prevent people from attempting to and actually being able to access care.

Why Project LETS?

Project LETS ("Let's End the Stigma") believes that we are the experts of our own narratives and lived experiences, and the solution to problems lies in services delivered by peers, for peers. We are composed of mentally ill, disabled, and neurodivergent individuals who lift each other and surrounding communities up in the hopes of achieving more accessible and culturally competent mental healthcare. Our model is built on trust, partnership, mutual decision-making, and transparency. We actively work to give power back to the students we work with, and therefore make it a top priority to create a safe place for students to talk about heavily feared and stigmatized topics.

I founded Project LETS in 2009, following the suicide of my friend and peer, Brittany Marie Petrocca. Initially, our work was focused on high school-based awareness—but quickly developed into advocacy-based programming and service delivery. In 2013, after incorporating as a nonprofit and launching the Project LETS International Crisis Line, our team realized immediate crisis intervention was only one small piece of the puzzle. We began researching programs and interventions that sought to connect those in crisis to longer term, follow-up care. In early 2014, Project LETS began offering one-on-one peer-counseling services to individuals from all over the world. Following the success of this model, and a conversation held with a student at Brown University, the Peer Mental Health Advocate (PMHA) program was born.

One day, I was helping to connect a struggling student to university resources. The next week, she asked whether I could possibly connect her to someone who was in recovery from an eating disorder. Though she saw a therapist and nutritionist, she said, "*There are so many other hours in the week. And I'd really like to see how someone else is surviving.*" After that day, I connected her to another student I knew in recovery, and their relationship became an important model for us. After that, I started building our curricular model so we could make these connections on a much larger scale at Brown.

As an organization, we prioritize the concept and core value of disability justice: We look at and recognize the intersecting histories of supremacy, colonialism, capitalism, gender oppression, and ableism, and really understanding how people's bodies and minds are labeled unproductive or disposable. In our PMHA program, we pair students with lived experiences with students who are struggling. They are doing one-on-one emotional-support work, peer counseling, but also advocacy work. A PMHA will show up to a meeting on your behalf, talk to the administrator, make phone calls for you, call your insurance company, and/or do background research. Advocates do a lot of the nitty-gritty advocacy and logistical work that is so hard for people who are struggling. We work with folks to remind them about their appointments or help them figure out the logistics of medical leave.

The core of our training curriculum comes from state-level Certified Peer Recovery Specialist (CPRS) training and Intentional Peer Support (IPS). From here, we derive the job responsibilities, ethics, and main roles of a peer supporter (Box 14.1). Additional training components were developed by the Project LETS Team, and work to prioritize a social-Justice lens and antioppression framework as well as social models of disability and history of psychiatry.

Impact/Results/Outcomes: How Do We Measure Success?

"I think the bottom line is you have to organize. And I think that's the same path a lot of groups have had to use to get heard, to get seen, to get care, to get something to happen for them." —Will Meek, Brown University, Director of Counseling and Psychological Services

---

Box 14.1 Main Responsibilities of PMHAs

What are the main responsibilities of PMHAs?

- Create personalized safety/relapse prevention plans.
- Send reminders about medication and appointments.
- Cultivate your peers' ability to make informed, independent choices.
- Help your peers identify and build on their strengths.
- Support your peer in accessing help/resources and learning how to interact with the healthcare system.
- Answer questions about mental illness to develop confidence and reduce stress.
- Provide support in times of struggle and crisis.
- Provide information relating to coping mechanisms and how to maintain healing.
- Assist your peers in gaining information and support from the community to make their goals a reality.

PMHA, peer mental health advocates.

Source: Project LETS. (2018). *Project LETS: 2018 Update.* [Internal Document]. Brown University, Providence, RI.

Since officially launching our pilot program at Brown University in 2015, Project LETS has trained 200+ PMHAs across multiple universities, and connected over 140 student peers with PMHAs. We have 105+ direct leaders across 20+ campus chapters throughout the United States who have engaged in various critical advocacy and educational programming outside of our direct peer counseling model.

Peers feel that they have gained skills in critical areas. With regard to the post evaluation taken at the 6-month mark:

- Ninety percent of peers report an increase in their knowledge of, and ability to utilize, coping skills.
- Sixty percent of students report an increase in their quality of life.
- Sixty-five percent of students report an increase in their ability to manage self-destructive behaviors/suicidal thoughts.
- Seventy percent report feeling more confident in their ability to handle crises.
- Sixty percent report an increase in their help-seeking behaviors.

We measure our success through the effectiveness of individual PMHA–peer relationships, as well as the demand for our program. We track the adhesion of a specific program by evaluating the volume of applications from individuals who want to work as a PMHA (and their demographic characteristics), and applications from students who want to work with a PMHA.

We monitor the effectiveness of our training and programming by evaluating PMHA training pre/posttest, initial PMHA requests, peer's preevaluations, bimonthly check-ins/evaluation surveys (peers using the program and PMHAs) and notes/documentation from our PMHAs. We measure key metrics such as changes in quality of life and behavioral health, help-seeking behaviors, crisis response, size of support system, coping skills-building, self-destructive behaviors/suicidal ideation or attempts, and self-worth/self-esteem. We also compare how folks rate their feelings of agency, safety, and power in PMHA relationships versus institutional, medicalized, and/or state-sanctioned "support" in addition to quality of care.

Without PMHAs, students are more likely to drop out of their academic programs. Some students will never seek professional help, but they will talk to a peer. When students connect with trained peers, they are more likely to stay in school. We help students get connected to professional resources and navigate a system they would have never gotten to in the first place.

As shown in Figure 14.8, our PMHA–peer relationships are having a marked impact in three main areas: **crisis preparation** (20% has a crisis plan before, compared to 95%); **increase in help-seeking behaviors/comfort** using university and community resources (51%–80%); and a **decrease in how their mental health issues impact** their ability to "function" (67%–40%). Additionally, in our pre-evaluation measurements, 73% of students listed a friend or pet as their primary form of mental healthcare/support. At the 6-month mark, 65% of individuals listed their PMHA or a professional/community resource as their primary form of support.

Here are some samples of feedback from peers using our program:

- *"I'm no longer scared of entering places on campus that trigger me. Even just creating a safety plan has been really reassuring. I'm better asking for help when I need it and knowing the language I need to talk about what I'm going through."*

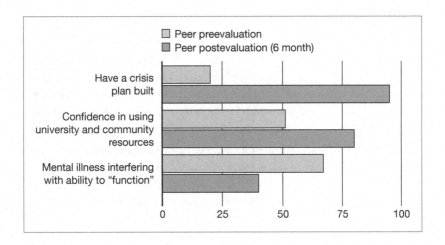

Figure 14.8 PMHA peer pre- and postevaluation.
PMHA, peer mental health advocate.

- *"I think I learned a lot about how to be more interdependent, when before I used to be very unwilling to ask for any sort of help. I also created a crisis plan and with the help of my PMHA began to realize a lot more about my thinking patterns and behaviors."*

- *"When I worked with my PMHA, I was able to regulate my studies and manage myself better. I was more conscious of the medical leave reapplication deadlines, therefore able to successfully submit to the university before the deadline. This was integral in me returning to Brown. Though I was seeing a therapist, my PMHA was useful in pinpointing academic and emotional issues I had in the past at Brown and how to deal with those in the future (especially as it relates to my first-generation identity). My PMHA also connected me with a student who successfully returned from leave, which was incredibly helpful."*

What we did not expect was how impactful the PMHA training process and curriculum itself would be for our students. Upon training evaluation, we found that:

- Ninety-three percent feel more confident in their ability to help themselves with their mental health struggles.

- Ninety-four percent feel more confident in their ability to help others with their mental health struggles.

- Eighty-six percent felt more confident in their ability to navigate Brown University's and the community's resources.

Here are some samples of feedback from our 2016 cohort:

- *"Overall, this training has made me realize the lack of an effective support system I had when I was at my lower points of my mental health, and it has prompted me to journal more in order to reflect on the topics discussed in training in relation to my own life. PMHA training helped me reframe and concretize my own recovery narrative and my relationship to self-care, and has reminded me of the power of warmth and nonjudgment in all my inter-actions, with friends, family, and strangers."*

- *"I learned that my relapses are part of me . . . a part of me that I must embrace and take responsibility for. I learned that when recounting my own experience I often tell my story from a second-person perspective, in an attempt to disentangle myself from the pain. This is something I have been able to catch and change, and in doing so I have experienced much less cognitive dissonance. I also learned that I had a substance use disorder, and I still experience cravings, intrusive thoughts, and drastic mood swings. Acknowledging these aspects of my psyche has allowed for more personal growth."*

- *"I learned new ways to consider my own 'recovery story', how to interact with myself when dealing with my own symptoms (be more forgiving), and about ways to seek help/maintain a more positive attitude and approach (be less helpless). I also feel drastically more prepared to deal with a crisis situation should I find myself in one—something that I know from personal experience is of the utmost importance."*

What we've found to be most incredible is the impact that PMHA–peer relationships also have on the PMHA. A series of quotes from Dana, a peer—and Lacy, her PMHA (who worked together for 2+ years) follows:

- *"I was skeptical that anything could help, but I finally resorted to applying for a PMHA through Project LETS. From our first meeting, Lacy (my peer mental health advocate) has cared for me with such kindness and an understanding that I have yet to find in anyone else. She genuinely affirms my feelings because she, too, lives through similar challenges. We fuel each other to carry on despite our struggles, and I now know that I never have to struggle alone."*—Dana, peer

- *"It is difficult to explain exactly how powerful my experience working with Dana has been. There have been times when I've struggled to leave my room, to feed myself, to begin my day, but if Dana needed to meet with me, there was almost a reserve that I could tap into that can only be described as the strength of community care. Dana has cared for me every bit as much as I have cared for her; I don't think I've left a meeting with her without feeling more restored, hopeful, and better prepared to care for myself."*—Lacy, PMHA

PMHAs like Lacy can provide skills to help their peers more easily navigate the mental healthcare system and offer consistent social support in which they can be honest about their experiences. The partnership and bond developed helps break down internalized stigma for both individuals, highlighting the immense power in that "me, too," moment, especially when you're dealing with a topic that so often makes people feel very vulnerable. It attributes value to the peer counselor's experiences with mental illness, and allows the PMHAs to use the experiential knowledge they've gained to make a positive change in somebody else's life. This is unique because so often we're told our mental illnesses are only something to overcome, and aren't anything to be proud of.

We also began measuring the number of peers (individuals using our program) who then applied to become PMHAs. To date, we have trained 16 peers to become PMHAs—which to the Project LETS team is an incredible sign of impact. A student who was once in a position of feeling scared, isolated, and without resources now feels he or she can pass along information, be a mentor for and advocate for another individual. What could be better than that?

- *"I had an incredible PMHA. Her impact made me want to impact someone else the same way by offering my time, expertise, and resources. I hope to gain a few new friends on campus and a sense of impact as both a mentor and an activist."*

- *"Having a PMHA to talk to, who was much closer in age than a psychologist, was really beneficial because they understood firsthand about the difficulties. It felt great to finally be able to talk to someone that I could consider a friend about my mental illness particularly because I had never told anyone outside of my family. I really want to help others and guide them through college as my PMHA did for me."*

- *"I understand the impacts a PMHA can have on a student who is struggling, as mine did when I was struggling with my own mental health. I believe I have a lot to offer and share—and I also believe I have so much to learn from my potential future peers."*

How Can Other Organizations Apply Our Style?

Over the years, we have increased our reliance on quantitative measurements, which are absolutely essential to measure impact. We have also continued to use qualitative measurements, storytelling, narrative sharing, and open-ended feedback that is then coded, using technologies such as NVivo. It is essential to integrate both quantitative and qualitative measurements into an impact assessment. Without both, you will never truly get the full picture.

It has been important for us to be creative in terms of *where* and *how* we are making impact. For example, it is of critical importance for Project LETS to prioritize working with the most marginalized, targeted, and at-risk members of our communities—most often, LGBTQ+ BIPOC (Black, indigenous, people of color) with highly stigmatized illnesses. To this end, we also monitor the percentage of multiple marginalized folks who served as an indicator of program accessibility—ensuring we are not primarily serving cisgender, heterosexual, White folks with depression or anxiety. Here is a look at our "illness category" breakdown from spring 2018—and our demographic change from fall 2017 to spring 2018 at Brown University (looking at indicators of POC, LGBTQ+ folks, and students who are the first generation in their families to go to college applying to be PMHAs in Figures 14.9 and 14.10).

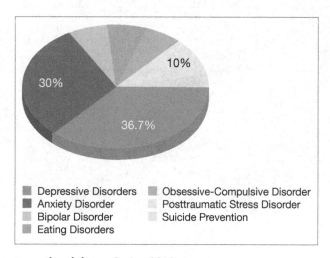

Figure 14.9 Illness category breakdown: Spring 2018.

Source: Data from Project LETS. (2018). *Project LETS: 2018 Update.* [Internal Document]. Brown University, Providence, RI.

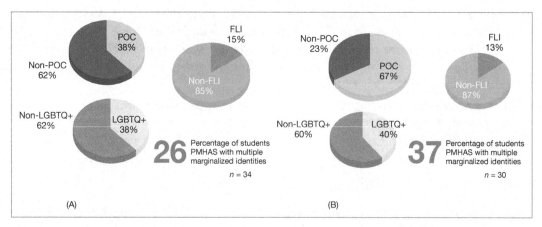

Figure 14.10 Demographic change among students applying to be PMHAs: (A) fall 2017, (B) spring 2018.

FLI, first-generation and/or low-income; PMHA, peer mental health advocate; POC, people of color.

Source: Data from Project LETS. (2018). *Project LETS: 2018 Update.* [Internal Document]. Brown University, Providence, RI.

EXHIBIT 14.1 **Project LETS Testimonial**

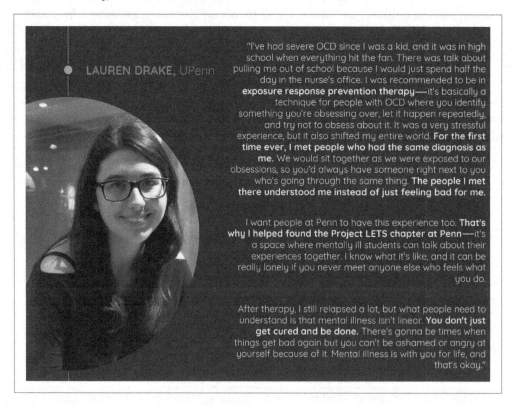

LAUREN DRAKE, UPenn

"I've had severe OCD since I was a kid, and it was in high school when everything hit the fan. There was talk about pulling me out of school because I would just spend half the day in the nurse's office. I was recommended to be in **exposure response prevention therapy**—it's basically a technique for people with OCD where you identify something you're obsessing over, let it happen repeatedly, and try not to obsess about it. It was a very stressful experience, but it also shifted my entire world. **For the first time ever, I met people who had the same diagnosis as me.** We would sit together as we were exposed to our obsessions, so you'd always have someone right next to you who's going through the same thing. **The people I met there understood me instead of just feeling bad for me.**

I want people at Penn to have this experience too. **That's why I helped found the Project LETS chapter at Penn**—it's a space where mentally ill students can talk about their experiences together. I know what it's like, and it can be really lonely if you never meet anyone else who feels what you do.

After therapy, I still relapsed a lot, but what people need to understand is that mental illness isn't linear. **You don't just get cured and be done.** There's gonna be times when things get bad again but you can't be ashamed or angry at yourself because of it. Mental illness is with you for life, and that's okay."

OCD, obsessive-compulsive disorder.

Source: Data from Project LETS. (2018). *Project LETS: 2018 Update.* [Internal Document]. Brown University, Providence, RI.

HOW CONNECTING CHAMPIONS MEASURES INNOVATION

By Sidney Kushner, Executive Director & Founder, Connecting Champions

What's the Problem?

Approximately 15,780 children are diagnosed with cancer every year in the United States. Although nearly 85% are surviving medically (American Childhood Cancer Organization, n.d.), almost two thirds of these children have serious, long-term psychosocial effects that can last decades after treatment. Compared to their noncancer peers, children with cancer have lower graduation rates, higher rates of chronic depression, and up to two times the rate of suicide. Research indicates that many child cancer patients face severe loneliness, heightened psychological distress, issues with self-concept and self-esteem, body-image issues, and identity-formation issues (Bruce, 2006; Cantrell & Ruble, 2011). Long-term social support is the backbone of a healthy transition away from clinical treatment but is one of the most lacking resources in healthcare (Stam, Grootenhuis, & Last, 2005). As families and studies suggest, cancer isn't just an attack on one's health; it's an attack on one's childhood. That's why the nonprofit Connecting Champions was created.

Why Connecting Champions?

When Sidney Kushner, Connecting Champions' founder, was a 16-year-old in high school, his friend was diagnosed with a rare cancer. She was immediately pulled out of school and, over the next 2 years, he was only able to share periodic updates throughout her cancer journey. One question that kept ringing through Sidney's mind was, "What can I do to be a helpful friend right now for someone who's clearly going through such a difficult journey?" His friend passed away a year-and-a-half later, but that question stayed with him as he enrolled at Brown University to study applied mathematics and biology.

Outside of his classes, he shadowed doctors and volunteered with children who have cancer. He met Jenny, a 9-year-old cancer patient who'd recently braved a tough cycle of chemotherapy. When Sidney saw her in the hospital, Jenny had been out of school for months and it was time for the next step of her journey—a bone marrow transplant. Jenny was terrified.

When they first met, Sidney asked Jenny, "What do you want to be when you grow up?" Her eyes immediately lit up as she said she wanted to be a dancer. He could tell, in that moment, Jenny totally forgot about cancer, and was just a kid again. Though their time together that day was cheerful, when it was time for Sidney to leave, Jenny became very serious: "I'm afraid my friends will forget about me because I have cancer." Hearing that, from a 9-year-old girl, was heartbreaking. Being out of school for so long, away from her friends, no longer with hair, and not able to dance—Jenny was afraid that she would be forgotten. That fear of falling off the map is pervasive in pediatric oncology. Connecting Champions hears it from many kids, parents, doctors, and hospital staff. It's echoed throughout research papers. When it comes to childhood cancer, an essential piece to the puzzle is missing.

Jenny inspired Sidney to find it.

Setting medical school aside, he turned to social entrepreneurship. "My grandma was a social worker, and she is my hero. I wanted to be just like her," he said, smiling. He founded

Connecting Champions in 2011 during his sophomore year at Brown and launched a pilot program in New England in 2012. After graduating in 2013, he moved the organization's headquarters to Pittsburgh, his hometown. Today, over 90% of child cancer patients in the region are referred to Connecting Champions. Ninety-seven percent of children are achieving positive developmental outcomes. The organization's outcomes-driven program is making waves in the field of pediatric oncology, and national expansion is on the horizon.

What Is Connecting Champions?

Connecting Champions is a mentoring organization for children with cancer that centers around the question, "What do you want to be when you grow up?" By providing a mentor through the cancer journey and transition back into the community, Connecting Champions proven model bridges the developmental gap between kids with cancer and their peers. As a continuously learning organization, every one of their initiatives can be traced back to a need expressed by a family, hospital staff member, or published research study.

As Chief Pediatric Oncologist Linda McAllister (Universiy of Pittsburgh Medical Center [UPMC] Children's Hospital of Pittsburgh) shared, Connecting Champions built "initiatives that significantly improve the quality of life for our patients." In 2015, it offered a historic partnership, integrating Connecting Champions' innovative child-development approach into the hospital care team. Children's Hospital included the organization in its budget, making Connecting Champions the first nonhospital organization to ever receive such support. Connecting Champions' program staff is composed of elementary educators—individuals expert in understanding the developmental needs of children of all ages. With their background in child development, they created three quantitative and qualitative rubrics to assess developmental challenges and drive outcomes not otherwise achieved in pediatric oncology. The program staff works with the child, parents, and hospital staff for up to 6 weeks to complete an initial assessment, establishing a baseline before setting a developmental goal. They then find a mentor in the child's field of interest and foster a developmentally significant friendship throughout the cancer journey.

With his background in applied mathematics, Sidney built outcomes-reporting software that collects data daily and automatically aggregates outcomes for every child. As a low-cost, deep-impact nonprofit, the organization's investment in outcomes allows it to drive impact competitive with much larger organizations. Connecting Champions has the rare ability to provide virtually unlimited hours of support (historically as many as 300) for children who critically need it. This unprecedented amount of care—especially within a healthcare setting—allows the organization to gather information about each child that no one else can or does in the hospital. By doing so, the hospital staff also rely on their data and expertise to better treat each child.

Instead of walking into the room asking the child about cancer or performing procedures, Connecting Champions' staff are often the only people walking into the child's room as friends first who visit the children regularly (weekly, monthly, etc.) to facilitate positive developmental moments. These range from cooking a meal with a local head chef, to chatting about what to study in college, to finding Waldo together during the long hours of treatment. One of the teens, Chloe, loved baseball but didn't feel she was in a place to think about what she wanted to study in college. Connecting Champions paired her with Ty Brooks, then assistant to the general manager of the Pittsburgh Pirates. Three years later, Chloe enrolled in Fordham University's School of Sports Business to become a baseball executive like Ty. Their friendship continues long after Chloe beat cancer, and Chloe continued to pursue her passion to become a baseball executive.

Results/Outcomes

Since 2013, Connecting Champions has paired over 130 children with mentors from 35 different careers—ballerinas, space technologists, chefs, train conductors, ghost hunters, and many in between. Parents have shared how Connecting Champions helps their children beat depression, find self-esteem, create plans for life after cancer, and build the confidence to take their hats off in public. After years researching in the field, Connecting Champions identified three core developmental challenges that kids with cancer and their families expressed (Figure 14.11).

1. **Family coping and parent support:** The ability for children and their families to effectively cope with the medical, social, and emotional challenges of the disease

2. **Having essential social and developmental experiences:** The ability for a child to continue reaching the developmental milestones he or she should be reaching had there been no cancer diagnosis

3. **Developing a postcancer life plan:** The ability for children to be prepared to reintegrate into school (primary, secondary, college), activities, social groups, and the community upon being declared cancer free

Through an initial developmental assessment (used as a baseline) and regular 3-month progress reports, Connecting Champions applies its quantitative and qualitative rubrics to assess the three main developmental challenges faced by Connecting Champions. Each outcome area is rated on a scale of 0 to 3, with 0 indicating no developmental need present and three indicating severe developmental need present.

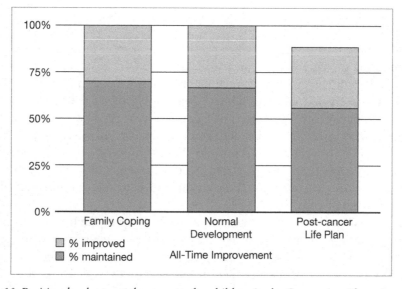

Figure 14.11 Positive developmental outcomes for children in the Connecting Champions program.

Research suggests that, when a child is diagnosed with cancer, development not only freezes, but often reverses. However:

- Ninety-six percent of children in Connecting Champions' program experienced "no regression" in the developmental areas listed earlier.
- Sixty-five percent of children in the program "improved" developmentally.

These overwhelmingly positive outcomes led UPMC to develop its historic partnership with the organization. Other children's hospitals around the country have put together implementation teams to bring Connecting Champions to their patients in the coming years. As one 17-year-old girl in the program sums it up, "[my mentors in Connecting Champions] gifted me not only their friendship but also a whole new outlook on life. To be quite honest, they gave me my will to live back. They gave me hope when there seemed to be no use in having any anymore."

 CALL TO ACTION

So often kids are asked the exact same questions: "How are you feeling? What did you do today?" A good question is a gift, especially during times of isolation from friends and normalcy.

Write down three creative questions for a 5-year-old, three for a 12-year-old, and three for a 17-year-old (e.g., "If you could have anything big or small right now, what would it be? What was the most exciting part of your week? If your feelings were like the weather, what weather would they be?").

 SUMMARY

Through these three powerful stories, we hope you've learned how innovation makes an impact on bettering so many lives in the healthcare world. It doesn't have to be complicated or complex. It doesn't have to always include technology, Food and Drug Administration (FDA) approvals, years in a lab with clinical trials, molecules bending in all sorts of new ways, or even a plethora of patents. The common denominator to all these stories is people—people who understand and deliver on the power of systems-level approaches. If you don't focus on the real critical customers' needs and have the right people working with customers to solve those needs, you can safely assume your ROI^2 won't be good—neither your return on investment (ROInvestment) nor your return on impact (ROImpact), which go hand in hand.

Connecting Champions is a great illustration of ROI^2. Many cancer treatments focus on medical outputs, such as the number of patients treated, percentage of patients in remission, mortality rates, recurrences, and so on. Clearly, these are critical metrics and ones that directly feed into the ROInvestment of the treatment to patients and the pharmaceutical firms. Connecting Champions focuses on other critical metrics, ones that give children receiving cancer treatment and their families a better quality of life such as the ability to cope better, the opportunity to continue reaching key developmental milestones, and the resources to develop a postcancer life plan. These metrics matter for achieving a positive ROImpact, which greatly impacts not only the child and family but also the ROInvestment of the medical treatment itself.

All three stories demonstrate that determining ROI is critical to both kinds of ROI. The best measures of innovation factor in both kinds of ROI. ROImpact and ROInvestment look like a college kid with obsessive-compulsive disorder (OCD), depression, anxiety, and so on, who is able to stay in school, define success on her or his own terms, graduate and positively impact others' lives; a family who is eating healthy foods, reducing blood pressure and sugars, and keeping family members out of the hospital; a young kid with cancer who gets to pursue her passion alongside her mentor, a world-famous chef. As you pursue your organizational innovations, spend the time upfront to identify the key metrics for ROI^2 success. It will make all the difference—especially in the lives of those you care for.

> *"Somebody once told me, 'Manage the top line, and the bottom line will follow.' What's the top line? It's things like, why are we doing this in the first place? What's our strategy? What are customers saying? How responsive are we? Do we have the best products and the best people? Those are the kind of questions you have to focus on."* —Steve Jobs

🔑 KEY TAKEAWAY POINTS

■ Innovation and the measurement of innovation do not have to be highly technical or complex.

■ When measuring innovation, consider both the return on investment and the return on impact.

■ Don't rely on existing metrics; create your own indicators to assess exploratory innovation.

■ Consider how learning can improve the way the existing model works and act as a springboard onto new models.

■ The power behind measuring any outcome is asking the right question.

REFERENCES

American Childhood Cancer Organization. (n.d.). US Childhood cancer statistics. Retrieved from https://www.acco.org/us-childhood-cancer-statistics/

Bruce, M. (2006). A systematic and conceptual review of posttraumatic stress in childhood cancer survivors and their parents. *Clinical Psychology Review, 26,* 233–256. doi:10.1016/j.cpr.2005.10.002

Cantrell, M. A., & Ruble, K. (2011). Multidisciplinary care in pediatric oncology. *Journal of Multidisciplinary Healthcare, 4,* 171–181. doi:10.2147/JMDH.S7108

Credit Suisse. (2017). Corporate longevity: Index turnover & corporate performance. Retrieved from https://plus.credit-suisse.com/rpc4/ravDocView?docid=V6y0SB2AF-WEr1ce

National Alliance on Mental Illness. (2012). College students speak: A survey report on mental health. Retrieved from https://www.nami.org/About-NAMI/Publications-Reports/Survey -Reports/College-Students-Speak_A-Survey-Report-on-Mental-H.pdf

Project LETS. (2018). *Project LETS: 2018 Update*. [Internal Document]. Brown University, Providence, RI.

Stam, H., Grootenhuis, M., & Last, B. (2005). The course of life of survivors of childhood cancer. *Psychooncology, 14,* 227–238.

15

Design Thinking for Healthcare Leadership and Innovation

Jess Roberts and Suratha Elango

"Have no fear of perfection—you'll never reach it." —Salvador Dali

LEARNING OBJECTIVES

- Define *design thinking* and describe its role in healthcare leadership, innovation, and practice.
- Develop an understanding of how design thinking relates to, and complements, other effective management and practice approaches.
- Develop comfort in and a way to navigate ambiguity and unknowns.
- Describe strategies for successful implementation of design principles and practices within your own practice/organization.

INTRODUCTION

Design thinking is an action-oriented problem-solving framework. As such, let's start with a quick exercise.

CALL TO ACTION

Take 2 minutes and list as many uses as you can think of for a paper clip. Don't overthink the request, simply list anything that comes to your mind (and don't look ahead).

So, how many did you come up with? This alternative-uses test is a relatively common way to gauge an individual's creativity and ability to think divergently. According to a study by Sir Ken Robinson, the majority of people will come up with 10 to 15 ideas (Abbasi, 2011). If you came up with more than 15 ideas, you are very much in the minority as a longitudinal study done by George Land in 1968 found that although 98% of kindergarteners scored at a genius level on a similar test, only 2% of adults were able to do the same (Land, 2011).

At the core of design thinking, or human-centered design, is the ability to reframe persistent challenges and their potential solutions, in other words build a competency for creativity. In fact, it could be argued that the greatest threat to addressing the most persistent 21st-century problems in healthcare is not a lack of interest, resources, or will, but instead a chronic lack of creativity. Tim Brown of IDEO, who brought design thinking to the masses in a 2008 *Harvard Business Review (HBR)* article, noted, "thinking like a designer can transform the way you develop products, services, processes and even strategy" (Brown, 2008, p. 85). Although design thinking isn't a magic bullet, it is well suited to systematically and collectively address complex problems because (adapted from Raising Places, 2018):

Design is a structure for the unknown.

It is a rigorous and iterative process for creating new insights around persistent problems by safely learning your way forward.

Design facilitates shared language.

It is an approach that starts with compelling, human-centered challenges that are grounded in the lived experiences of those most familiar with the problem, enabling diverse groups to develop shared understanding, language, and action.

Design allows for shared ownership.

It uses a framework to ensure shared power and decision-making with those who are most familiar with the problem and who have most at stake in addressing it. Design processes include both grassroots and grasstops perspectives.

Design makes the abstract tangible.

It uses a set of tools and practices to quickly and safely test assumptions and concepts in the real lives of real people.

Design thinking is not a new *concept* in healthcare, but its *practice* has struggled to gain traction because of significant regulation, burnout, and strict hierarchical management structures. A recent *New England Journal of Medicine (NEJM)* Catalyst survey found that although the vast majority (95%) of respondents "consider design thinking to be useful for the health care industry, its principles are not widely applied" (Compton-Phillips & Mohta, 2018). This chapter draws lessons from those at the cutting edge of applying design thinking in healthcare and public health practice to offer tangible and implementable lessons that can be applied in your practice and organizations.

"If I had an hour to solve a problem, I would spend the first fifty-five minutes determining the proper question to ask, for once I know the proper question, I could solve the problem in less than five minutes." —Albert Einstein

The Problem Is the Problem

Probably the biggest misconception of innovation is that it is the result of grand ideas leaping fully formed from the mind of a genius—think Steve Jobs. However, most of the breakthroughs throughout human history were the result of someone thinking differently about a problem, not the solutions (Fisher & Roberts, 2017a). Design thinking tends to place equal, if not more, emphasis on the problems than on the solutions. Unfortunately, we have become quite good in healthcare at elegantly solving the wrong problems over, and over, and over (Fisher & Roberts, 2017a). The most effective way to get to new and better solutions is to start with new and better questions or problems.

For problems that are clearly defined and simply need more efficient solutions, then design thinking probably isn't the most effective approach. As Tom Fisher notes, "design thinking is useful for when we need a paradigm shift, for instance when something is fundamentally broken about a service" (Kalaichandran, 2017). In design, we call these types of problems, *wicked problems* or those problems that are not solvable in the traditional sense because there is more than one viable solution and the problem itself is constantly changing. In an *HBR* piece, Snowden and Boone noted the following differences, "In a complicated context, at least one right answer exists. In a complex context, however, right answers cannot be ferreted out" (Snowden & Boone, 2007). In addition, they note that complicated contexts are the "domain of experts," whereas complex contexts are the "domain of emergence" (Snowden & Boone, 2007).

The biggest barrier for many in healthcare is that there is rarely any time or focus on exploring the problem at hand, and when there is, most will mistake complex problems for complicated problems, thinking that more expertise or resource is what has been missing. But as Snowden and Boone describe, complex contexts require an approach well suited for emergence and are the key difference between a design orientation and an improvement orientation (Exhibit 15.1).

EXHIBIT 15.1 Differences in Improvement (Complicated) and Design (Complex) Methods

improvement complicated	design complex
Prioritizes evaluation of **limited set of possible solutions**	Prioritizes **comprehensive understanding** of underlying problems
Well suited to address problems that have **predictable solutions**	Well suited to address problems that have **unpredictable solutions (wicked problems)**
Promotes consensus building **(convergent)**	Promotes opposing ideas and debate **(divergent)**
Aims to uncover what is **important to consumers** within a particular experience	Aims to uncover what is **important to consumers** in their everyday lives
Empathy research focuses on **what people** *think* to reveal improved outcomes	Empathy research focuses on **what people** *feel* to reveal new/disruptive outcomes

Source: Roberts, J. P., Fisher, T. R., Trowbridge, M. J., & Bent, C. (2016). A design thinking framework for healthcare management and innovation. *Healthcare, 4*(1), 11–14. doi:10.1016/j.hjdsi.2015.12.002

Illustration

Recently, a large Midwestern health system was in the process of building a new clinic that would specialize in the needs of young mothers and adolescent children. Prior to hiring a design consultant, this health system had spent the previous 4 years in a traditional planning process, hiring consultants to facilitate strategy exercises and market research. The approach taken by this health system (those outlined under an "improvement" in Exhibit 15.1), namely, bringing together the "experts" across the system, resulted in ideas such as valet parking, joint appointment times for mothers and children, and offering robes and tea to mothers in the exam room. Although these ideas were well-intended efforts that could improve efficiency and clinical experience, they were created under a couple of flawed assumptions that all young mothers (a) saw themselves as active patients, (b) the reason they were not utilizing primary care was because they simply desired increased comfort and convenience while at the clinic, and (c) mothers and their children were seen as separate patient populations rather than part of a familial unit. The board of directors for this health system was not comfortable with this conclusion, which prompted engagement of a design-thinking consultant.

In taking a design approach, namely, better understanding the values and needs of real mothers in the real world (not what a room full of mainly older men healthcare leaders think young mothers want), several previously unidentified insights emerged very quickly:

1. Mothers, even those dealing with their own health concerns, saw themselves first and foremost as caregiver and almost never as a patient. Their healthcare needs, specifically preventive, are last to be attended to, if they are at all.

2. Not one mother was seeking a better clinic; in fact, all were looking for the best ways to avoid the clinic at all together. The last thing most wanted to do was to try to schedule something into an already impossible schedule and drag two or three other healthy children to the clinic, where they are most likely to contract an illness.

3. Most mothers identified how helpful the health system was in navigating new parenthood. For example, many cited a nursing help line they could call when they had questions about their infant's health—a high fever, for example. The nurse was able to (a) normalize the high fever, (b) offer information on what needs to be done (treatment), and (c) offer guidance on what to watch for in case the child's health didn't improve. The insight was, as one respondent suggested, "why can't we have a similar hotline for issues with my adolescent." Most noted the need for help in navigating the mental health concerns facing adolescents, from bullying to puberty.

At the end of this 2-month design approach (yes only 2 months of a 4-year process), the health system board decided it did not make economic or customer-value sense to build the clinic and terminated the project in lieu of prototyping ideas grounded in the insights outlined earlier. This is just one short example that demonstrates the value (in this instance, not spending millions of dollars) of asking different questions of different people in different ways to get at new insights and underscores the importance of aligning an approach built for complex problems when faced with complex problems in the first place. No amount of effort to solve the wrong problem will lead to a viable solution, and, we contend that it is one of the greatest sources of waste in the healthcare system today (Fisher & Roberts, 2017a).

DESIGN-THINKING PRINCIPLES

Design-Thinking Framework

Design, above all else, is a process that cannot function under the same constraints that have been built around more linear and quantitative approaches in healthcare. Design thinking requires a different ecosystem, one that allows for and embeds empathetic engagement, radical collaboration, and rapid prototyping (Roberts et al., 2016).

Empathetic Engagement

Empathetic engagement prompts teams to focus on developing a deep and diverse understanding of the explicit and latent needs, experiences, and values of a particular stakeholder group. We know more about many health/healthcare problems than at any other time in human history, yet many problems persist and even continue to get worse because understanding a problem at an abstract level is very different than understanding it through the eyes, minds, stomachs, and hearts of those living it every day. However, there is an important distinction between empathetic *engagement* and empathetic *thinking*. Some research shows that by thinking empathetically, we actually become less empathetic because we will apply our own experiences and world views on an abstract population (Berinato, 2015). This principle cannot be overemphasized enough and is the most critical aspect of design thinking in healthcare and is foundational to breakthrough thinking.

Radical Collaboration

Radical collaboration recognizes that no one discipline alone can systematically address complex issues, precisely because they exist across and at the intersections of disciplines and sectors, not within them. Healthcare is well known for collaboration, but it tends to occur with the same people using the same approaches to address the same problems. (Albert Einstein offers a definition for this approach.) Instead, radical collaboration is about being intentional about fostering creativity. Contrary to popular belief, creativity is not about new ideas; it is about combining existing ideas and experiences in new ways. As such, the most effective, if not only, way to build creativity into an effort is to bring people together that represent a diversity of thinking, experiences, culture, and perspectives.

Rapid Prototyping

Design offers an action-oriented problem-solving framework that moves from a "thinking-to-do" orientation to one of "doing-to-think," or prototyping. Rather than fully deploying a few theory-only ideas, testing many rough ideas (and even questions) in rapid iteration aims to generate and test multiple alternative assumptions and divergent strategies before selecting the most promising, or even reframing your original problem. Prototyping allows ideas to get into the real lives of real people rather than become fully formed initiatives isolated from those who will ultimately determine their success (top-down approach). Many are familiar with piloting, but there are a couple of key differences in concept and application. Pilots are intended to test a (often top-down) hypothesis to be true or false, and occurs over a long period of time with a significant number of "subjects." Prototyping, on the other hand, is intended to learn something new and occurs over very short periods of time (sprints) with only a few participants and will often engage those same participants in redesign of the prototype in real time.

Design Thinking and Systems Thinking

Complex issues continue to persist because they cannot be deconstructed and isolated like parts of a machine. Instead, they exist and adapt within larger dynamic systems that "can only be understood as an integrated whole" (Anderson, Crabtree, Steele, & McDaniel, 2005, p. 3). Although there is no universal approach to systems-level problem-solving, many have outlined the approaches that are *not* working well. As Anderson et al. note, "Most available techniques have us break a system into smaller bits, study the bits and when we believe that we understand the bits we put them all back together again and draw some conclusions about the whole" (Anderson et al., 2005, p. 2). In addition, "reductionist approaches yield limited insights in the context of dynamic systems" (Diez Roux, 2011). Many have called for more emergent approaches, especially when working with populations that are chronically underrepresented with more traditional methods. This, however, has been difficult to move beyond the abstract, as formal systems-level approaches tend to be highly complex and inaccessible to those outside the fields of system or complexity science.

Although most approaches tend to operate within silos, design thinking yields increased systematic understanding of a problem and its possible solutions because it starts, and is driven by key stakeholder's lived experience(s), which cut across sectoral, social, geographical, and political boundaries. In fact, by grounding problems in the human experience, system elements as well as their interactions and interdependencies become increasingly visible and tangible. In this way, design thinking has the ability to better understand and humanize the complexities of a system, but not overcomplicate the system to a degree that stakeholders become paralyzed to do anything about it. In fact, we argue that an exploratory and iterative approach, like that of design thinking, is perhaps the only reasonable way to safely learn about and intervene within a complex system. In citing Duncan Green's writing on systems thinking, Vexler noted that, "working in complex circumstances requires an iterative, collaborative and flexible approach," one more like parenting, which is "about trial and error, and endless testing of assumptions about right and wrong, a constant adaptation to the evolving nature of the child" (Vexler, 2017).

Power, Privilege, and Equality

The most overlooked aspect of any improvement or innovation strategy in healthcare is the immense level of disparity in power and privilege, which only contributes to the United States suffering from one of the largest health disparities on the globe (Hero, Zaslavsky, & Blendon, 2017). There is a big difference between complicated and complex problems, and relying on the expert-driven approach to the latter tends to reinforce and strengthen existing inequalities—you cannot expect those who have benefited most from a system to be the ones to change it. Simply having the opportunity to address issues impacting those other than yourself places you at a unique and significant position of power and privilege. George Aye outlines several questions to pose to your design team (and yourself) as you begin any change effort to ensure power structure is fully understood; "1) How does the world see you? 2) How far ahead can you plan; and 3) How predictable does the world feel" (Aye, 2018)?

Traditional approaches, as outlined by Aye, tend to place you as "expert" in a position of power and those you are engaging with at a place of vulnerability—oftentimes the same communities that have been traumatized by this disproportionate power structure in the past (Aye, 2018). In short, it is completely different to understand a problem from a place of expertise and privilege than it is to live with it on a daily basis, and this is why authentic empathetic engagement is not just a good design practice, it is disqualifying if not part of an improvement or innovation effort. In this way, the design process itself needs to live squarely within the space and with the people most impacted by the problems you aim to address, not within conference rooms, the C-suite, or an "innovation center."

Design Thinking Is Not Magic

If there has been one negative associated with the growing awareness and practice of design thinking, it has been the proliferation of design as an add-on practice (often in the form of a half-day workshop) that will fix all that ails an organization or community (Fisher & Roberts, 2017b). The reality is that this surface application of design has more potential to be detrimental to the organization or community than it does to benefit them.

The best way to understand design thinking is as an upstream complement to other practices such as Lean, Six Sigma, Agile, and controlled research. Although there is a lot to mastering the design process, the good news is that you do not have to be a master's or PhD-level designer to effectively practice design thinking. Many in healthcare are already good at key design principles such as empathetically understanding a problem (empathetic engagement), creative collaboration (radical collaboration), and trying something on the fly (prototyping). However, having an understanding of design skills and tools is not sufficient to ensure effective practice. What is most needed is a rigor and infrastructure to organize and guide these skills and tools in day-to-day practice and innovation.

PROCESS

Design-Studio Structure

Even with the best of intentions, design thinking is ineffective if not deployed under different rules and expectations than those regulating traditional operations. John Kotter noted the need for two complementary systems: (a) the traditional hierarchical, management system for day-to-day operations; and (b) a networked, leadership system for vision, agility, and the ability to avoid future disruptions (Kotter, 2012). In identifying the need for a complementary networked system, Kotter was essentially describing the need for organizations and leaders to have and grow a capacity for design thinking. Although there is no shortage of design-thinking tools and approaches, what is almost always missing is the structure for practicing it—a design-studio structure.

Studios offer a balance of divergent exploration and convergent synthesis essential for uncovering new insights and more important, turning them into real-world change that benefits society. In this way, the studio structure can be an important enhancement to approaches such as social innovation labs (Hassan, 2014) and collective impact models (Kania & Kramer, 2011). The studio structure uses an iterative sequence of individual and/ or team research (or development, depending on where you are in the design process) *sprints* followed by stakeholder *feedback sessions*, followed again by research/development sprints, and so on. These feedback sessions, called *pin ups* in the design world, allow design teams to visually share (usually by pinning or taping them up on a wall) and receive real-time feedback on their questions, ideas, barriers, and predictions for the future from a broad cross-section of stakeholders. It is with this feedback that the design teams create their next research and/or development sprint. The phrase *back to the drawing board* literally came from this process, as it allows you to incorporate feedback from those looking at your work with fresh eyes.

As you can see, this structure is quite different from most management processes that focus on quickly arriving at a "solution" (usually with limited stakeholder input), implementing that idea over a long time period and then, and only then, sharing your results with key stakeholders when they have little or no opportunity to inform the effort. Finally, and perhaps most important, a studio approach allows design teams to break from simply *seeking input* from stakeholders to *directly engaging* them in the process, where they have an active and equitable opportunity to design and drive the change that will directly impact their daily lives. By flipping the power structure inherent in many patient/community engagement efforts, the design-studio approach can offer meaningful and tangible opportunities to foster what Arnstein describes as "citizen power" (Arnstein, 1969).

Putting It All Together: The Rhythm of Design

As described earlier in this chapter, design cannot be boiled down to a linear process, precisely because the problems that design thinking is best suited for are not linear. Although most problem-solving techniques tend to focus on convergence only (getting to the right answer as fast as possible), the design process places equal emphasis on divergence and exploration. Figure 15.1 illustrates an end-to-end design process that, although having a general sequence of work, should be understood as an iterative approach that will likely move back and forth across phases many times over the course of a single project, or even suggest the need for an entirely new project. Although the descriptions that follow offer a number of approaches and specific tools, it is not an exhaustive list, and you should not feel beholden to do only what is described here. Instead, pay particular attention to the intent of each phase and find the approaches and tools that work best for you and the problem ecosystem you are working within.

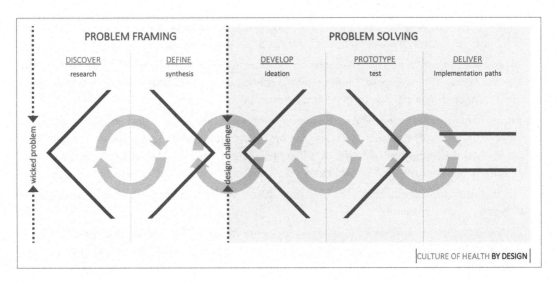

Figure 15.1 Iterative design process.

DISCOVERY PHASE (DIVERGENCE)

Overview

The discovery phase is foundational to the rest of the design process and must start with gaining a broad understanding of the institutional and community knowledge around a particular problem (what is already known about the problem). By grounding yourself and your team in existing knowledge, the appropriate "start point" for further investigation will emerge and help you avoid doing harm, such as not being aware of historical trauma in a particular community or patient population. Once aware of the context you are entering into, the discovery phase places significant emphasis on the lived experience of those most impacted by and with the most at stake in addressing the problem as well as better understanding the reality for those who have the most influence over the design and operations of the system (identifying the influenced and influencers). Your efforts should be biased toward quality over quantity and in engaging in diverse experiences and perspectives (think snowball sampling). The focus of this phase is not to extract what you think you want from stakeholders, but to explore with them to uncover unexpected insights—these nuggets are the key to reframing your problem(s) in the next phase.

Approach and Tools

- Research existing institutional, community, and historical context and knowledge. What is (and is not) known about this problem?
- Define who your stakeholders are, both those who are influenced by a problem as well as those who can influence the outcome(s). Be sure to pay particular attention to who might be missing—those voice(s) that are usually overlooked.

- Uncover the lived experiences of your stakeholders. Explore stakeholder relationships, behaviors, motivations, beliefs, hopes, and needs through various cultural probes.
- Avoid focus groups and patient–caregiver advisory councils. Although they can offer valuable feedback, they are your "super-users" and not usually reflective of those who may be most impacted by a particular problem, or even know it exists.
- Brainstorm questions, not ideas. Research shows that brainstorming solutions does not work (Chamorro-Premuzic, 2015), so try brainstorming questions to ask your stakeholders instead. Ask questions that prompt broader insights such as "Describe the last time you genuinely felt healthy" or "What brings you joy?" or "What are you most fearful of?"
- Get outside your institution and engage one-on-one with those you seek insight from (where they live, work, and play).
- Facilitate contextual observations: How do your stakeholders make decisions, navigate health challenges, and exist on a daily basis (this approach will often yield insights that stakeholders cannot articulate)?

CALL TO ACTION

Interview a senior leader at your organization as well as your organization's primary patient/client/stakeholder. Say: "Describe the last time you genuinely felt healthy/well. What about that time in particular made you feel healthy/well?" How did their responses compare? How did they differ? How were they similar? Why do you think that is?

DEFINE PHASE (CONVERGENCE)

Overview

Only after you have gained insight into the lived experiences of those most impacted by a particular problem can you begin to frame it. This phase is when you will unpack and synthesize your "discovery-phase" findings into a compelling, yet tangible problem statement. Your problem statement should recognize the systemic nature of the problem and be framed in a way that is human centric and promotes divergent ideation. It is important to note that you are unlikely to arrive at a consensus problem statement here, but the goal is to generate a good-enough framing and design criteria (definitions of success) for the next phase. Remember, the design process is not linear and may require that you reframe your problem numerous times before arriving at an idea that generates the most compelling solutions. Correctly framing your problem is the most difficult, yet most critical, part of the design process as it creates vision and principles for the remainder of your effort.

Approach and Tools

- Visually map the problem ecosystem, as this process requires us to understand the problem in entirely new and more comprehensive ways (Nelson, Reed, & Walling, 1976). This can be accomplished in a variety of ways, but creating a simple journey or experience map is an effective way of organizing the problem around an individual/set of individual's experience(s).

- Identify the key leverage points within the problem map. Leverage points can include: (a) pent-up energy for change—energy disrupting the status quo or trying to reorganize for new patterns/behaviors to emerge; (b) bright spots—where positive change is already happening; and (c) ripple effects—strong factors/dynamics that could potentially affect many other subsequent factors/dynamics (Booth, Roumani, & Mohr, 2017).

- Frame and reframe your problem. Be sure to create a problem statement that is human centered and that concerns preferred experiences or behaviors rather than a tool or program (think verbs not nouns). A proven method for creating an effective problem statement is with a how might wee (HMW) statement as it asks **how** (not what), **might** (not a directive), and **we** (as a collective) address a particular issue. These statements should be narrow enough that they lend direction, but broad enough that they allow for exploration and a diverse set of ideas (Stanford University d.school, 2018). An example of an HMW statement might be something like, "HMW ensure that patients with diabetes *are confident* in their own self-care"—the key question is how we design for confidence, not create another checklist or education brochure for a patient who is already overwhelmed.

- Articulate key design principles (what would success look like and from whose perspective) based on your HMW statement.

 CALL TO ACTION

Over the next month, sit down with one of your patients/clients/users and create a short journey map describing their experience caring for a loved one (child, neighbor, parent)— what are the most rewarding and difficult parts of this experience? Develop an HMW question that responds to their concerns/experience.

DEVELOP PHASE (DIVERGENCE)

Overview

The intent of this phase is to come up with creative ways of addressing the problem statement (HMW statement) created in the "define phase." Remember that the best way to come up with the most viable and creative ideas is to draw on the collective wisdom and creativity of a diverse set of stakeholders, so find ways that draw on that diversity rather than looking to build universal consensus. This is once again a divergence phase, you will want to explore a broad range of ideas (both in quantity and diversity) instead of focusing on a singular best solution (Stanford University d.school, 2018). As with defining a problem statement, aim for good enough as you will be able to test your assumptions and questions in the next phase.

Approach and Tools

- Avoid product-centric thinking and focus solutions on stakeholder experiences and behaviors.
- Avoid groupthink and brainstorming by allowing for individual and small-group reflection and exploration (see the section "Design-Studio Structure").
- Amplify assets: Focus on what you/your stakeholders *do* have; this ensures solutions that are creative, viable, and sustainable.
- Radical constraints: Make your most challenging constraints or barriers even more challenging can liberate your thinking from what is probable to what is possible.
- Analogous scenarios: Discover entirely new ways to meet complex and persistent needs by investigating how other industries or sectors have approached similar problems. Look for analogies, as you are unlikely to find fully baked transferable best practices. For example, what would the Airbnb model of healthcare look like?
- Ultimate failure: Developing what you feel would be the least effective solution (the biggest failure) can open new insights into what an alternatively effective solution might look/function like.
- Just as you did to better understand the problem, visually map the solution ecosystem. Create a journey or experience map of your solution. What resources, relationships, programs, spaces, and/or tools will be needed and how might your stakeholder interact with them?

 CALL TO ACTION

Reflect on one of your organization's recent initiatives. What was the problem they are/were looking to solve? Now create the ultimate failure solution to that problem. How does it look different and/or similar to what the organization is doing/has done? Why do you think that is? How might you redesign the original initiative?

PROTOTYPE PHASE (CONVERGENCE)

Overview

You are ready for the prototype phase when you are able to test the assumptions, questions, and ideas you developed in the previous phase. This phase will help you/your team clarify and home in on the most viable and meaningful solutions to the problems as defined by those who will be most impacted by the solution. Remember that prototyping is about learning something new about the problem, its solution, or your stakeholders (doing-to-think), not testing a hypothesis. Prototyping can take many forms and can be used to test concepts, tools, or even experiences and should be done in *quick* and *cheap* ways (think minutes and two to three people—remember the difference between piloting and prototyping; Stanford University d.school, 2018). The key is to keep the prototypes really simple and test them in the real lives of real people, not in a conference room, because simply asking someone whether he or she likes your idea in the abstract will result in false feedback, which although making you feel good, does little to inform your ideas.

Approach and Tools

- Make ideas tangible. They should involve something people can see, touch, and experience. A great early-stage prototype could be the "future state" journey map you created in the development stage. Ask your stakeholders to react to the idea, specifically calling out the parts of the experience they think would be most valuable and the ones they think would be least valuable and why.

- Avoid focus groups or asking people whether they "like" an idea as most will respond positively to whatever you offer them, even if it does not address the issues that are most impacting them.

- Engage in user-driven prototyping: Instead of creating something for stakeholders to respond to, engage them in the prototyping process (Roberts et al., 2016).

- Identify variables: Instead of prototyping full-scale solutions, it is often more effective to identify particular variables for testing (Roberts et al., 2016).

 CALL TO ACTION

The next time your team gets "stuck" trying to agree on a solution to a particular problem, create a high-level journey or experience map showing how your stakeholder's problem will be addressed for each viable solution. Then get it in front of three to five of your stakeholders and get their feedback on what part of the experience is most important and most directly addresses their concerns/problems and why. Ask them what/how they would change it—let them draw on the map.

DELIVERY PHASE (IMPLEMENT AND EVOLVE)

Overview

In order for any solution to be valuable to your stakeholders, it must be implementable and able to adapt to changing stakeholder needs and environments. Implementation must be desirable (meet needs) as well as economically and culturally feasible. Although there is no one way to ensure project or initiative success, the best approach may be *to not* see your work as static, one-time projects or initiatives at all, but as organic and ongoing movements. The design process laid out in this chapter helps ensure sustainability and long-term success in that it follows principles of successful healthcare and public health efforts: (a) they are guided by and respond to the systemic nature of complex problems; (b) they are co-designed with, and of, the community (context-specific solutions); (c) they are fiercely asset-oriented (leveraging what is available); and (d) they are a beginning, not an end product. The delivery phase, in fact all phases, is most effective when design thinking is integrated into staff's and leader's day-to-day practice and why this chapter has outlined it as a "translatable practice framework that can be learned and embedded into the DNA of an organization," instead of a stock set of tools or practices (Roberts et al., 2016, p. 12).

Approach and Tools

- Explore unlikely partnerships. Create unique value propositions and funding mechanisms by looking beyond the usual suspects. For example, if your team has developed ways to better support individuals managing their diabetes, look at partnering with local employers as they lose real dollars when their employees (or those being cared for by their employees) cannot manage their diabetes.

- Complete a business model canvas (Greenwald, 2012). Although your end game may not be a business, looking at your idea as a business opportunity has great potential to ensure your work has a healthy mix of desirability and feasibility and is a great way to identify possible partnership opportunities.

- Look for ripe environments. Remember, context matters greatly. Look for those contexts that are a good fit for the solution(s) your team has developed and tested. One of the most effective ways to grow acceptance of and participation in change is to create small, visible wins (Amabile & Kramer, 2011).

CASE STUDY

Background

Hurricane Harvey hit the Greater Houston area on August 25, 2017, damaging over 200,000 homes and apartment buildings with historic flooding. Texas Children's Hospital is the largest child health provider in the region, with over 3.7 million patient encounters in 2017 through its three hospital campuses and over 50 clinics across the region, and over 438,000 patients in its health plan. In Harvey's aftermath, the Section of Public Health Pediatrics (SPHP) at Texas Children's Hospital was fortunate enough to receive some funding to address the social needs of impacted families. Given this is a systems-level challenge with impacts far beyond the health system complicated by the complexity that follows a disaster, the SPHP looked to design thinking to provide needed structure to navigate the unknown.

Deep Empathy

To ground and give direction to their own efforts, as well as to help create shared language across our diverse group, the SPHP found deep-empathy interviews with affected residents an essential starting point. These narratives illustrated significant financial challenges facing families before and especially after Harvey, the difficulties of accessing resources and navigating an incredibly complex system, and ultimately leading to immense *feelings of hopelessness and abandonment*. It became clear that any solution would have to help navigate and access information that would help empower families rather than feel like it was submitting them to additional layers of bureaucracy. Through traditional exploratory efforts, most hospitals stay within traditional clinic boundaries and roles. By probing deeper into the core needs of the patients and communities they hoped to positively impact, the SPHP was forced to step outside its walls and focus on how the problems were actually being experienced by those most impacted by them, not just how they showed up in the clinic.

Radical Collaboration

The very process of facilitated cross-sector conversations grounded in a common interest (client experience) generated important insights. The SPHP at Texas Children's Hospital partnered with the local Long Term Recovery Committee (LTRC), which includes representation from the Federal Emergency Management Agency; the Red Cross; city, county, large and small nonprofits; home-repair agencies; and grassroots organizations. It is unique for a health system to engage with and facilitate such a broad set of stakeholders, but as was discovered in the empathy work, home repairs, transportation services, and access to schools had at least equal, if not more, impact on the community member's ability to not just survive but thrive, especially when those communities are on the economic fringe. Furthermore, it's not often that "expert" organizations and grassroots organizations discuss problems together in the same room. Through this process of convening radical collaboration studios, each organization realized it was challenged by similar difficulties within a complex system ("The process is the punishment"). The organizations also came to understand that sometimes they cause those challenges ("Most of our organizations operate with a 'screen-out' procedure. How can we all try to be 'screen-in' organizations instead?"). But ultimately the organizations were working toward the same end ("We need a streamlined process")—a way for community members to find and navigate resources (formal and informal) they could trust, which can only be defined by the individual and his or her unique situation.

Rapid Prototyping

The need for up-to-date information for both residents as well as those helping them comes up regularly but remains a significant challenge as resources and services are constantly changing. A hard-hit and underserved pilot community was identified, and the notion of a one-page "road map" visualizing resources for different topics specific to this community seemed of value and relatively feasible to create in a short time period. The *process* of creating this road map was critical in and of itself. Identifying which organizations to list was enlightening—in reality many previously active organizations no longer had funding and so the list of 30 organizations whittled down to 10. An initial prototype (Figure 15.2) in the format of a road map received feedback that residents were all in different stages and had different needs. There was no one path that would be representative of the needs of them all. Therefore, the workgroup shifted to more of a "guide," laying out each area of need and placing relevant organization(s) in buckets (Figure 15.3). Feedback has shown that this low-tech and cheap prototype meets the most basic, yet overwhelming question for most families, "Where do I start?" More surprising is that many listed organizations were not aware of each other! The next challenge the SPHP and LTRC workgroup are prototyping is what happens *after* residents reach out to these services/organizations.

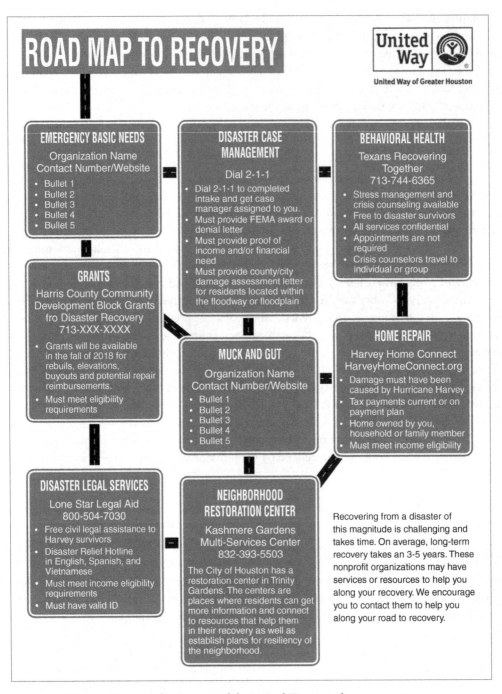

Figure 15.2 Initial prototype of the United Way's road map to recovery.

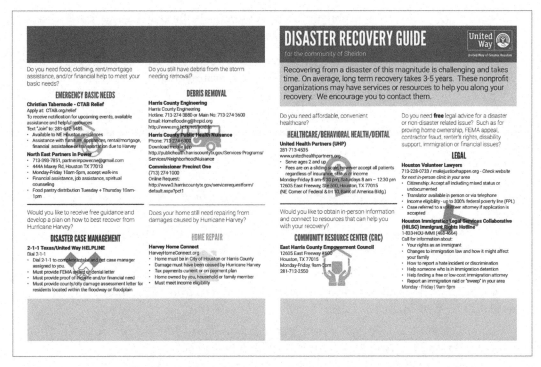

Figure 15.3 Disaster recovery guide for the United Way.

🔑 KEY TAKEAWAY POINTS

■ Twenty-first-century problems are systemic and dynamic and are not "solvable" in the traditional sense, and their solution requires an entirely new generation of practitioners and leaders, one that is fluent in design thinking.

■ Design is for those problems not well understood and/or those that continue to persist over time regardless of the efforts to address them in the past.

■ It is not good enough to ask people about their problems, the design process must be driven by those most impacted by and with the most at stake in addressing the problem (empathetic engagement).

■ New questions, not answers, are the most likely way to yield new thinking and breakthrough solutions.

■ There is no universal "10-step" process for problem-solving; instead, it is an iterative process of divergence and convergence.

■ Divergence in opinions and experiences, not consensus, is the only way to foster creativity (radical collaboration).

■ Just start. The universal commonality across all breakthroughs is that they started somewhere, which almost always was not the "right" place (rapid prototyping).

REFERENCES

Abbasi, K. (2011). A riot of divergent thinking. *Journal of the Royal Society of Medicine, 104*(10), 391. doi:10.1258/jrsm.2011.11k038

Amabile, T., & Kramer, S. J. (2011, May). The power of small wins. *Harvard Business Review.* Retrieved from https://hbr.org/2011/05/the-power-of-small-wins

Anderson, R. A., Crabtree, B. F., Steele, D. J., & McDaniel, R. R., Jr. (2005). Case study research: The view from complexity science. *Qualitative Health Research, 15*(5), 669–685. doi:10.1177/1049732305275208

Arnstein, S. R. (1969). A ladder of citizen participation. *Journal of the American Institute of Planners, 35*(4), 216–224. doi:10.1080/01944366908977225

Aye, G. (Producer). (2018). The designer's weakness: Understanding the role of power. *South By Southwest.* Retrieved from https://vimeo.com/260803001

Berinato, S. (2015, March). Putting yourself in the customer's shoes doesn't work: An interview with Johannes Hattula. *Harvard Business Review.* Retrieved from https://hbr.org/2015/03/putting-yourself-in-the-customers-shoes-doesnt-work

Booth, T., Roumani, N., & Mohr, J. (Producer). (2017). Design thinking for the social sector. *Design Thinking.* (Live-streamed webinar from Stanford Social Innovation Review, December 6, 2017)

Brown, T. (2008). Design thinking. *Harvard Business Review, 86*(6), 84–92, 141.

Chamorro-Premuzic, T. (2015, March). Why group brainstorming is a waste of time. *Harvard Business Review.* Retrieved from https://hbr.org/2015/03/why-group-brainstorming -is-a-waste-of-time

Compton-Phillips, A., & Mohta, N. S. (2018, June). Care redesign survey: How design thinking can transform health care. *NEJM Catalyst.* Retrieved from https://catalyst.nejm.org/ design-thinking-transform-health-care/

Diez Roux, A. V. (2011). Complex systems thinking and current impasses in health disparities research. *American Journal of Public Health, 101*(9), 1627–1634. doi:10.2105/ AJPH.2011.300149

Fisher, T. R., & Roberts, J. P. (2017a). Biggest threat to health? Solving the wrong problems. Retrieved from https://www.huffingtonpost.com/entry/biggest-threat-to-health-solving-the -wrong-problems_us_59682c53e4b06a2c8edb4576

Fisher, T. R., & Roberts, J. P. (2017b). Rethinking design thinking. Retrieved from https://www .huffingtonpost.com/entry/rethinking-design-thinking_us_589b504ce4b061551b3e066a

Greenwald, T. (2012, January). Business model canvas: A simple tool for designing innovative business models. *Forbes*. Retrieved from https://www.forbes.com/sites/tedgreenwald/ 2012/01/31/business-model-canvas-a-simple-tool-for-designing-innovative-business -models/#4d8e0b5c16a7

Hassan, Z. (2014, May). The social labs revolution: A new approach to solving our most complex challenges. *Stanford Social Innovation Review*. Retrieved from https://ssir.org/articles/ entry/the_social_labs_revolution_a_new_approach_to_solving_our_most_complex_chall

Hero, J. O., Zaslavsky, A. M., & Blendon, R. J. (2017). The United States leads other nations in differences by income in perceptions of health and health care. *Health Affairs, 36*(6), 1032–1040. doi:10.1377/hlthaff.2017.0006

Kalaichandran, A. (2017). Design thinking for doctors and nurses. *The New York Times*. Retrieved from https://www.nytimes.com/2017/08/03/well/live/design-thinking-for-doctors- and-nurses.html

Kania, J., & Kramer, M. (2011, Winter). Collective impact. *Stanford Social Innovation Review*. Retrieved from https://ssir.org/articles/entry/collective_impact

Kotter, J. P. (2012). Accelerate! *Harvard Business Review, 90*(11), 44–52, 54–48, 149.

Land, G. (2011). The failure of success. *TEDx*. Retrieved from https://www.youtube.com/ watch?v=ZfKMq-rYtnc&feature=youtu.be&t=5m29s

Nelson, D. L., Reed, V. S., & Walling, J. R. (1976). Pictorial superiority effect. *Journal of Experimental Psychology Human Learning and Memory, 2*(5), 523–528. doi:10.1037/ 0278-7393.2.5.523

Raising Places. (2018). Our approach. Retrieved from https://raisingplaces.org/www.raising places.org/our-purpose.html

Roberts, J. P., Fisher, T. R., Trowbridge, M. J., & Bent, C. (2016). A design thinking frame-work for healthcare management and innovation. *Healthcare, 4*(1), 11–14. doi:10.1016/j. hjdsi.2015.12.002

Snowden, D. J., & Boone, M. E. (2007, November). A leader's framework for decision making. *Harvard Business Review*. Retrieved from https://hbr.org/2007/11/a-leaders -framework-for-decision-making

Stanford University d.school. (2018). An introduction to design thinking: Process guide. Retrieved from https://dschool-old.stanford.edu/sandbox/groups/designresources/wiki/36873/ attachments/74b3d/ModeGuideBOOTCAMP2010L.pdf

Vexler, D. (2017, June). What exactly do we mean by systems? *Stanford Social Innovation Review*. Retrieved from https://ssir.org/articles/entry/what_exactly_do_we_mean_by_systems

Negotiating Complex Systems

Dan Weberg

"I cannot say whether things will get better if we change; what I can say is they must change if they are to get better." —Georg C. Lichtenburg

LEARNING OBJECTIVES

- Describe three characteristics of complex systems.
- Discuss four types of innovation culture in organizations.
- Apply three strategies to negotiate complex systems change.

INTRODUCTION

To create meaningful innovation in organizations, leaders must understand how to negotiate through the whitewater of complex systems. To navigate complex systems, leaders must first challenge their own conventional assumptions of how organizations work, how things truly get done, and who really has influence to execute innovation. In complex systems, the whole is greater than the sum of its parts (Burke, 2017). The connections and relationships among people, teams, information, and technology hold significant value in the success and adaptability of organizations. High-performing organizations are not simply a compilation of high-performing individuals. Rather, high-performing organizations consist of a range of skills, diverse thought, and talents, but have a highly tuned system of connection that drives adaptability, resiliency, and focus to achieve greatness. There is little argument that healthcare organizations are complex systems and that the healthcare system as a whole is a complex system made up of complex systems. This chapter discusses practical ways leaders can use information, facilitation, and risk-taking to influence change in complex systems.

THREE CONCEPTS OF COMPLEX SYSTEMS

Complexity science is a fascinating group of theories that explain how organizations, and the people inside them, interact to provide value to the world. Some theories that combine to create complexity science include graph theory, theoretical biology, and systems thinking

(Hatch, 2018). Many of these theories are complex by themselves, let alone combined, and create some confusion for many leaders who want to adopt their principles. The good news is that you can negotiate and influence complex systems without a comprehensive understanding of all of the underlying theory. However, there are three concepts of complex systems that any leader in healthcare should understand.

Networks Are More Powerful Than Hierarchy

Complexity science research has demonstrated that organizations consist of two power structures. First, as many leaders are well aware, organizations have a hierarchical matrix of front-line leaders, middle managers, directors, executives, and boards of directors. This hierarchy is what is known as the *formal power structure*. That is, the people in the hierarchy have clearly defined levels of authority to execute the business of the organization. The formal power structure creates stability in the organization and clears pathways for predictable actions, such as finances, human resources, policy, and safety. These actions keep the core functions of the organization intact and provide consistency that is needed for the management of day-to-day tasks.

CALL TO ACTION

Reflect on innovations at your place of work. How many successful innovations were driven from the top-down (formal network) versus the informal network?

Research has shown that the formal structure is needed to keep the lights on but is actually very bad at creating innovation or change. The hierarchy is overstructured and rigid and does not allow the deviation and risk-taking that is needed for meaningful change. This does not mean that your boss cannot create meaningful change; it simply means that formal power structures are not optimally arranged to lead adaptive changes such as innovation.

Every complex system also has an **informal network,** the interconnected relationships that span across titles, people, teams, and departments (Ward et al., 2014). The informal network reflects that friendships, personal relationships, hallway interactions, and political climate drive much of the work in organizations. It is through the informal network that change and innovation actually occur. As a formal or informal leader in a complex system, you must be aware of the informal network and its power in relation to the hierarchy (Figure 16.1).

Because complex systems mimic living organisms, let us illustrate the hierarchy and the informal network using a simplified physiologic example. Think about the human body as a complex system (because it is). Your bones are like an organization's hierarchy: They are needed for structure and support. Bones also are inflexible and break relatively easily. They also take significant time to adapt to stress and heal from injury or loss. Organizational hierarchies are exactly the same. Now, think of the human body's cardiovascular (CV) system. When subjected to stressors, such as exercise, it is able to adapt quickly, easily, and fluidly. The CV system continually adapts and can become more efficient over relatively short amounts of time. The CV system also translates multiple inputs from hormones, nerves, electricity, and pressures into coordinated pumping efforts. Even when parts of the system are dysfunctional (i.e., dysrhythmias), it can adapt (although not optimally over the long term) to maintain its

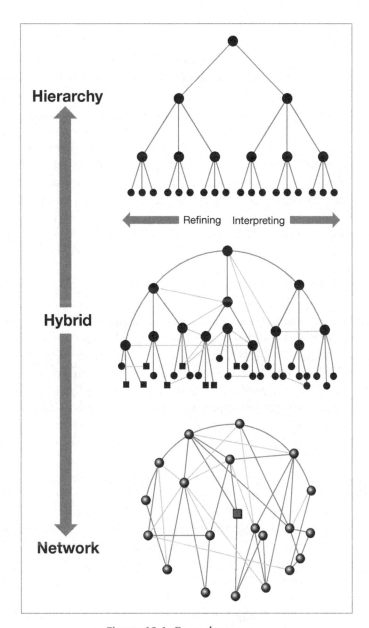

Figure 16.1 Control structures.

function and sustain life. Organizations' informal networks are very similar to the CV system. Leaders wishing to create innovation and system-level change should understand and engage the informal network and the hierarchy. Many times, innovators only attempt change through official channels and are dismissed, rejected, or otherwise ignored. This is because the hierarchy is not structured to adapt to dramatic changes from the norm. Leaders wishing to depart from the status quo should look to the informal network as a source of change and collaboration and utilize the hierarchy for resources such as money, time, sponsorship, and other operational needs that the informal network may not have full access to.

Information Is the Currency of Influence

As discussed, formal titles are only one small part of how the system is influenced. Much more powerful than a vice president is the currency of information, which can be used to both build innovation capacity or to completely reduce the ability for teams to innovate. For example, teams with the right information at the right time can make informed decisions about changes that will impact their work. Meanwhile, teams that do not have access to relevant and transparent information will not make informed decisions. Because complex systems are adaptive, teams without the necessary information to do their jobs will subsequently fill out the information with inaccurate stories and misinformation. This is not done in malice, but is a product of human nature. Humans generally do not like ambiguity in organizations as it reflects a risk to psychological safety. Fear of losing one's employment, changes to scheduling, stressing about new norms and power dynamics all originate when information about a change is not disseminated well. Over time, these stories and misinformation can become perceived as fact and people act believing that they are fully informed.

For leaders, this is good news. It means, in complex systems, you can have significant influence to create change simply by gathering information and sharing it in a meaningful way. One tangible example of this in action is with evidence-based practice. Curating valid and reliable evidence to support the need for change is overwhelmingly more successful long term than those innovators who simply brainstorm ideas without an evidence review. Furthermore, those leaders who also gather opinions, approvals, insights, and support from their contacts throughout the informal network before they approach the formal hierarchy are much more successful than those leaders who only follow the chain of command. This is because complex systems are changed through engagement of the system, not the linear influence of a single person. Therefore, to be a successful leader in a complex system, you must use information to initiate change in multiple places across the system because everything is interconnected.

For example, although you might want to create a change in the admission process for an ED, you will need to not only catalyze the ED to adopt the change, you will also need to influence the receiving hospital units, the physician hospitalists, the registration teams, the financial teams, and the environmental services workers to be totally successful. Simply changing the process in the ED will not be successful because of the interdependent nature of complex systems. To influence all these systems, you need to gather information and translate it into the process, outcomes, and evidence for change. This is because a change in one part of the system ripples and impacts the rest of the system in unpredictable ways. The more a leader is able to anticipate where the ripples of change will impact the most, the better that leader will be at catalyzing system change.

Predictability Is Limited

The third concept of complex systems is that predictability of change is limited. Unlike a complex system, in a complicated system, you can more easily understand the cause-and-effect nature of a pressure on the system. For example, a car engine is a complicated system, but it is predictable. When you push on the gas pedal, complicated responses are created but they are predictable and result in the engine speeding up and the car moving forward. If that car engine was somehow a complex system, pressing the gas pedal might inflate the right rear tire, recline your seat, and turn the lights on. This is because a complex system is connected and interdependent in a matrix and networked design. It is called complex because it is impossible to fully map or understand all of the factors and connections within that system.

CALL TO ACTION

Reflect on a change you have experienced lately. What ripple effects occurred from that change that you did not predict? List both positive and negative impacts of the change and where they occurred in the organization. What does this tell you about the connections of the network?

If we reflect back on the previous emergency room admission example, some of the connections where the change will have an impact can be anticipated (not predicted). However, once the change is implemented, many other impacts will be uncovered. For example, the new admission process may significantly quicken the movement of the patients from the ED to the admitting floor, thus decompressing the ED waiting room and creating staffing issues in the ED due to lack of patients, but subsequently this may lead to a nightmare for the hospitalists and transport teams.

All this is to say that even the most experienced healthcare leaders cannot predict the impact of any given change in a complex system. Leaders must build their networks, test ideas regularly, and gather information routinely to see the patterns that will help inform them of how a change might play out. Ultimately, a leader who gathers and shares the right information at the right time to both the hierarchy and his or her informal network will be best positioned to anticipate and prepare for the unpredictable impact of change and innovation in a complex system.

THREE WAYS TO INFLUENCE COMPLEX SYSTEMS

Now that the main social and structural components of a complex system have been established, it is time to provide guidance on how to influence those systems. Although there are many ways to influence systems, this section will focus specifically on common areas of struggle in creating innovative change. To be specific, we discuss the impact of the right information at the right time, facilitating ground-up innovation, and challenging the status quo.

Right Information at the Right Time

The problem: A lack of transparent and accessible information leads to ineffective, misguided, and inappropriate decision-making. Many of us have heard of "water cooler conversations." Those are informal interactions between team members that spread rumors, gossip, and fragments of information quicker than any formal memo or email chain. These informal social interactions are a foundation of how the informal network communicates around the structure of an organization. During times of change and innovation, these informal discussions can have significant influence on the success of the initiative and can either support or undermine the leader's ability to influence change.

There are two ways leaders create conditions in their teams that may lead to negative "water cooler" conversations, thus undermining their innovation efforts. First, leaders restrict information from getting to the teams. Second, leaders provide irrelevant information to their teams. Let us explore the consequences of both actions.

There are many reasons leaders might restrict information from teams. Many times, it stems from good intentions or a desire to protect their teams. For example, when budget cuts might be imminent for the department, the manager may not want to scare her team by sharing specifics related to the dollar amount, timing, or initial reaction of senior leadership. In complex systems, however, information is rarely ever a secret. Because of the complex interconnected relationships among people, information flows around the artificial blocks set up by the hierarchy and reaches the teams in a fragmented and potentially misrepresented fashion. Using our budget cut example, the administrative assistant (AA) for the department may be friends with the chief financial officer's assistant. They talk in the hallway and share the budget cut implications. Your department's AA then shares that information with her friend on the team, and so on and so on. This process is much like the game Telephone you may have played as a kid. The more the information is shared down the line, the more fragmented it becomes, making it different from the actual message. The fragmented message can sometimes vary dramatically from the original message and create more stress, fear, confusion, and reaction in teams than the original and complete information ever would have.

The solution: Enable better decision-making through transparent information sharing. Sharing transparently may sound easy, but it represents a significant portion of the leader's work. The solution is not simply to share information with your team, but to also set up systems so that you, as the leader, do not have to always manage that information flow (Table 16.1). If staff continually rely on you for information, this will create a bottleneck as your priorities shift. The work of the innovation leader in a complex network is to set up ways for teams to get the right information at the right time without having to rely on a single individual.

One mistake leaders make as they work on becoming more transparent is that they tend to share blindly all the information they have without providing context. For example, a manager might share the entire department budget in an effort to engage the team in finding ways to save money. This usually does not work as the entire department budget is not the right information or relevant information for frontline staff engaged in the change process. A better solution would be for the manager to share specific supply-related costs or overtime information as these are two areas the staff have direct influence over changing. It is helpful for the leader to

TABLE 16.1 Tools for Sharing Information Among Team Members

Tool	Impact to Information Flow
Shared storage drive	Allows easy access to updated documents and files for review
Team wiki site	Allows anyone to update information and ask questions about that information in a transparent way
Chat systems (Slack, Skype, etc.)	Allow real-time interaction of team members to clarify, confirm, or deny information as it is received

also provide the context around the information, too. In our supply example, simply sharing the budget spreadsheet is not enough. The leader should explain his or her hypothesis as to why costs are high and what the information means. This allows the frontline staff to understand some of the system factors influencing the issue and create better informed solutions with the rest of the team.

Finally, make information easy to find. One study showed that nurses spend around 30% of their shift hunting for information or people. This is non-value-added work and is a great example of wasting a team's energy in the pursuit of information to make decisions. Leaders should work to find structures and methods to support information flow directly to the people who need it easily. This can be done by implementing technology to connect people faster, such as secure text messaging, or setting up information databases that have user interfaces and search capabilities that reflect the needs of the frontline staff. This allows team members to have the right information at the right time and make the right decision with the right information.

CASE STUDY: RIGHT INFORMATION AT THE RIGHT TIME

One large community hospital was having issues in how patients moved through the system after having surgery. Patients would leave the operating room and recover in the post-anesthesia care unit (PACU). From there, they were moved to a room in the hospital to further recover. The process for moving the patient from unit to unit was challenging. All communication was run through a single person in the bed placement office. This person held three cell phones and placed hundreds of calls a day to determine what beds were clear, which patients needed to be moved, and what staffing was available in the area. The process was a restrictive one and did not account for the complexity of the issue it was trying to solve.

The chief nurse recognized the issue and tasked the bed placement office, nurse managers, and an innovation facilitation team to create a better solution. After weeks of ethnographic research in which frontline staff, environmental services, patients, physicians, administrators, and others were engaged in problem-solving and prototyping, the teams realized that the primary reason patients were not moving between units efficiently was because the teams receiving the patient, cleaning the rooms, and planning the placements did not have access to real-time actionable information.

The teams worked to create a system that provided access to the relevant information the different teams needed to improve the movement of patients throughout the hospital. Instead of creating one large dashboard displaying all the patients, the teams took a complex systems approach and created custom screens for each stakeholder. Environmental services had a custom dashboard that showed the rooms needing to be cleaned and automatically organized them by priority in real time. The PACU could see which patients were coming out of surgery and what hospital rooms they needed before they even left the operating room. The nursing floors could see which patients would need rooms and various information that would allow the nurses and managers to more efficiently place the patient. The information was freed from the bed placement leaders' phone and opened for people to problem solve in real time as issues arose.

This work allowed the bed placement managers to focus on the entire hospital and not spend their days fighting every fire that arose in the process. In all, the opening of relevant information at the right time allowed teams to be more efficient, communicate more effectively, and improve the patient experience.

Ground-Up Innovation

The problem: Top-down solutions restrict engagement, decrease innovation adoption rates, and build a culture of reliance rather than innovation. Problem-solving in complex organizations is most successful when it occurs at the point closest to the problem (Davidson, Weberg, Malloch, & Porter-O'Grady, 2016). For example, if there are issues related to patient care, nurses at the bedside should be solving those issues, not the director or chief nurse who is three or four hierarchal layers removed. When formal leaders do not view their organization as an adaptive complex system, they tend to dictate solutions that are formed in conference rooms rather than engaging the people closest to the problem for answers. When top-down solutions are proposed and handed down, they are usually not good fits to the actual work occurring at the point of service, nor do they resonate with the people doing the work.

The solution: Successful leaders of complex systems take a different approach. They look for sources of problems, work to bring them to the surface, and then engage the team to solve those issues.

Facilitating difficult conversations about what is not working well on a team is not an easy task. It takes vulnerability, transparency, and a willingness by the leader to give up the fallacy that leaders have all the answers.

> In cultures where leaders solve all the problems of the team, cultures of reliance are created.

This means that the team stops problem-solving and instead brings every issue to the leader for resolution. Although the leader may feel good as he or she puts out the proverbial fires, over time his or her team will become lower and lower performing and unable or unwilling to solve issues themselves.

Leaders can look in many places for sources of issues to bring them to the attention of the teams. One of the most useful places to look is for systematic work-arounds. Work-arounds are processes that team members develop that do not follow normal operating procedures to make their work easier, more efficient, and oftentimes more practical. I once heard a new-graduate nurse say, "I cannot wait to graduate! I look forward to developing work-arounds to poorly designed processes." In healthcare, work-arounds exist in almost every aspect of care. This is because processes are designed for predictable events and, in healthcare, there are often unpredictable issues that require creative solutions to overcome. Knowledge workers, such as nurses, physicians, and other health professions create new ways of work to deliver safe and effective care to their patients. Many times, leaders can see work-arounds that are more efficient and effective than the policies currently in place. Leaders can work to recognize these work-arounds and, instead of punishing staff for deviating from the norm, use the opportunity to identify broken parts of the complex system.

For example, at one large hospital, leaders were very frustrated that their medication bar-code scan rates were lower than expected. They held leadership meetings to reprimand low-performing units. Finally, the chief nurse decided to shadow some of the staff nurses and found that the cord on the scanner did not reach the patients. Nurses were still checking the medications in the system but could not comply with the scanning. The chief nurse quickly identified that the work-around was safe and began to fix the system issue of short cords.

 CALL TO ACTION

At your next workday, count how many work-arounds you notice. Write them down and categorize them as helpful or harmful to the system. Are there any that could be a source of innovation for your organization?

Caveat: Not all work-arounds are safe and effective. The point of this discussion is not to say you should celebrate all deviation from the norm but rather for the leader to look for places where very smart people have adapted new ways of work to provide better and safer care. Leaders should keep an open mind when looking at deviation in the system. Sometimes these deviations help uncover an issue with the system and may be the source of amazing solutions that can help the complex system adapt.

Challenging the System

The problem: Blindly accepting the status quo leads to stagnation of culture, ideas, work, and people. Let us take a moment to remember that complex systems mimic living organisms. That means that they require movement, adaptation, and connection to survive. When organizations maintain the status quo, they are reducing all three of those things. Can you think of anything that is alive that does not move in some way, that cannot adapt or is not connected to another living thing? Organizations that only maintain the status quo quickly become irrelevant in their industry, and leaders who maintain the status quo quickly become ineffective.

The mistake many leaders make when working to create innovation and change within their teams is that they focus on trying to convince those who cannot be convinced (small minority of laggards) rather than focusing energy on the majority of the team, who will actively engage in the process.

For example, a manager is leading a routine staff meeting and begins describing some changes that are occurring on the unit. One or two vocal staff members speak up against the changes in a disruptive fashion. The ineffective leader then spends the rest of the meeting attempting to convince those two staff members rather than engaging the rest of the department in the changes. In short, this is a misuse of the leader's energy.

The solution: Using our example of the disruptive staff meeting, we can provide two ways that the leader could better influence the team around a change. **The first solution is for the leader to handle the disruption from the perspective of a complex system.** The disruption is a needed aspect of the change. It provides information to the leader that the change is challenging the values and assumptions of the team. However, catering to all of the concerns of the few disruptors rarely works while in large meetings. Instead, the leader could thank the team members for their concern and reframe the question to engage the rest of the team. Handle disruption and negative feedback with an eye for the overall system. Ask yourself, "How can I translate this information into something that moves the work forward?" Say, for example, "Thank you for your feedback. I would like to hear from the rest of the team if there are things we should consider related to this change." This creates a safe place for others to speak up and provides valuable information to the leader about things to consider in the change process.

Second, **leaders should focus less on the "negatoids" and more on the people who will adapt and change.** Rogers (2010) researched the way innovations are adopted in teams and populations. Since publication of his seminal text, over 2,000 studies have been conducted across multiple industries looking at the diffusion of innovations. From all of this evidence, Rogers created the "s-curve" of innovation adoption. Basically, he found that roughly 84% of people will adopt innovations that show value in their work or lives. This means that only 16% of people will not adopt and Rogers called them *Laggards*. The problem is that leaders in complex systems routinely spend the majority of their energy trying to change the 16% and forget that their energy would be better spent focusing on the 84% who will change.

Characteristics of Early Adopters

- They adopt the latest technology first.
- They use the latest evidence in their practice.
- They continually proposes solutions to team issues.
- They are willing to try unproven solutions.
- They are comfortable with failure.
- They have a history of adapting quickly to new situations.

Diffusion of innovations helps leaders focus on the 84% even further by suggesting that leaders trying to create change must convince the early adopters in the group first. Early adopters are those team members who are willing to evaluate new things before others. They make up roughly 13% of teams. Leaders can identify and cultivate **early adopters** by looking for team members who adopt new technology when it is released, constantly review the latest changes in practices, or continually propose solutions to problems.

Leaders can influence complex systems in a variety of ways if they focus on building connections, gathering and sharing information, and engaging the changeable team members. This is not easy work. Leaders must continually assess and challenge the status quo to keep their teams moving forward and their system working at an adaptable capacity. Leaders need to challenge with evidence, be bold, take risks, and create a legacy.

CALL TO ACTION

Mapping the Complex System

Creating mind maps is a great way to help leaders understand all the complex relationships that occur. Figure 16.2 shows an example of a mind map that you could use to map out key stakeholders and how they may impact a change project.

Instructions:

1. In the center bubble, type your change-project title.

2. In the dark gray bubbles, you should list the teams, departments, or people who you anticipate will be impacted by your change project.

3. Use the pink and red bubbles to anticipate the positive (pink) and negative (red) or neutral (gray) impact they may have. For example, you might list willingness to adopt as a positive impact but the need for financial resources from that team as something that might cause resistance to the change.

4. Finally, in the white space, begin noting the leadership behaviors that you will use to remove the negative reactions or flip neutral reactions to positive ones.

As you move along your change journey, you should continually update this map to help provide a road map for you to address issues and anticipate the system-level changes that occur in complex organizations.

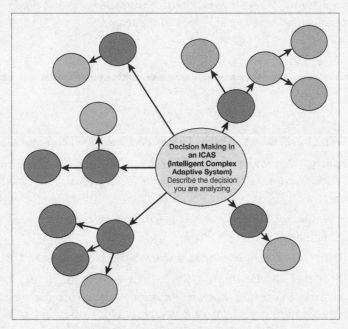

Figure 16.2 Decision-making in an ICAS.

ICAS, intelligent, complex adaptive system.

🔖 CONCLUSIONS

Leaders wishing to challenge the status quo need to keep the complex system in mind. This means they need to focus on engaging their teams with the right information, facilitate ground-up innovation, and challenge the status quo. The work of the leader in supporting innovation is not easy. Leaders must be bold, risk failure, and challenge by using evidence.

🔑 KEY TAKEAWAY POINTS

- Complex systems require different leadership skills to influence team members.

- Complex systems are interdependent, interrelated, and more than the sum or their parts.

- The results of change in complex systems are not predictable.

- Leaders can influence change in complex systems through sharing information, facilitating ground-up innovation, and challenging the status quo.

- To anticipate change in complex systems, the use of mind mapping can help leaders anticipate where change will occur and work to be proactive in addressing issues.

- Leading in complex systems requires leaders to build and maintain strong relationships across the system, not just in their own departments.

- The work of the successful leader is to facilitate conversations of what does not work, to listen intently, and to value the voice and solutions of the team.

REFERENCES

Burke, W. W. (2017). *Organization change: Theory and practice.* Thousand Oaks, CA: Sage.

Davidson, S., Weberg, D., Malloch, K., & Porter-O'Grady, T. (2016). *Leadership for evidence-based innovation in nursing and health professions.* Burlington, MA: Jones & Bartlett Learning.

Hatch, M. J. (2018). *Organization theory: Modern, symbolic, and postmodern perspectives.* Oxford, England: Oxford University Press.

Rogers, E. M. (2010). *Diffusion of innovations.* New York, NY: Simon and Schuster.

Ward, V., West, R., Smith, S., McDermott, S., Keen, J., Pawson, R., & House, A. (2014). The role of informal networks in creating knowledge among health-care managers: A prospective case study. *Health Services and Delivery Research, 2*(12), 1–132. doi:10.3310/hsdr02120

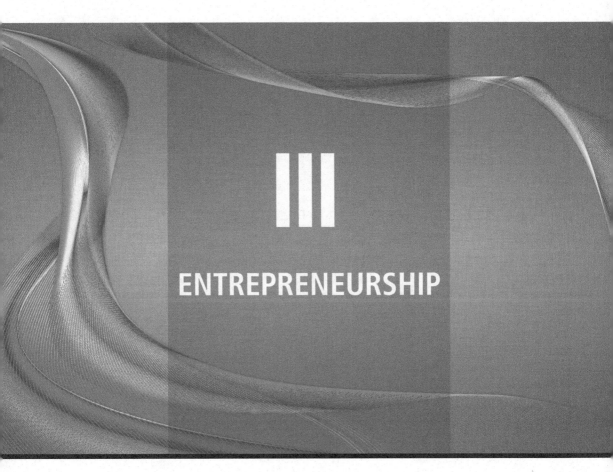

III

ENTREPRENEURSHIP

Entrepreneurship in Healthcare

Tim Raderstorf

"The greater danger for most of us lies not in setting our aim too high and falling short, but in setting our aim too low and achieving our mark."—Michelangelo

LEARNING OBJECTIVES

- Understand the need for entrepreneurial leadership in healthcare.
- Examine the foundations of entrepreneurship through the evidenced-based entrepreneurial learning concepts.
- Apply entrepreneurial concepts to healthcare settings.
- Inspire the reader to change behaviors and adopt entrepreneurial principles into his or her healthcare role.

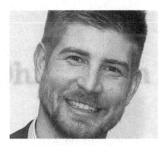

*Editor's Note: Please note this chapter is written in the first person by **Tim Raderstorf**. Dr. Raderstorf is the chief innovation officer at The Ohio State University. He is also the founder of Quality Health Communications, a healthcare IT (information technology) company that communicates the right clinical information to the right clinician at the right time. He was previously the founding chief innovation officer of the healthcare startup Mindful Management. Tim co-founded his first business, a small real-estate company, in 2008 and has been addicted to entrepreneurship ever since. **Here's Tim.***

INTRODUCTION

Still feeling great after 16 chapters on leadership and innovation? That content is pretty powerful and mastery of those concepts will surely lead to a more fulfilling career in the future. Even though some of the concepts were new and others a little foreign, I hope it wasn't too much of a stretch to draw a direct line from those concepts, to how they are applicable to your work as a healthcare professional. Perhaps after reading those chapters you may have even conceived a few new ideas to impact your organization. And that's wonderful, because in this next section we are going to discuss a concept that may not be as familiar to you, but one that is equally as impactful in advancing healthcare. A concept that may help you turn those new ideas into action: entrepreneurship.

By this time you probably have realized that this textbook is pretty unique in both its content and its delivery. You will notice things get a little different in this last section of the book as it is written by individuals who are living and working in the entrepreneurial trenches. You'll hear firsthand from experts on what's worked, what hasn't, and how they believe you can become a better healthcare provider by learning from their journeys. This final section of the book is broken down into nine chapters, with this first chapter being the heaviest in content. You will start first with exploring entrepreneurial concepts; how they have been taught and adapted in healthcare and beyond. Admittedly these concepts are not all-encompassing. You may not run into them on every entrepreneurial journey, nor may they be the helpful resource you need for your particular situation, but integrating these concepts into my professional practice, whether as a bedside RN, clinic manager, chief innovation officer, or healthcare IT entrepreneur, has improved the outcomes for the patients and providers with whom I have interacted.

The following chapters cover business model development, financing your ideas, and showcase businesses that have successfully navigated the entrepreneurial journey. You'll be inspired by healthcare leaders who have started businesses in their garages and grown into companies that generate over $100,000,000 annually. You'll hear from the nurse who invented the first implantable port, clinicians who have founded successful software companies, and practitioners who own their own practices. Whether you are inspired or intimidated by these concepts, before you dive into this section, you are encouraged to reflect back on Chapter 2, Important Lessons Learned From a Personal Leadership, Innovation, and Entrepreneurial Journey, and the breadth of the issues dismantling our nation's healthcare system. Something needs to be done. That something could start with you. Are you ready?

A CASE FOR ENTREPRENEURSHIP IN HEALTHCARE

In my frequent travels throughout the country presenting on entrepreneurship in healthcare, I often hear two common responses from healthcare professionals when we start discussions on entrepreneurship:

1. "I didn't get into healthcare for the money."

2. "I'm just a (insert healthcare profession here), I leave that stuff to the business experts." (Sidenote—The phrase "I'm just a nurse" is my least favorite sentence ever uttered in the history of the world.)

What is often lost on these individuals at the beginning of our discussions is that entrepreneurship takes many forms. Entrepreneurship isn't always about making more money. Much like innovation, entrepreneurial principles in healthcare are about creating more value. Properly integrating innovation and entrepreneurship principles into healthcare provides more value and less cost for patients, and greater job satisfaction for providers (Warmelink et al., 2015). Embracing these principles will give you the opportunity to have a greater impact on healthcare,

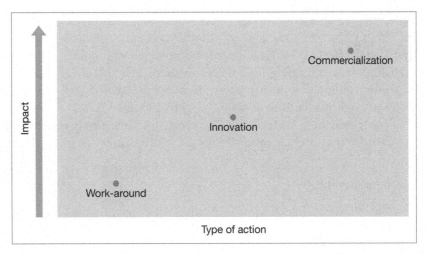

Figure 17.1 Potential for impact in healthcare.

and as leaders we must be aware that true healthcare impact does not occur within organization but within our communities, nation, and the world. It is my belief that the only way to have a broad impact on healthcare is through the principles of entrepreneurship and commercialization. *Commercialization* is defined here as the process of taking products, services, or solutions to the market so that they can be purchased and consumed by another entity.

Some of you may be pretty uncomfortable with my approach. Maybe you are even thinking exactly what others have said to me, " *I am not in healthcare for the money.*" But bear with me here as I believe we can align our values pretty quickly on this concept. You got into healthcare to help others and impact your organization, community, and maybe even the world. I am fully aligned with you in that statement. We are both all about impact in healthcare. But if we really dive deep into how we can impact others, it quickly becomes clear that the only way to integrate our ideas/solutions into healthcare is to ensure that they are sellable and consumable by a healthcare organization. Clearly stated, if you can't sell it, they can't use it.

Think about it. What goods, services, or solutions does your team use on a daily basis that do not cost the patient money? When I ask that question at conferences, people often respond, "The care and compassion that we provide at the bedside." And although as providers we do an excellent job at delivering care and compassion, that care and compassion is very costly to the patient. Just ask to see his or her most recent healthcare bill.

So as you navigate your way through this engaging and exciting section on entrepreneurship, I challenge you to think of the impact on your practice and how you can increase the level of impact you have on your organization, community, and beyond (Figure 17.1).

ENTREPRENEURIAL CONCEPTS

Entrepreneurship is commonly viewed as someone who opens a retail store at your local mall, a respiratory therapist who develops a new intubation device, or a nurse practitioner who starts his or her own practice. But there are also many principles of entrepreneurship that can be applied to the bedside, or to managing a team of healthcare providers. In this chapter, we are going to examine 15 core concepts of entrepreneurship, and directly apply them to life as a clinician. These 15 concepts are adapted from 13 concepts initially identified by Morris, Webb, Fu, and Singhal (2013). Two additional concepts, managing uncertainty from David Ochi, and my addition of reframing failure take us to an even 15. We will dive deeply into most of these concepts, though there are a few like *Guerrilla Skills* and *Resource Leveraging* that are already (though maybe unknowingly) deeply ingrained into healthcare leadership, and thus we will only skim their surface. I've also taken some liberties in rearranging Morris's concepts into an order that I feel is more closely aligned to our work in healthcare (Morris et al., 2013):

1. Recognizing opportunity
2. Assessing opportunity
3. Managing uncertainty
4. Mitigating and managing risk
5. Envisioning the future
6. Creative problem-solving
7. Innovation—creating new value
8. Planning/modeling when nothing exists
9. Resource leveraging
10. Guerilla Skills
11. Building and leveraging a network
12. Stay focus and yet adapt from learned experience.
13. Tenacity/perseverance
14. Self-efficacy
15. Resilience and reframing failure

You will notice that some of the concepts closely mirror healthcare processes like ADPIE (assess, diagnose, plan, implement, evaluate) and PDSA (plan, do, study, act). Whether you choose to use them at the bedside or apply them to start your own business, applying these entrepreneurial concepts is beneficial in both improving patient outcomes and developing your professional career.

Entrepreneurial Concept 1: Recognizing Opportunity

Recognizing opportunity is the core concept of our current healthcare system. The opportunities to prevent, heal, or soothe are central to daily practice. As a healthcare leader, engaging with bedside clinicians is perhaps the most efficient way to recognize opportunity as they are aligned with the current needs of their healthcare system. In entrepreneurship, *opportunity* is often synonymous with the terms *pain point* and *problem*. A pain point is a process, service, product, solution, policy, or anything else that inflicts some type of "pain" on the user. An example of a pain point would be the amount of time clinicians spend charting in the electronic health record (EHR) rather than spending that time at the bedside taking care of patients. In enterprise, recognizing opportunity is seen through a professional's ability to identify changing conditions or opportunities that other individuals have failed to capitalize upon to create profit or value for their business (Morris et al., 2013).

Healthcare providers often use opportunity recognition when perceiving changes in the patient's condition to create new value and improve health outcomes. With the United States ranking top in healthcare spending (Organisation for Economic Co-operation and Development, 2018), but 34th in life expectancy outcomes (World Health Organization, 2018), opportunity abounds. Traditional opportunities have been seen through providers recognizing a lack of healthcare providers in a community and starting their own practice. Other healthcare providers recognize opportunity through the misuse of commonly prescribed treatments. For example, ENTvantage DX is a product that was developed to address the opportunity of reducing the number of antibiotics that are prescribed to patients with viral infections. This point-of-care test was developed by an ear, nose and throat (ENT) physician because he did not have a timely method to determine whether his patients presenting with potential upper respiratory infections would benefit from antibiotic treatment. His new tool allowed him to quickly diagnose the patient's infection as either viral or bacterial and determine, with the patient in the room, whether antibiotics would be helpful or harmful for that patient. Antibiotic resistance has been identified as an area of concern in healthcare for decades, yet it took the insights of a bedside clinician to recognize the opportunity and utilize the concepts that will be discussed further in this chapter to improve the quality of care and patient outcomes.

 CALL TO ACTION

What opportunities do you see in your organization? Make a list of these opportunities. Concepts 2 through 15 will teach you what to do with that list!

Entrepreneurial Concept 2: Assessing Opportunity

Those who are best at assessing opportunity have the skill set to both evaluate opportunities and determine the potential return on investment (ROI) or impact to the world (Morris et al., 2013). With assessment as the first step in the ADPIE (assessment, diagnosis, planning, implementation, and evaluation) process, assessing opportunity is a concept that should come naturally to most healthcare professionals. Whether determining if a patient's infection is viral or bacterial, or ruling out febrile neutropenia for a patient with cancer, providers continually assess the situation and determine which options would lead to the best outcomes. Assessing opportunity through an entrepreneurial lens is exactly the same. You must determine what the ROI will be from acting upon an opportunity. It is important to consider that there is a different ROI for every person or group involved. The patient's ROI will be different than the organization's ROI or the practitioner's ROI.

In Chapter 15, Design Thinking for Healthcare Leadership and Innovation, you learned about measuring the ROI in innovation. The concepts highlighted there provide a framework for you to assess the potential opportunity for your innovative or entrepreneurial endeavors. When assessing opportunity, remember two factors that burgeoning entrepreneurs sometimes forget:

1. The status quo always exists as competition. Your opportunity must create a better outcome than what people achieve from maintaining current practice.

2. You must always consider the opportunity cost and ask yourself "What will happen if I do not act?"

Entrepreneurial Concept 3: Managing Uncertainty

Oftentimes when people think of entrepreneurs, they think of people who took great risks; people who worked out of a garage or took a second mortgage out on their home to finance their business. And although managing risk is discussed in Concept 4, leaders and entrepreneurs must first master the management of uncertainty. You may be wondering what the difference is between the two? Risk is something that can be calculated. Uncertainly lies in the unknown. David Ochi, New Ventures Director at the University of California, Irvine's ANTrepreneur Center, recently clarified this concept in a way that made it crystal clear to me through this hypothetical game. Let's give it a try and see what you think.

> Imagine a candy jar filled with 100 pieces of candy that are of exactly the same shape and size. The only difference between the candy is that 50 pieces are wrapped in silver and 50 pieces are wrapped in gold. You have the opportunity to blindly pull out one piece of candy from the jar. If that piece of candy is wrapped in a gold wrapper, you win $10,000. Given this information, how much money would you be willing to pay to play this game? (Write that down now.)

> Now imagine the exact same scenario with one key difference. This time the jar is still filled with 100 pieces of candy, but you are unaware of the ratio of silver to gold pieces. It could be 50:50, it could be 18:82, or maybe even all of the candy is silver or gold. Again if you pull out a piece of candy that is wrapped in gold, you win $10,000. How much money would you be willing to pay to play this version of the game? (Write that down now.)

These two scenarios highlight the difference between risk and uncertainty. You likely were willing to spend much more to play the game in scenario 1, where you were able to calculate that you had a 50% chance of winning $10,000. In scenario 2, no calculations were able to be made. You were uncertain of your odds and therefore were likely to pay much less, or maybe even abstain from the game.

THOUGHT-PROVOKING QUESTION OF THE PAGE: How often as a healthcare professional do you teeter between managing risk versus managing uncertainty?

Entrepreneurial Concept 4: Mitigating and Managing Risk

When it comes to managing or mitigating risk, the skilled leader must have the ability to take action to achieve one of two outcomes:

1. Decrease the likelihood of a risk actually occurring.

2. Decrease the impact of a risk if it were to occur.

Again if you think back to the candy game example outlined in Concept 3, managing risk was relatively simple to do when all external parameters were identified. If you were able to calculate that there was a 90% chance that you would pull out a golden-wrapped piece of candy, you can be fairly confident in your ability to identify the opportunity, calculate its cost, and determine the risks involved in both engaging in the game or not engaging in the game.

Risk and uncertainly abound in healthcare and in entrepreneurship. A bedside manager may need to determine the risks involved in hiring travel nurses during an extended staffing shortage. There is ample evidence surrounding the effectiveness of travel nurses and the impact of poor staffing ratios on patient outcomes. The manager can, with relative certainty, determine the risks involved by not meeting typical staffing ratios. That same nurse manager must also deal with the uncertainty of how long this staffing shortage will take place and if/when it will occur again. The success of the leader is determined by his or her understanding that what is required is not to control the risk or uncertainty but rather to recognize that risk and uncertainty can only be managed, not controlled. He or she must embrace what he or she cannot control. This is an uncomfortable position for many leaders and entrepreneurs, but the success of the leader lies in his or her ability to become comfortable with being uncomfortable.

Other than managing uncertainty, there perhaps is no entrepreneurial concept more aligned to daily healthcare practice than in mitigating and managing risk. Yet this concept is one that needs much attention from healthcare professionals due to the unintended harm caused by our healthcare system. Each year in the United States, approximately 400,000 people die due to preventable healthcare errors (Makary & Daniel, 2016). That is the equivalent of eight fully loaded 737 jet airliners crashing and killing every passenger on board, every day. This example highlights both the need for healthcare professionals to increase their skills for mitigating and managing risk and also a hefty entrepreneurial opportunity for healthcare professionals who are willing to tackle the daunting challenge of medical errors.

Entrepreneurial Concept 5: Envisioning the Future

Envisioning the future is actually a two-part concept. The first part of envisioning the future stems from the ability to recognize what future states may look like. For example, Elon Musk envisioned a future where gasoline was no longer used to power automobiles and founded Tesla. When Tesla began accepting orders for the Model 3 in 2016, they received nearly 200,000 requests in the first 24 hours.

The second component of envisioning the future is the ability to communicate your vision in a way that others can understand and endorse it (Morris et al., 2013). For example, electric vehicles have recently began to pop-up all over the marketplace in the last decade, with companies like Tesla releasing their more affordable Model 3 and Volvo changing their strategic vision by removing conventional engines from all vehicles by 2019. But the electric vehicle actually had many false starts leading up to this more recent wide-stream adoption. The first was during the early 1900s as electric vehicles competed with the Model T for market share. Of course, the Model T won this battle. Again in 1990, there was an upsurge in electric vehicle production, with General Motors (GM) making the EV1, an all-electric vehicle with a range of 80 miles. Low gas prices and a booming economy are credited as contributing factors to the lack of sales for the vehicle (Department of Energy, 2014). Elon Musk's success at Tesla showcases his team's ability to not only envision the future, but better communicate their vision than GM and other electronic vehicle companies of the past.

When providers take a step back from the bedside, it can be a little easier to see the trends evolving in healthcare. Because healthcare is subject to an extremely lengthy time between the publication of research and its adoption to the bedside (did you know that it takes on average 17 years for healthcare research to reach the bedside? [Balas & Boren, 2000]), leaders may benefit from taking a look back to publications from 10 to 15 years ago to determine what new procedures and technologies will be integrated into practice in the near future.

The good news is that this glaring weakness can be leveraged to achieve success. If a leader is able to identify emerging technological trends that have yet to be applied to healthcare settings, that leader can then capitalize on this opportunity. Need an example? Think about text messaging in hospitals. Text messaging became a mainstream method of communication around 2005. While industries outside of healthcare were able to leverage this new communication method, healthcare struggled to widely adopt HIPAA-compliant text messaging platforms until almost a decade later. As a result, improved team communication leads to improved patient outcomes.

The critical condition of patients and overwhelming volume of individuals seeking care can make it challenging for providers to look beyond the next few hours, let alone envision the future. But mastery of this concept by leaders is essential if healthcare is going to evolve into the next generation of care delivery.

 CALL TO ACTION

Dr. Melnyk, the co-author of this book, regularly challenges her colleagues to envision the future, but she does this in a very inspiring way. She asks "If I was your fairy godmother and could ensure that you cannot fail in your work, what would you do in the next 5 years?" This question unknowingly requires the individual to look to the future envision what a successful healthcare provider would look like. You answered this question in Chapter 1, Making the Case for Evidence-Based Leadership and Innovation, now I encourage you to tackle this from an entrepreneurial lens. Knowing what you know about the future of healthcare, what would you change in the next 5 years if you knew you could not fail? Write that down and reflect on your progress on the first day of every month.

Entrepreneurial Concept 6: Creative Problem-Solving

"Fall in love with the problem, not the solution." —Kareen Hanson

Morris et al. (2013) identify creative problem-solving as an individual's ability to connect products, services, or solutions that were previously unrelated, resulting in the creation of new/useful outcomes. There is nothing foreign about this concept to healthcare professionals. Creative problem-solving is the foundation of our work. As a nurse and Chief Innovation Officer, I cannot count the number of times I have seen respiratory therapists reach into their carts to modify ventilator tubing to meet the unique needs of their patients, or nurses use tongue depressors and medical tape to create a myriad of healthcare prototypes. The trick to successful creative problem-solving in healthcare is to balance creativity with current practice. It can be challenging to implement new services in healthcare that require substantial behavioral change from providers. The creative healthcare problem solver understands this and often develops solutions that allow for incremental behavioral change to improve patient outcomes. This is not to say that disruptive innovations are not possible in healthcare, but those seeking to disrupt healthcare may be better suited to focus on solutions that do not involve significant behavioral change.

Within creative problem-solving, healthcare providers and entrepreneurs alike must consider the *problem–solution statement*. In Concept 1, we identified opportunity as *the problem*. Now in Concept 6, we pair of that problem with a solution through creative problem-solving. A problem–solution statement recognizes the problem–opportunity and states a creative solution to address the problem. Using the previous example of ENT Advantage, their *problem–solution statement* might look something like this:

Problem: Patients are often prescribed antibiotic medications without evidence that the treatment will be effective.

Solution: A point-of-care nasal swab test that will identify if patients with upper respiratory infection complaints will benefit from antibiotic therapy within 15 minutes of receiving the test.

CALL TO ACTION

Create a "Wall of Pain" for your unit/department/organization. Dedicate a white board as a location for team members to identify "Pain Points" in the workplace. Sit down with three to five of your colleagues and determine which statement on the "Wall of Pain" is the worst pain point your team faces at work each day? Together develop a solution for that problem and take that idea to whomever you directly report. Ask them what you need to do to put your solution into practice. (Then figure out how you can commercialize it to maximize your impact!)

Entrepreneurial Concept 7: Creating New Value

The concept of creating new value is certainly not foreign to you at this point. You examined multiple processes of innovation in the second section of this book and now are hopefully beginning to draw parallels between innovation in healthcare and entrepreneurship in healthcare. Morris et al. (2013) explore value creation through one's capabilities to develop new products services and/or business models that meet two criteria. These products, services, or business models must provide enough benefit to the user(s) so that the user is willing to pay an amount greater than the cost to produce the products, services, or business models *and* the products, services, or business models must make more than they spend (revenues must exceed costs).

It's easy to confuse these concepts as being the same, but there is an important distinction between them. The successful entrepreneur can create market demand to increase revenue, but must also be cost conscious when making spending decisions to ensure the sustainability of the product/service/or solution. Whether you are making a lot of money and spending a little, or you are making a little money and are spending even less, you must have a positive relationship between what money comes in, and what goes out.

Entrepreneurial Concept 8: Planning/Modeling When Nothing Exists

Perhaps one of the greatest challenges to entrepreneurship in healthcare or healthcare leaders is how to plan or model when there is no benchmark from which to measure your idea. This concept does not present for all types of entrepreneurship; for example, if you were to purchase a franchise of a yoga studio or gym, there would be plenty of competitors in similar communities for you to benchmark your company against. But if you are going to take on one of the most challenging aspects of entrepreneurship and create a new category of product service or solution, you may find yourself in a situation where your idea stands alone. At this point, there are three main components to consider. The first is that every product always has a benchmark, and that benchmark is the status quo. Customers always have the option to continue to behave as they currently do and not adopt your product.

As an example, let's again look to the invention of the automobile. While there were many individuals attempting to commercialize the automobile at the turn of the 20th century, those entrepreneurs did not have a universal understanding of what automotive travel would look like. The category in which they were displacing was traveling by horseback or horse and buggy, which was widely adopted buy most of the developed world at the time. If they stayed within their own category, automotive entrepreneurs would have likely developed more comfortable saddles or developed products that would minimize the amount of maintenance needed for buggies. Instead, they proceeded with creating a new category and thus only had the status quo upon which to benchmark.

The second component of planning and modeling when nothing currently exists, and perhaps the most critical component of entrepreneurship, is that the entrepreneur must always *listen* to their customer. Henry Ford is famously quoted as saying, "If I asked people what they wanted, they would've said faster horses." And while there is debate over whether Henry Ford actually said these words, this comment has been a point of debate throughout entrepreneurial circles for the past century. Many agree with this quote and believe that customers are unable to verbalize their needs. However, many others like myself believe that the customers' ability to verbalize their needs is based on the questions that are being asked. If Ford I Had asked, "What would make your transportation experience better?" He very well may have gotten a response such as "Faster Horses." The key here is that listening to customers doesn't always mean incorporating their feedback, but rather gathering insights by asking clarifying questions to determine what you believe is best for your venture.

This information would be incredibly valuable to any entrepreneur or innovator who adheres to the third important component to *Planning/Modeling When Nothing Exists*, which is always challenge assumptions. When the question was asked, Ford would also need to consider what assumptions lie behind the question. Was it implied that the new technology would only be applicable to a horse travel? Is the inventor only thinking of advancements to horse travel or is he/she considering all methods of travel? When an answer is received, does the inventor focus on the word horse or the word faster? An inventor who challenges assumptions would focus on the word "faster" and search for methods to increase the speed of any type of individualized travel. Perhaps Ford later challenged assumptions and asked, "As the speed of your horse is an issue, if I created a carriage that could safely transport you in a quarter of the time it currently takes to travel in your existing carriage, would that be of interest to you?"

Entrepreneurial Concept 9: Resource Leveraging

Regardless of your role, resources surround you. From medical tape and tongue depressors, to fellow colleagues, resources are everywhere you turn. The simple fact about what separates those who are excellent at leveraging resources from the rest is their ability to recognize the opportunity and asking for *help*. I could go on and on about leveraging resources (and do a bit in the next concept on Guerilla Skills), but I purposely want to keep this section lean and encourage you to *start asking for what you need to be successful*. It may be the only thing that keeps you from success.

Entrepreneurial Concept 10: Guerrilla Skills

Perhaps you are working in organization with limited funds or are employed in a field where resources are not as comparable as other fields. (Any nonprofit workers out there?) If you find yourself in such a scenario, guerrilla skills can help you achieve success. Guerrilla skills are another concept that should be very familiar to healthcare leaders as they work to get the job done. Morris et al. (2013) define guerrilla skills as one's ability to take advantage of his or her surroundings and employ unconventional and low-cost tactics that have not been employed by competitors. Those with guerilla skills are able to do more with less to get the job done. From managing patient needs during staffing shortages to reallocating resources during budget cuts, healthcare leaders are accustomed to guerrilla tactics and can translate this skill for entrepreneurial success.

Entrepreneurial Concept 11: Building and Leveraging a Network

Building and leveraging a network can be a challenge for healthcare professionals as it often requires the individual to reach beyond the traditional limits of his or her professional network. As healthcare professionals tend to run in closer circles within their unit/department/organization, we would greatly benefit from extending beyond our comfort zones to connect with new individuals. This in turn provides more resources to leverage for our patients and businesses. There are *two* key components to this entrepreneurial concept. It is not enough to build a large network, but you must be able to leverage the resources included within that network as well.

Leverage is an interesting concept that's come up twice now in these entrepreneurial concepts and something that we should dive a little bit deeper into. To be able to apply leverage, one must have some type of asset, force, and or power that he/she is able to utilize to help achieve an outcome he/she desires. When leveraging your network, ask yourself, "What asset do I bring that could help the individual with whom I am trying to network?" For example, when I was just starting to make the planned transition from healthcare quality to healthcare innovation, I knew that my journey of commercializing a healthcare IT platform was an experience that few other healthcare providers had. And though it is sometimes fun to be on the cutting edge and a leader in innovation, I quickly recognized it was more important for me to set the groundwork for other healthcare professionals to follow for their own entrepreneurial journey. I knew that if I was going to have a broad and lasting impact, I would also need to look beyond my own organization, identify other pathways to influence, and encourage other healthcare providers to engage in entrepreneurial activities.

At that time in my career, my professional network was relatively small and isolated to my own geographic area. In the year prior to making my professional transition, I had attended the nursing innovation Summit at the Cleveland Clinic. During one of the breakout sessions, I introduced myself to the event organizer and thanked him for setting up the summit. Still new to building my professional network, I did not think to reach out to him until months later. When I finally did, we ended up having an hour-long conversation on healthcare innovation and how we can better deliver innovation content to our colleagues. By the end of the call, he had asked me to speak at the summit in the upcoming year, and I have since spoken at that summit three times. My performances speaking at these summits have led to securing other speaking invitations at conferences across the country. If I had not reached out to him and leveraged my network, I am confident that my speaking career would have taken a less impactful path and more importantly, far fewer healthcare professionals would not have been exposed to the concepts of innovation and entrepreneurship.

Entrepreneurial Concept 12: Stay Focused and Yet Adapt From Learned Experiences

One question that is commonly asked by investors and mentors is whether or not the team or individual is "coachable." Coachability refers to the individual's ability to receive feedback from experts, customers, and/or product testing and apply feedback to improve his/her solution. This does not mean that the entrepreneur or leader must always take the advice of others, but that the entrepreneur must be willing to consider that advice and determine if they believe suggested changes are the right solution for their team. As your coachability increases, so too does your ability to learn from experience and apply those lessons to improve your business.

The majority of leadership and entrepreneurship is trial and error. Being honest with yourself about the data you receive regarding your product services or solutions will help you improve your business and better address an unmet need. To be successful, one must recognize that numbers can be manipulated, but they never truly lie. Trying to change your interpretation of data only allows you to operate under false assumptions. Instead of looking for a way to "spin" the data in your favor, ask what you can learn from the data to improve your business.

Tim's Thoughts on How to Demonstrate Coachability

I'm going to assume that many of you have seen the television show *Shark Tank*. For those of you have not seen the show, it is a reality TV series where entrepreneurs pitch their ideas for businesses to a panel of investors who then decide if they would like to invest in the entrepreneur's business. As you can imagine, this is often an anxiety-producing event for the entrepreneurs and sometimes this leads to tears being shed. Emotion is not a bad thing to bring into entrepreneurship. There is however a noticeable difference between the entrepreneurs who let emotion move them to tears on the show and still get funded versus those who cry on the show and do not get funded. What is often detrimental to those who end up

(continued)

(*continued*)

showcasing emotion is their inability to receive feedback from the judges. These entrepreneurs are missing the main purpose of pitching their ideas: to receive feedback about your idea from individuals with expertise. When receiving feedback from individuals, there is only one true response that an entrepreneur or leadership provides: "Thank you for your feedback. That's something for me to take back to my team to discuss." Again this doesn't mean that you must take every piece of advice you receive from experts. You will likely receive conflicting advice more often than you'll receive similar advice. Stay focused on solving your problem and stay open to receiving feedback from others. If you cannot master this skill, it is likely that you won't receive the resources needed for success.

Entrepreneurial Concept 13: Tenacity/Perseverance

The biggest challenge in entrepreneurship (and in many times in healthcare) is knowing when to count your losses and give up in the face of insurmountable odds. The entrepreneurial world distinguishes itself through the fact that there are three simple answers that you can receive when pitching or selling your product, service or solution to customers or investors. The best answer is, of course, "Yes." A "yes" means that your company is meeting an unmet need for your customer base. It means that you are more likely to achieve the outcomes that you set out to accomplish.

One may think that "Maybe" is the next best answer you can receive, but in the entrepreneurial world "maybe" means not "right now" and "right now" is the only time that matters for entrepreneurs. It also could mean that you may not be meeting the unmet need *or* that the timing of your idea does not match the current needs of the customer. Or maybe even both.

This ambiguity between unmet needs and poor timing causes entrepreneurs to regularly teeter between potential solutions. A much better answer to maybe is "No." While it is difficult to hear "no" and learn that you're not meeting the need or the desired timing of the customer, you can be certain one of those is the case. This certainty will allow you to amend your product, service, or solution to better meet the customers' needs. This process of changing or iterating your product service or solution is often referred to as a *pivot* or *pivoting*. Pivoting is the practice of successful entrepreneurs who focus on solving the problem. The solution will likely look very different from the start of the project to what eventually becomes the final solution. (We'll further examine two of my favorite "pivots" in Concept 15.)

In entrepreneurship, even the best solutions hear a "no" much more frequently than they hear a "yes." Being told that your product service or solution doesn't have a chance is a rite of passage; a badge of honor for entrepreneurs to wear on their sleeves. They hear a "no" and they keep the pedal down, looking for better solutions, better customers, better outcomes. But at what cost? At what point do you decide to proceed as planned, pivot to a more aligned opportunity, or move on to something else? Most entrepreneurs will tell you that the truth is there's no magic rule. Set parameters at the start of your business that define under what circumstances would your business no longer be successful. These parameters may be something like *customers are unwilling to pay for my product, service, or solution at a price point that is profitable*. Another parameter could be the simple fact that you're no longer enjoying the work. Running an assessment of your parameters on a quarterly basis will provide you with an ongoing trend of where your business stands and will allow for an objective decision to be made if you are questioning if it's time to explore other opportunities.

CALL TO ACTION

How do you determine when it's time to persevere versus pivot versus move on through challenging situations at work? Create an assessment tool that will help you determine how to make these decisions. Develop 5 to 10 "yes or no" questions and answer them on a quarterly basis.

Entrepreneurial Concept 14: Self-Efficacy

A universal truth about entrepreneurship is that the person who is leading the entrepreneurial effort is the most important piece of technology for that business. This leader must demonstrate confidence in his/her ability to lead the initiative forward. Buy-in must be captured from investors, customers, and colleagues, but most importantly, the entrepreneur himself/herself. There are thousands of books on self-efficacy and developing confidence and I am certainly not the expert in this field. My recommendation for those who are seeking further development of your self-efficacy skills is to read religiously, but not on how to develop self-efficacy skills. Rather I believe you should focus upon your technology, the field in which it exists, and who most often engages with it. Being a world-class expert in these three views will assist you in conveying confidence and showcasing the leader within (remember that from Chapter 3, Understanding and Developing Yourself As a Leader?). If you can achieve that status and still receive feedback that customers or inventors don't believe in your skills, then it may be time to jump into reading some of those great self-efficacy development books.

Entrepreneurial Concept 15: Resilience and Reframing Failure

Estimates show that about one-third of businesses fail within the first year of founding and only half are still in operation at 5 years (Small Business Association, 2012). With such high failure rates, a healthy respect for failure is key to maintaining resiliency. This respect will allow the entrepreneur or leader to effectively manage stress and potentially thrive during unpredictable scenarios and uncertainty. I was recently reminded of the importance of resiliency and reframing failure while listening to a podcast (Raz & Butterfield, 2018) with Stuart Butterfield, the founder of Flickr *and* Slack (yes that is an "and"). Both Flickr and Slack were not the intended businesses that Stuart and his team sought out to build. Stewart and his team twice failed to develop a massively multiplayer online role-playing game. After their first failed attempt, his team recognized that the file sharing component used within the gameplay could be utilized to share digital picture files on the Internet. This company eventually became Flickr, a widely successful picture-sharing webpage that was sold to Yahoo! and is still in production today.

With a successful exit under his belt following his first big pivot, Butterfield returned to his dream of developing a massively multiplayer online role-playing game. The second time around, he was able to lean on his reputation as a successful entrepreneur and found it much easier to obtain the resources he believed his team needed to be successful. Yet even with all of these added resources, the team was again unable to successfully develop the video game they set out to create. He had to fire all but four of his employees and was beginning to lose his reputation as a capable entrepreneur. But lightning stuck once again as Stuart and his team found a diamond hiding in plain sight. The internal software his team had developed to help with communication as they rapidly built out the video game was actually a platform that had multiple applications on the enterprise software market. Suddenly a new, much larger application existed for this software. It is now known as Slack and currently valued at over $5.1 billion (Nusca, 2017).

SUMMARY

That certainly was a lot of information to digest, and I recognize that for many of you these are entirely new ideas, terms, and phrases. My hope is that you now see the 15 entrepreneurial concepts as a potential pathway for you to increase your impact on healthcare. I suspect there were many that allowed you to draw parallels to your current work, and develop a few new ideas on how you can become a leader. As you put these concepts into practice, maintain focus on the status quo as a key competitor, listen to your customers, and always challenge assumptions.

🔑 KEY TAKEAWAY POINTS

- Become comfortable with being uncomfortable.

- The only way to have a wide-reaching impact in healthcare is to be able to sell your solutions to healthcare organizations. If they can't buy it, they can't use it.

- To succeed as a leader and an entrepreneur, you must listen to your customers, users, colleagues, and yourself. Use a reliable assessment tool to determine whose advice to follow.

- Healthcare must be able to make money to provide continued services to the community. Wouldn't it be best if you, a healthcare leader, were one of the people who determined how that happens?

- Those who ask for help often receive it. Leverage the word "help" often.

REFERENCES

Balas, E., & Boren, S. (2000). Managing clinical knowledge for health care improvement. *Yearbook of Medical Informatics*, (1), 65–70. doi:10.1055/s-0038-1637943

Department of Energy. (2014). *The history of the electric car*. Retrieved from https://www.energy.gov/articles/history-electric-car

Makary, M. A., & Daniel, M. (2016). Medical error—The third leading cause of death in the US. *BMJ, 353*, i2139. doi:10.1136/bmj.i2139

Morris, M. H., Webb, J. W., Fu, J., & Singhal, S. (2013). A competency-based perspective on entrepreneurship education: Conceptual and empirical insights. *Journal of Small Business Management, 51*, 352–369. doi:10.1111/jsbm.12023

Nusca, A. (2017). Slack raises $250 million; tops $5 billion valuation. *Fortune*. Retrieved from http://fortune.com/2017/09/17/slack-raise-valuation/

Organisation for Economic Co-operation and Development. (2018). *Spending on health: Latest trends*. Retrieved from http://www.oecd.org/health/health-systems/Health-Spending-Latest-Trends-Brief.pdf

Raz, G., & Butterfield, S. (2018). *How I built this with Guy Raz: Slack & Flicker: Steward Butterfield*. Podcast retrieved from https://www.npr.org/2018/07/27/633164558/slack-flickr-stewart-butterfield

Small Business Association. (2012). *Do economic or industry factors affect business survival?* Retrieved from https://www.sba.gov/sites/default/files/Business-Survival.pdf

Warmelink, J. C., Hoijtink, K., Noppers, M., Wiegers, T. A., de Cock, T. P., Klomp, T., & Hutton, E. K. (2015). An explorative study of factors contributing to the job satisfaction of primary care midwives. *Midwifery, 31*(4), 482–488. doi:10.1016/j.midw.2014.12.003

World Health Organization. (2018). *Life expectancy and healthy life expectancy data by country*. Retrieved from http://apps.who.int/gho/data/view.main.SDG2016LEXv?lang=en

Identifying Opportunities to Innovate and Create Your Niche

David Putrino

"The best innovators make themselves vulnerable enough to create, but are then emotionally resilient enough to manage the feedback that is returned when they share their creativity." —David Putrino

LEARNING OBJECTIVES

- Identify key behavioral features that differentiate innovators from noninnovators.
- Understand the role of creativity in producing innovation.
- Acknowledge that creativity is a skill set that can be taught and developed.
- Respect the role of risk in the innovation mind-set and process.
- Identify when key opportunities to innovate present themselves.
- Identify common barriers to innovation and how to overcome them.

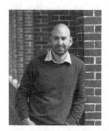

*Editor's note: This chapter is written in the first person in order to best capture **David Putrino**'s personal experience in finding his own niche in healthcare. **Here's David.***

INTRODUCTION

When I was about 8 years old, my older brother came to me with a proposal. It was a typically blistering hot summer's weekend in Perth, Western Australia. We were all in the house trying to escape the heat, sitting in our living room on the cold tile floor watching bad TV, and trying anything we could to distract ourselves from the heat. I was playing with my brand new remote-control car. I'd only had it a few days, but it was *the coolest*. None of the other kids on the street were allowed near it: it was all mine. My brother had been watching me mess around with the car for a while now. Maybe he had an idea, or maybe the sound of the crappy little toy car engine working overtime had finally gotten to him, but he sat up and said,

"I can make that thing go faster."

I eyed him skeptically. He was 7 years older than me, and he already had a bit of a reputation in the family for being a tinkerer. Talented with electronics, but his strike rate was kinda 50/50: Things went bad as often as they went well. I was intrigued, but suspicious, "What would you do with it?" This was my *treasure* I wasn't going to just hand it over.

"I told you—I'm going to make it go faster. Way faster. It will be so much better!"

I shook my head. I knew him too well for that to work. "No, Gino." Yes, my brother's name is *Gino Putrino*, but let's move past that, "You need to tell me exactly what you're going to do."

"You won't understand."

"Ok, then you can't have my car."

Long sigh.

He sat me down and explained how my car worked. How there was a motor that made the wheels of my car turn every time I turned the knob on my remote control. He showed me how that motor was powered by a 9-volt battery on the underside of the car, and that if we removed the battery, the car didn't work. Then he told me his theory: "The car goes pretty slow because the 9-volt battery is that strong but imagine if we could plug it in to a really strong power source. It. Would. Be. So. Cool."

My 8-year-old brain was sold. If I'm being really honest, he had had me at "I can make that thing go faster," but good sense had dictated that I at least put up some token resistance. I asked him where we were going to find a strong power supply, and, as if by magic, he produced one of Dad's old extension cords that Gino had already cannibalized for the express purpose of allowing him to connect things to a house's power outlets that under no circumstances should ever be connected to our house's power outlets. One end of the extension cord had a plug, and the other end had three wires: positive, negative, and ground. He attached the positive wire to the positive battery contact, the negative to the negative, and just stuck the grounding wire to a random bit of the car chassis with duct tape. He plugged the other end of the extension cord into the wall, flipped on the switch, and indicated for me to use the remote to propel the car forward. I must have turned the knob a millimeter and the car streaked forward like a bat out of hell. We looked at each other, elated,

"It's work—"

We never even got the chance to finish the sentence. My little car's motor began to feel the consequences of taking on way too much juice all at once: first, it started smoking and then, with very little further warning, erupted into a fireball. Right on my mother's living-room rug. We put the fire out and surveyed the consequences of our little experiment. The rug was ruined, my prized remote-control car was a twisted blob of smoldering plastic, and we were both in a ton of trouble with Mum. So, in the moment, I probably couldn't have told you that our collaboration was exactly a "success" … but over the years I've gotten more mileage from the story than I ever would from the toy car, so I guess that on some level I'm ahead, right?

I know what you're thinking: This book is all about health, so why on Earth is this guy talking about blowing up toy cars? Well, this chapter is all about innovation. More specific, we are here to focus on how to identify "your moment"—the moment you take off your "health professional" cap and strap on your "health innovator" jetpack. My childhood story about accidentally blowing things up with my brother is an example of not letting an opportunity for innovation pass. When my brother asked to mess with my toy car, I absolutely could have told him no, and there would have been a very predictable end to the story: "and then I played with the remote-control car until I was tired of it a week later. The end."

Instead, I decided to accept the risk that was associated with the innovation: I *may* get a way better toy, or I may destroy my favorite toy in the process. That decision turned out to absolutely bite my brother and I on the ass, but the upside was that we didn't create a sizable fire, it wasn't an expensive rug, our parents got over it quickly (they thought it was pretty funny, actually). All things considered, we sustained our disaster quite well. Could it have been worse? Sure—one of us could have been electrocuted, the other could have inhaled toxic plastic fumes (maybe I did and none of this chapter will make sense!). But here is the first fact that you need to internalize as a potential innovator—*innovation is risk*. There is no way around that, and every second you spend trying to de-risk a project takes you further away from innovation. Keeping in mind that I am going to ask you to suspend disbelief for the duration of this chapter and be ready at a moment's notice to destroy a young child's favorite toy, let's delve into how to identify opportunities for innovation.

INNOVATION IS RISK

There is no way around this statement. I'm often asked by large companies to sit with their board and discuss innovation, and I cannot tell you the number of board rooms that I have sat in, surrounded by demographically homogenous individuals being told,
"We need more innovation!"[1]

The problem is that it feels wise to individuals running large companies to shy away from innovation because spending money on a truly innovative idea often feels too risky, and large corporations are simply not risk tolerant. They are told by their board to maximize profits and only invest in risk that has a high probability of return. Now, many (even most) large companies will proudly tell you that they have an "innovation fund" but what they don't tell you is that the innovation fund is usually viciously guarded by the least innovative person in the company: someone who will obsessively de-risk every idea presented until the company is no longer funding innovation, it is funding a "sound, well-vetted investment opportunity." In short, there is a reason that legends about innovation feature a disheveled genius working out of a garage. This is the most commonly encountered ecosystem that is 100% risk tolerant. This disheveled genius then goes on to disrupt a major industry and put a bunch of large companies out of business because, while the large companies were making money doing things the way they had always been done (because that was the safest way of running the business), the disheveled genius came along and tested an idea that had no data behind it, no reason to work other than it made sense that it would. Underestimating this type of innovator is how powerful companies fail.

---

[1] I was once even told, "We need to *purchase* more innovation. David, how do we purchase innovation?" ☺

Hospitals and healthcare systems are, ostensibly, large companies. Regardless of whether you're living in a country that has a largely privatized healthcare system like the United States or some socialized medicine utopia like Sweden, innovation is difficult in healthcare. In both cases, healthcare companies are run like large, inflexible companies: They are desperately trying to provide the highest standard of evidence-based care for the lowest possible cost. Most investments in new services or technologies are geared toward improving operational efficiency within the organization. Unfortunately, that doesn't leave a whole lot of budget left over for investing. In short, innovation in healthcare is so rare, it is celebrated when it happens.

THE INNOVATION MIND-SET

Innovation in healthcare is tough, but it is possible. The next step is to start to understand how to become an innovator. Innovation is most definitely a process, and it starts with adopting the right mind-set. When it comes to leadership in innovation, we can have quotes for days—Simon Sinek says, "*Start with why.*" Jeff Bezos preaches, "*It's not an experiment if you know it's going to work.*" Steve Jobs told us "*Innovation distinguishes leaders from followers.*" If you had to distill the wisdom of a thousand innovators down to one message, my favorite would have to be from the legendary American economist Theodore Levitt, who said, "*Creativity is thinking up new things, innovation is **doing** new things.*" We all have ideas, and it's always fun to sit around a table with a couple of drinks and talk about all the ways that we can change the world. The thing that separates innovators from everybody else is that after everyone has had their fun imagining "what if," they take the crazy idea and run with it. To be very clear from the outset: This is not an open invitation to be irresponsible or unethical with patient care, or to convince people to take risks with their health so you can test out an unvalidated technology. In healthcare, no matter what, there are still lines that we don't cross. Don't worry, though—there is still no shortage of ethical ways to innovate in healthcare.

For all the reasons we discussed earlier in the chapter, innovation is tough in healthcare. There is very little incentive to make it happen, so innovators usually have to make it happen on their own, which requires a very special mind-set. If you truly believe in your project, you have to be willing to fight for it: work nights and weekends, build something without overintellectualizing what you're doing, and have the fortitude to ignore all the people telling you that your idea is crazy, bad or wrong. Noninnovators *love* telling innovators that they're crazy and they love watching an innovator fail … probably because it makes them feel better about not being innovators. Elon Musk tells us "*If things are not failing, you are not innovating enough.*" So be ready for failure by embracing the idea that the process of innovation, the very action of creating something that has never existed before and maybe doesn't even have a reason to exist, is a high-failure game. What you learn with each failure is why we innovate, and what allows you to become an expert in the new space that you have created. Sometimes (most of the time) your innovation won't go anywhere at all, but the crucial part of an innovator's mind-set is finding the activation energy to take idle talk about an idea and transform it to meaningful action.

Diversity Fosters Creativity and Innovation

I tend to give a lot of talks and contribute to a lot of courses about innovation. A question that routinely comes up is: "*if you had unlimited resources and could run the perfect innovation course what would it look like?"* Here I am at the front of a conference room banging on about this intangible, almost mystical quality that other people have divined in me, and people get excited. They want to know: *How do we teach innovation? How can we do what you do?*

Let's start by rejecting some conventional wisdom about creativity and innovation. As a society, we love to lump people into different categories—you're a "creative," you're "right-brained" and other such nonsense. Very early on in life, we instill the notion into the populace that certain cognitive features *can't be taught*, and creativity tends to be one of those things. The reason that this is a problematic attitude is because it leads to kind of a cultish reaction to having *"creatives"* around. I can't tell you the number of times I have watched on as a company has brought on a "design guru": not a solid human-centered designer with a good head on his or her shoulders, no, no, no—a design *guru*. The guru is outrageously expensive, mutters wistfully about his or her time at IDEO and spends most of this or her time chasing your development team around speaking in parables and faulty metaphors, and of course, becomes outraged if anyone questions his or her gospel. Meanwhile, because he or she is spending so much money on the guru, an ordinarily intellectually curious, nonsense-resistant CEO bows and scrapes, nods knowingly as the designer makes meaningless assertions (so as not to be outed as a "noncreative") and say yes to objectively bad decisions. As I watch on in horror, I have seen companies rapidly burn through sizable design budgets on the words of a charlatan only to be left with nothing.

I'm not trying to say that designers and design thinking is bad or unnecessary. On the contrary, I have worked with some brilliant designers in my career. People who are wonderfully creative, process-driven, and essential to successful completion of a project. The point here is not to say negative things about the profession of design, but rather to highlight what happens when we fetishize concepts like creativity. We see the same in many fields and it contributes to the proliferation of questionable professions such as faith healers, telephone psychics, and other purveyors of snake oil.

As we have established that creativity is a teachable concept, how do we go about fostering it? We know that diversity is a key element in creating unique, groundbreaking work. Richard Freeman, an economist from Harvard University, showed that academics who only published within their own specific research groups published papers that were less widely cited and less likely to be published in high-impact journals than individuals who published with a wide network of collaborators (Freeman & Huang, 2014). Are you reading this correctly? Yes. By simply being part of a team that is made up of members from a broad range of research, ethnic, and cultural backgrounds, you significantly increase the probability of your work being more prestigious and paradigm shifting. It runs deeper than this, though. Social psychologist Adam Galinsky tells us that one of the easiest ways to become more creative is to live abroad (Leung, Maddux, Galinsky, & Chiu, 2008; Maddux & Galinsky, 2009), and one of the strongest stimuli for long-lasting creativity is to marry someone who is of another ethnicity, Now, to be clear, there are lots of concepts at play that can confound these findings—the most obvious being that maybe people who engage in these behaviors are individuals who already have traits that self-select for them being more creative in the first place. However, as more research is completed, the evidence is certainly building up: Diversity fosters creativity.

A great example of this comes from studying the history of food preparation. Before the invention of refrigeration, every culture had the same problem to solve: preventing food spoilage. Yet, every culture came up with a fantastically diverse way of preserving its food that often formed a fundamental cornerstone of its cuisine. If you were trying to solve this problem from scratch, I'm sure most of you would agree that having team members from multiple ethnic backgrounds would likely lead to the largest number of actionable strategies to solve your problem and maybe even place you in a position to think of one that no one else had ever thought of before. As this applies to ethnic diversity, so it applies to occupational diversity.

Look no further than the ever-expanding field of digital health. Every day we are seeing new and exciting examples of technologies that could revolutionize healthcare because clinicians are starting to interact with computer scientists, engineers, and entrepreneurs at an unprecedented rate. To summarize, creativity is a precursor to innovation and if you want to train yourself to be more creative, the first step is to purposefully spend time interacting with people who are outside of your profession and culture.

 CALL TO ACTION

Attend a Conference Not in Your Field

Many of us have to attend the same old conferences every year. We usually come back with a bunch of cool ideas and inspirations, but they are usually held within a very narrow field. My first call to action is to skip one of your regular conferences and attend a conference outside of your field. Maybe you're exploring virtual reality in healthcare? Go to a visual effects conference. Using video games for physical therapy? Attend a gaming conference. If you have no budget to attend conferences, then go online to your local meet-up website and look for public talks to attend. Go anywhere that you may be able to get a new idea or fresh perspective.

For those of us who maybe can't take a year off to travel the world or might find it slightly inconvenient to rush off and marry someone from a distant culture, please don't panic. There are other ways to train, promote, or stimulate creativity. A powerful exercise is to attempt to frame your problem as a set of generalizable components. You see, we like to think that many of the problems are unique to our field. However, if you think outside of the box a little, you can often classify your problem more generally than that.

On a previous project of mine, we were tasked with helping a company to develop low-cost rehabilitation robotics for kids with cerebral palsy. I remember thinking at the beginning of the project that it was an insurmountable task, but after working with some engineers, we saw that many of the problems were rather tractable: Writing code to control actuators was pretty straightforward, and precisely tracking the end positions of the robotic segments seemed like it would be easily achievable as well.

However, the biggest problem was finding a device that was strong enough to firmly move a child's limb, but gentle enough to not cause joint or bone pain. Not only was it remarkably difficult to find such an actuator, finding one that was tested to a level of scrutiny that would be acceptable to the Food and Drug Administration (FDA) seemed to be nearly impossible. It was a hard problem, but we had our parameters in place: We wanted an exhaustively tested actuator that was capable of moving with significant amounts of force and precision. We couldn't find anything suitable in the medical world that wasn't going to cost us an arm and a leg, so we looked outside of our field for professions that may have solved this problem. Before too long, we came across a potential solution in the automotive industry. Specifically, the actuators that car companies use to operate the automatic sunroof mechanism for cars that have that feature fit our specifications *perfectly*. Not only that, but the degree of testing and regulatory procedure that these actuators had to pass through to be suitable for the automotive industry far exceeded that of the FDA, so we were in luck there as well. We found our actuators and used them to successfully build the first generation of the robotic device.

The point of this story is that at first we thought we had a medical engineering problem to solve, but once we opened ourselves up to the possibility that another field had already solved our problem for us, we found a perfect solution almost immediately.

Another great example of this concept can be found in the field of biomimicry. In her TED (technology, entertainment, design) Talk (www.youtube.com/watch?v=k_GFq12w5WU), Janine Benyus, who is one of the most influential thinkers in the field of biomimicry, reminds us that *"natural organisms have managed to do everything that we want to do without guzzling fossil fuels, polluting the planet or mortgaging the future."* Dr. Benyus and her team routinely work with innovators to help them extract elegant solutions to their problems from nature. They find solutions to complex problems that leverage sustainable, local materials that have been in common usage by nature for millions, if not billions, of years. With this in mind, I would remind you that although it might not be feasible to spend a year in a different country, it is absolutely feasible to attend a conference that is a nontraditional scene for a health professional. You might just meet some people who have already solved your problem for you.

 CALL TO ACTION

Visit a different department within your own hospital: People working in different hospital departments rarely speak. Hospitals are busy places, though, so we rarely get the opportunity to discuss difficulties that may be common to all of us. Reach out to a friend in another department and ask to shadow him or her. Be on the lookout for problems that your department needs to solve that don't appear to be a problem for your colleague. If you find something, ask your friend why it isn't a problem for his or her department. What did they do differently than your department did? Is their solution transferrable to your group?

IDENTIFYING YOUR OPPORTUNITY TO INNOVATE AND OVERCOMING COMMON BARRIERS

One of the most powerful motivators for innovation in healthcare is need. It may sound simplistic, but if you're experiencing the healthcare system regularly, as either a consumer or a worker, identifying your personal opportunity for innovation may be as simple as identifying the thing each day that is making your life the hardest. This is true whether you're an outsider looking into the healthcare system thinking "I can do better," or the most highly trained and specialized surgeon in the world looking at a surgical instrument you use every day thinking "I can do better."

Regardless of whether we're talking about a big innovation or a small innovation, the first step in finding your opportunity to innovate is to identify the thing that you most want to change about the situation you're observing. In his book, *Not Impossible: The Art and Joy of Doing*

What Couldn't Be Done, innovator Mick Ebeling (2017) refers to this process as "identifying the absurd." That is, identifying a problem, process, or situation that seems wrong on a fundamental level. We've all experienced this in one form or another: that feeling you get when you look at the way that something is being done and think "surely we could be doing better than this." What separates innovators from non innovators is when an innovator experiences that feeling, he or she is compelled to act.

Our anti-innovation instinct (or probably more apt to label it our "anti-effort" instinct) is to fatalistically do nothing: "*There must be a reason for doing it this way that is above my pay grade.*" "*How could I possibly fix this? I don't have the resources.*" "*The system is broken,*" and so on. There are a million reasons *not to* innovate and every one of them is seductive because it is always easier to do things the way they have always been done. I often hear from people that they are not working in an environment that is conducive to innovation—the old, "my boss won't let me spend time on that" excuse. Most good innovation starts outside of work hours because it starts as a passion project that keeps you up at night. This is what keeps pure innovation so authentic and hard to fake: If you aren't willing to work after hours to solve a problem that is bothering you, then I'm sorry to say that you probably haven't yet found your opportunity to innovate. One of the key ingredients to identifying your personal opportunity to innovate is passion: Solving the problem (at least at the beginning of the project!) must not feel like work, it *must* feel like play.

CALL TO ACTION

Commit to solving a common problem at your hospital: Every workplace has problems: something you wish worked better, a common complaint from patients, or a simple process inefficiency that doesn't make sense but costs everyone a lot of time every day. My call to action is simple: find one problem that you think you can solve and make a commitment to creating some sort of simple prototype, process, or protocol that will fix the problem.

Who Pays?

I'm going to address this barrier to healthcare innovation first because it is the one that I hate the most. I've seen this play out so many times: Someone is describing the details of a truly innovative method for improving the standard of care or patient experience or one of the million intangible aspects of interacting with a hospital system that needs fixing. The idea is simple and elegant, sometimes some pilot data show that it works: It's an idea that just makes sense. Everyone is nodding along, and then there is that one person in the room. Almost always wearing a suit, arms folded, who barks out (usually interrupting the presenter) those dreaded two words, "*Who pays?*" Everyone nods knowingly, the stricken innovator stammers and starts to babble—he or she thought he or she was here to present a blue-sky, creative idea to improve patient care or process, not to be grilled about revenue models. It is hard to watch.

Forget about the suit. Seriously. I rarely advise people to discount feedback out of hand, but in this case, I will call it out very clearly: Do not listen to the person asking you to provide some magical return on investment strategy (usually shortened to *ROI* by the business types) on an early innovative idea. One of the biggest lies, propagated again and again by people in the "business" of delivering healthcare, is that your healthcare innovation needs to immediately result in direct cost savings. This is total nonsense and it destroys innovation.

As an innovator, the best way to avoid your innovation from experiencing this fate is to delay speaking with your institution's business arm until you have something solid. This is controversial advice, but I think that it needs to be said, simply because hospital systems have not yet been adequately geared to support early innovation. You see, the "who pays" question is usually asked by the hospital/university tech transfer office; its job is to monetize innovation for the organization. As such, these individuals are only interested in working on your innovation if they see an easy way to get to an ROI. Now, it is not my intention to make the tech transfer office out to be a bunch of villains who want to destroy your beautiful idea, because that is not the case. The tech transfer office of an institution can be an incredibly useful and powerful core service if it is used appropriately. The real issue is that fostering innovation is still so new to healthcare institutions that they don't know how to manage innovators. The minute someone has an inkling of an idea, the standard advice is, "*go and talk to the tech transfer office.*"

This results in an unprepared and vulnerable innovator sharing a way-too-early idea with a bunch of people who are expecting to see a well-thought-out business plan. The resulting blood bath typically ruins everything: The idea goes nowhere, and the innovator who put him- or herself out there in the first place goes back to his or her workplace crestfallen, apathetic, and far less willing to take a risk with sharing his or her ideas in the future. A total lose–lose situation.

Please be careful with your early-innovation ideas—don't share them too early with the tech transfer office. Share them with allies within your department. If possible, start to collect some early feasibility data to show that your idea holds water and might indeed add value to the department. Be patient, log everything, and build your case. Always remember that creating early innovation is a completely separate process to creating a sustainable business model.

Embrace Your Harshest Frenemy

A common complaint from innovators is often that they *tried* to innovate, but the higher-ups didn't like the ideas, so they shut it all down. This can be a tough hurdle to navigate because it requires open and honest self-evaluation, and the ability to make some hard decisions. I wish I could tell you, "it's not you, it's them." That in every case, innovation fails because one of those fat cats upstairs couldn't understand your brilliant ideas. But I can't … sometimes it really is you. Occam's razor tells us that the simplest explanation is usually the best, and sometimes the simplest explanation for failed adoption of an innovation is not some conspiracy against the innovator. No, it was just that that the idea was lousy, or the plan to implement it was disorganized or unrealistic.

Successful innovators are rare because they need to be highly creative, but also completely open to constructive criticism of their own ideas. If you don't have a safe environment to share your ideas and receive constructive feedback, my advice is to approach the friend in your social circle who is the straightest shooter you know. That terrible monster who always, with painful transparency, tells people exactly what he or she thinks (we *all* have that one friend)—and share your idea. If this person likes it, you could be onto something. If he or she tells you that your idea is no good, listen, get all the horrible details from your friend, and then try to decide whether your idea can be reframed, or whether it is not worth pursuing.

A lot of early innovation meets failure at first and you should not be afraid or ashamed of it. Failure should be viewed as nothing more than a launchpad onto your next idea. Google X has a division of innovators, and they reward failure; every idea that is taken to completion is rewarded. This is a not as easy than it sounds, though. Innovators are often creatives and creatives are very sensitive. We do not live in a culture that values failure.

Personally, one of my biggest struggles is cutting through all the unhelpful emotions that come up when someone starts to poke holes in one of my ideas and to remain objective. It is hard for me to share risky ideas, so if someone shuts them down out of hand within minutes of me sharing I tend to clam up. When that happens, we're done with creativity for the day. This is a nasty side effect of the vulnerability that goes hand in hand with innovation and if you let it, it will ruin you.

Probably the best vulnerability researcher around, Brené Brown, reminds us in her TED talk that, "*vulnerability is the birthplace of innovation, creativity, and change*" (2010). Although this is absolutely true, remember that she also teaches us that the best innovators make themselves vulnerable enough to create, but are then emotionally resilient enough to manage the feedback that is returned when they share their creativity. Just make sure you are sharing your ideas with people who will be constructive to your vision. They don't need to agree with you, but you want them to be on your side.

Innovation Cannot Happen in a Toxic Environment

Sometimes your ideas will conceptually pass muster with everybody else, but they are legitimately being held back by a boss who is simply too ingrained in system-wide inertia to want to implement any sort of change. Unfortunately, this scenario can be rather common in the healthcare world, which still maintains a rather hierarchical leadership structure and extreme aversion to risk. Nine times out of 10, my advice to a committed innovator stuck in a situation like this is to leave. This is hard to hear, because your boss may not be that bad and your workplace might be great, just highly resistant to change. But let me unpack this just a little more: Risk-averse environments are inevitably toxic to innovators, and no matter what, as a general life rule, you should never stay in a toxic workplace. They impede personal and professional growth, they ruin reputations, and they are bad for morale and well-being (Housman & Minor, 2015). If you are a committed innovator, meaning that you love innovation and you want to continue developing that aspect of your professional persona, and you are in a workplace that is not conducive to innovation, then that workplace is going to be toxic for you. Your best career option is to get out. You can waste a lot of time and energy trying to change a workplace, or you can find one that suits your needs and career goals, allowing you to grow. I understand that this sounds like risky advice, but if there was ever a thing to get tattooed across your forehead, it should be "Innovation *is* risk." This is incredibly privileged advice. I have quit jobs that were a terrible fit for me as an innovator without a backup plan, but I'm also a healthy, White male with no kids, no student loans (I grew up in Australia where my college education cost very little) and no personal debt. About as privileged as you can get.

As a result, quitting was risky, but it was a *tolerable* risk—the only person who stood to get hurt was me and I calculated that I would be able to recover if things became intolerable. If this is not your situation, I still recommend leaving, but don't quit without a plan. We have, at our fingertips, a set of incredibly powerful (and free) tools: online and physical communities like

Meetup, LinkedIn, Facebook, Twitter, YouTube, Instagram, Snapchat, the list goes on and on. Become active in these communities—"out" yourself as an innovator and explore opportunities with like-minded people who will allow you to feel less isolated in your existing job while you search for your next step.

Innovation Happens Most Easily When You Have a Committed Community

This sounds obvious, but it is probably the hardest lesson that I have learned most often because every time I get it wrong, it has resulted in the death of my project. Unless you're a unicorn, no one can create great impactful health innovations alone, so it is almost a foregone conclusion that you will require a robust team to get your work done. Here is the most important piece when it comes to forming your team of innovators: Make sure your team is strongly aligned on the **mission,** and is **passionate** about making it happen. Innovation is rarely wellfunded or carefully planned—the most natural birthplace of innovation is when someone sees a problem that consumes him or her—he or she simply *must* solve it.

The next step is to form a team that can solve your problem and that is where things can get hairy. If you're entering a team like this, you need to be ready for some pain: long hours, low chances of success, and little to no pay. Unfortunately, what often happens is that as you're frantically reaching out to whomever is willing to work for free, you lose track of onboarding people who are passionate about your mission. Before you know it, you have a team full of well-meaning (usually), but ultimately unengaged individuals who won't have the necessary fire to put in the hard yards and get it done. This doesn't make them bad people; it just means that they aren't as committed as you to this cause. You deserve a team full of people who share your passion.

One of my first experiences with this problem happened just following one of the most widely televised and award-winning projects that I completed with Not Impossible Labs, Project Daniel (www.youtube.com/watch?v=ol19tt3VWhQ&t=84s). I had just started a new project that we hoped would be similarly disruptive. We had no shortage of volunteers after the success of our last project. I started working with a very talented programmer and I guess I was a bit naïve at the time because I didn't see the warning signs at all. I remember thinking that some of his comments were odd, because while I was obsessed with solving the next problem, he was obsessed with the next press release, the next award. Upon reflecting on the failure of that project, I realized that what this team member of mine was really doing was telling me why he was in the group.

I've since had similar experiences with team members who are obsessed with the money that will come out of the creation of an innovation, or are working on it because they're excited at the prospect of being thought of as an innovator, or a thousand other reasons. You can't fake authenticity when you're innovating. When you're going through the process of creating a thing that has never existed before, you need to have a room full of people who are just as excited as you about creating that thing for the right reasons. No other team of people is going to be resilient to the failures, the thousands of unpaid hours and sleepless nights that will be required to move your idea forward. I recognize that this is hard advice to follow: Innovators often feel isolated, precisely because they find it very difficult to find people as passionate as they are about a problem. If you are genuinely struggling to put together the team you need, then bootstrap your little heart out. What I mean by this is find some well-meaning volunteers and give them a tractable problem to solve that will move you to the next step.

One of my current projects, a wearable, vibrotactile technology that allows deaf people to experience music, began just like this. I had made some good progress on a basic prototype but was stalled and I knew that I needed a software engineer to get me to the next step, so I invited a friend over for beers. I knew he was overloaded with his own projects, so I wasn't going to ask him to commit to the project as a whole, but I explained one simple problem I was having that was stopping my rough prototype from working. We worked on it for a couple of hours (and a couple of beers) and he eventually found the bug in my code and we got the thing working. This first prototype was so crappy, but you know what? It gave me something to show around to people, and it eventually captured the attention and imagination of an amazing musician, inventor, and friend, Daniel Belquer. He took on the project with even more passion than I had for it, and it is now 100% his baby. Helpful volunteers who aren't fully committed to your vision can be crucial to your mission if you apply them to the problem in the right way.

CALL TO ACTION

Create an interdisciplinary think tank: Once you have found a problem that you want to solve, form a team of enthusiastic volunteers who represent *all of the stakeholders* who have the potential to be impacted by your solution—patients, doctors, allied health professionals, caregivers, everyone and anyone who is relevant to your problem. Begin having regular focus group meetings with them to discuss solving the problem. This won't be easy—people are very protective of their time—but persevere and your think tank will form.

CASE STUDY: WELLPATH

WellPATH is a project that I have been working on for around 5 years. It is a mobile application that we designed for the treatment of suicidal ideation and suicide prevention. This project began shortly after I had accepted my first faculty position at Cornell. I was a young investigator who had been tasked with building a telemedicine division for the Burke Medical Research Institute in White Plains. As I was getting to know my new colleagues and forming collaborations, I was introduced to a brilliant professor of psychology, Dimitris Kiosses. Not only is Dimitris a psychologist who was clinically active, but he is also a great scientist who has had a distinguished scientific career. Dimitris's area of expertise is to work with older adults who have severe, treatment-resistant depression. Many of Dimitris's patients are at significant risk of suicide—it is a sad, but often ignored fact that older adults are actually the subset of the population that has the highest risk of suicide. Not teens, not veterans, but our aging population. Along with some colleagues from Stanford and Johns Hopkins, Dimitris developed an innovative form of therapy to treat older adults who were vulnerable to suicide.

The therapy, called *problem adaptation therapy (PATH)*, is designed to identify specific daily events that trigger negative emotions that patients are unable to successfully regulate. After PATH-trained therapists have identified the problematic negative emotions and the environmental triggers that cause them, they design highly personalized strategies to help their patients regulate when the negative emotions emerge. Dimitris has shown in several studies that PATH can outperform conventional psychological techniques in reducing suicidal thoughts and ideation and reducing symptoms of depression (Kiosses, Arean, Teri, & Alexopoulos, 2010; Kiosses et al., 2015, 2017).

PATH is an exciting therapy that has the potential to significantly impact the suicide epidemic, but Dimitris was facing a problem. His elderly patients had difficulty remembering their PATH strategies, and his therapists didn't have a strong sense of how often their patients were performing their prescribed home exercises. He needed a way to deliver care remotely, to track progress over time, and to allow his patients an easy and convenient way to access their home exercises. A mutual colleague, Dr. Pasquale Fonzetti, was kind enough to connect us, and Dimitris explained his problem.

Every so often, an opportunity to innovate comes along that is very clear. Take this case at face value: What we had was a group of world-renowned experts on a specific problem who were *telling us* about a technological solution that they wish they had. They had neither the expertise nor the funding to make this solution happen, but they had made the crucial first step of speaking to someone outside of their field. I knew immediately that we had to help. Working on this project was not easy. Innovation is risk and risk is not tolerated well by academic institutions. Making a commitment to help on this project was questioned strongly by the senior leadership of my institution—why was I helping these people? I was hired to develop technological solutions for *stroke*, not *depression*—a project like this was nothing more than a distraction. Heaven forbid that anyone should step out of her or his silo, because it's not like I've ever heard of a stroke survivor being depressed or anything . . .

On our end, the undertaking was technically challenging because we had never worked on a psychology project before and Dimitris's team had never worked on a digital health project before, so we had to talk often and do our research. We spoke with as many potential stakeholders as we could think of: app developers, clinicians, people who were at risk of suicide, and people who had survived a suicidal attempt. Our goal was to capture everyone's opinions to make sure we were developing something that our community *wanted*, rather than something that *we assumed* that they wanted.

Despite all our research, we still made some rookie mistakes. For instance, because we had very little dedicated funding for the project, we partnered with an app development company to help us on the project. I think they smelled blood in the water and asked to be cut in for equity in the product (even though we were paying them for development of the initial proof-of-concept app) to cover future developments of the product over time. I know you are probably shaking your head at how naïve this sounds, but at the outset it really did seem like a reasonable deal. Spoiler alert: It turned out to be an unmitigated disaster.

Recall that earlier I spoke about how in the early stages of innovation it is crucial that you work with a community that is as passionate as you are about solving your problem. That was the main tenet that we violated here: While we were talking about creating something innovative and new that could potentially help our patients, they were talking about market size, widespread distribution, and subscription fees. These are fine conversations to have in the life cycle of a health technology product, but not when you're focusing on an initial innovative process. The company began to aggressively push us toward a go-to-market strategy with a product that was nowhere near ready for widespread use. We tried to explain the cardinal rule of health technology development: We aren't developing a *tech product*, we're developing *medicine*. Medicine must be rigorously tested before it is released to the public, especially in cases in which we are dealing with such a vulnerable population. Furthermore, we tried to explain that we wanted this app to be a *prescription app:* Something that would never be generically available on the app store, but rather available only to people who had had it prescribed by their therapist. But they wouldn't listen. The relationship began to deteriorate, and we had to make the difficult choice to leave the product we had developed with them behind and part ways with them.

I am not going to lie to you all, losing the development company was a hard hit to the project and we very nearly lost sight of the mission all together. Then the unthinkable happened: One of the first team members I ever hired in my lab and a dear friend to this day lost her father to suicide. We were a tight-knit team and a loss like this was devastating, but it also served to galvanize the team and turn the project around—there wasn't any doubt anymore—this terrible event had reminded us of what we had to do and why we had to do it.

We decided to continue with the app development on our own by any means necessary. I met a brilliant young volunteer programmer, Jacob Dunefsky. A high school student at the time, Jacob developed our first working prototype of the app—exactly what we asked for; it only worked in a protected offline mode so that we could control exactly who was accessing the app at any time and conduct some controlled clinical trials. Not long after that, we had deployed the app to an initial group of patients and clinicians in order to get an initial sense of how everything was working. Jacob worked tirelessly on a growing list of updates and modification requests from the therapists, but it was worth it: The pilot results were phenomenal. Through the dedicated and brilliant work of Dimitris and his clinicians, we had soon collected enough pilot data to capture the attention of some funding agencies and we were able to work our app into two separate National Institutes of Health grants for 5 years of funding. Fast forward 3 years into our clinical trials, and we've been able to present preliminary results in peer-reviewed journals and at international conferences showing that out of hundreds of app interactions, our users experience an average 40% reduction in the intensity of negative emotions within just a few minutes of initiating interaction with the app.

Thanks to the hard work of this passionate team of committed people, we are well on our way to proving that we have developed a method of providing personalized, point-of-care emotion regulation therapy for individuals who are at risk of suicide. This is novel, powerful, and has the potential to change the way we treat suicidal patients forever.

CONCLUSIONS

I hope that this chapter has given you a good sense of how to approach innovation in healthcare. If you take anything away from here, please let it be that anyone is capable of innovation. There is no specific qualification or special training required, just a willingness to think outside of the box, not accept the status quo, and to have a genuine passion for solving problems that people are experiencing. Let things happen organically—if you've identified a problem you want to solve, there are likely a lot of other people who are equally invested in solving it (unless you work in a *super* specialized field!). Seek those people out and make the time to sit down and work on a solution together because the best innovations come from a deeply diverse team. Finally, never lose your passion.

By and large, the healthcare industry is terrible at supporting innovative ideas. If I can promise you anything, it is that once you commit to a project, you need to find the resilience and grit within yourself to see it through. This means that the true innovators, the ones who really disrupt the field of medicine, have a level of authentic commitment to the cause that can't be faked or manufactured. Innovation in healthcare certainly is not easy, but if you get it right, you might just change a whole lot of lives.

CALL TO ACTION

A crucial step in the innovation process is approaching a problem with a highly analytical mind-set to identify the root cause of the problem. For instance, let's say you keep running out of sterile gauze in one of your surgical suites: Is this a staffing problem? A logistics problem? A surgical planning issue?

It's often easy to define the problem, while the cause remains elusive. Once you have identified the cause, there is a great innovation exercise that is often called "superhero versus supervillain." The process is very simple: your supervillain is the cause of your problem. To defeat your foe, you need to search for a superhero. In this case, your ideal superhero is a person, process, or thing that has been implemented somewhere else in the world to solve exactly the issue you're experiencing. Once you've found it, dust it off and apply it to your own ecosystem.

Look everywhere: Google, Google Scholar, podcasts, YouTube. You never know where you're going to find your superhero, but I promise you that somewhere, someone has faced your supervillain before. I know this might sound silly and simplistic, but the point of this exercise is to break down seemingly complex problems into far more tractable ones in a fun and engaging way. Go ahead and try it out with your supervillain.

KEY TAKEAWAY POINTS

■ Anyone is capable of innovation. There is no specific qualification or special training required, just a willingness to think outside of the box, not accept the status quo, and to have a genuine passion for solving problems that people are experiencing.

■ Let things happen organically—if you've identified a problem you want to solve, there are likely a lot of other people who are equally invested in solving it (unless you work in a *super* specialized field!).

■ Seek those people out and make the time to sit down and work on a solution together because the best innovations come from a deeply diverse team.

■ Never lose your passion.

REFERENCES

Brown, B. (2010). *The power of vulnerability.* [Video file]. Retrieved from https://www.ted .com/talks/brene_brown_on_vulnerability?language=en

Ebeling, M. (2017). *Not impossible: The art and joy of doing what couldn't be done.* New York, NY: Atria.

Freeman, R. B., & Huang, W. (2014). Collaboration: Strength in diversity. *Nature News, 513*(7518), 305. doi:10.1038/513305a

Housman, M., & Minor, D. (2015). *Toxic workers* (Working Paper 16-057). Retrieved from https://www.hbs.edu/faculty/Publication%20Files/16-057_d45c0b4f-fa19-49de-8f1b-4b12fe054fea.pdf

Kiosses, D. N., Arean, P. A., Teri, L., & Alexopoulos, G. S. (2010). Home-delivered problem adaptation therapy (PATH) for depressed, cognitively impaired, disabled elders: A preliminary study. *American Journal of Geriatric Psychiatry, 18*(11), 988–998. doi:10.1097/JGP.0b013e3181d6947d

Kiosses, D. N., Gross, J. J., Banerjee, S., Duberstein, P. R., Putrino, D., & Alexopoulos, G. S. (2017). Negative emotions and suicidal ideation during psychosocial treatments in older adults with major depression and cognitive impairment. *American Journal of Geriatric Psychiatry, 25*(6), 620–629. doi:10.1016/j.jagp.2017.01.011

Kiosses, D. N., Ravdin, L. D., Gross, J. J., Raue, P., Kotbi, N., & Alexopoulos, G. S. (2015). Problem adaptation therapy for older adults with major depression and cognitive impairment: A randomized clinical trial. *JAMA Psychiatry, 72*(1), 22–30. doi:10.1001/jamapsychiatry.2014

Leung, A. K. Y., Maddux, W. W., Galinsky, A. D., & Chiu, C. Y. (2008). Multicultural experience enhances creativity: The when and how. *American Psychologist, 63*(3), 169. doi:10.1037/0003-066x.63.3.169

Maddux, W. W., & Galinsky, A. D. (2009). Cultural borders and mental barriers: The relationship between living abroad and creativity. *Journal of Personality and Social Psychology, 96*(5), 1047. doi:10.1037/a0014861

Intrapreneurship, Business Models, and How Companies Make Money

Tim Raderstorf, Michelle Podlesni, Christine W. Meehan, Joseph Novello, and Pamala Wilson

"Don't tell us all the reasons this might not work. Tell us all the ways this could work." —John Wood

LEARNING OBJECTIVES

- Examine the concepts of intrapreneurship, entrepreneurship, and social entrepreneurship.
- Identify opportunities to be an intrapreneur in your current organization.
- Highlight the multiple business models that help entrepreneurs impact healthcare.
- Differentiate between entrepreneurship and social entrepreneurship.
- Identify local and global social entrepreneurship organizations that are currently active.

INTRODUCTION

After examining the core concepts of entrepreneurship in the previous chapter, you should have a clear vision of how healthcare leadership, innovation, and entrepreneurship are intertwined. In this chapter, we are going to discover the many different ways companies structure their businesses to make money and explain why it is import for healthcare leaders to understand these models through both the lens of entrepreneurship and intrapreneurship.

The word *intrapreneurship* may be foreign to you, though it is very likely that you have been serving as an intrapreneur for many years. Gifford and Elizabeth Pinchot (1978) are credited with coining the term *intrapreneurship*. An intrapreneur is an individual working in a large organization/corporation/health system who behaves like an entrepreneur. The majority of healthcare leaders apply entrepreneurial principles into large health systems, exemplifying intrapreneurship.

EXPLORING INTRAPRENEURSHIP

"You must do the thing you think you cannot do." —Eleanor Roosevelt

Many healthcare leaders will spend most of their careers working for an organization such as a hospital or healthcare company. In this environment, nurses and other healthcare professionals have always innovated, but as intrapreneurs, not entrepreneurs. Why the difference and is it important?

It is indeed very important as many healthcare professionals do not want to start an independent business from an idea that they have to improve a clinical service or device/technology. It is very risky and expensive. Many ideas for innovation should be developed for and in conjunction with a healthcare employer to minimize risk and maximize impact. This first section of this chapter explores how to be an intrapreneur within the organization you work for and how to benefit from this innovation opportunity.

> **CALL TO ACTION**
>
> Go to LinkedIn and Facebook and search for healthcare professionals who list innovation and entrepreneurship in their profiles. Make a list of the organizations that they work for and view their profiles. Send a connection request to those individuals who inspire you.

Revenue Generation as a Core Component of Intrapreneurship

"A wise person should have money in their head, not in their heart." —Jonathan Swift

Ideas for innovation and improvement come to us in our working environments as a result of needing or wanting to solve a healthcare problem. If clinicians are improving an organizational process or initiating a new service or have identified a technology opportunity while an employee, and this results in a financial benefit to the organization, then both the organization and the employee should benefit from this innovation. In general, clinicians do not think about generating revenue for our organizations, so it is important to begin to value what they do and any innovations they think of and develop.

The first step is to think about and do some "homework" about your idea or innovation before you bring it to your organization's attention. Write down exactly what the problem is that you are trying to solve and your solution. Have as much information about the problem and your solution as possible before you talk with administration.

Things to consider:

- What is the problem?
- What does it cost to keep doing it this way?
- How many people/patients does this problem affect?
- What is the current way of managing this problem (if at all)?

- What are the difficulties to putting your solution in place?
- Research to see whether this problem has been published in the literature and whether others are working on a solution.
- What is the cost of your solution? Who will pay for it?

These steps will sound very familiar after you read Chapter 20, Legal Considerations in Starting a Healthcare Business.

CALL TO ACTION

Take your innovation idea and write down the answers to the questions in the preceding list. Come up with another innovative idea and repeat the same exercise.

The second step is to identify who in administration is responsible to help foster innovative ideas from clinicians. It is to be hoped that fostering healthcare innovation starts with your departmental leadership and reaches all the way from the bedside to the C-suite. In some of the larger hospital organizations there may be a chief innovation officer who is responsible for helping clinicians turn ideas to actions. There may also be an Office for Innovation, which can help staff develop and implement their innovative ideas. It is important to identify key stakeholders and the supporters of innovation within your organization.

When you are a clinician intrapreneur within an organization you are part of a team and, therefore, all the team members will benefit from innovative changes. If your innovative idea is patentable, your organization should help to undertake this task, which can be costly and time-consuming. Because they are contributing to the success of the innovation, all parties will benefit from any success, financial or otherwise.

There may be an instance when your organization is not interested in your innovative idea. If you are still interested in developing it on your own, many organizations will give you a written release indicating that they have relinquished any rights to your innovation. Be sure to get that in writing before moving to independent development or sale of your idea/prototype to another organization (such as a medical device company).

CALL TO ACTION

Identify whether your organization has someone designated to handle new ideas and innovations. This could be in nursing administration, medical affairs, business office, and so on. Meet with that individual to learn more about potential collaborations.

There are many types of healthcare organizations in which nurses are employed and all of them provide an opportunity for nurses to be innovative (Box 19.1).

Box 19.1	Opportunities for Healthcare Innovation and Intrapreneurship (Sample)

Hospitals
Nursing homes
Rehabilitation providers
Urgent care
Retail clinics
Physician/NP/PA offices
Health insurance companies

NP, nurse practitioner; PA, physician assistant.

How to Think About Negotiating for Financial Benefit From an Innovation That You Created That Benefits Your Organization

It is absolutely okay for healthcare professionals to reap financial rewards for their intrapreneurial efforts. As an intrapreneur, you are often both making your organization more money and saving it money at the same time. Do not be afraid to ask your organization how it compensates employees for contributing to a healthier bottom line. Bonuses are regularly provided to physicians and C-suite executives for comparable contributions to the organization. Do your homework to see how much money your intrapreneurial initiatives are making the organization and, if you are feeling bold, ask for a percentage of that savings to be paid to you as a bonus.

Saving money for the organization is always harder to quantify; therefore, you may want to think about negotiating for a pay raise or bonus based on predetermined milestones.

Three opportunities for financial benefits to consider:

- Negotiating for a percentage of the revenue generated from a service or product developed under the hospital or organization's name and support
- Negotiating a pay raise as a result of achieving a financial or evidence-based milestone for the organization
- A promotion within the organization (with a salary increase and/or title change)

Other benefits to discuss in all the preceding scenarios include:

- Copyright recognition
- Authorship on articles or publications
- Name included on any patent application

 CALL TO ACTION

Do you know whether your hospital or organization made money last year or lost money? Hospitals are either for profit or nonprofit and have to report financial results regardless. Google your organization's financial results or annual report. Read it and note where the organization made money and where it lost money. Think about whether your innovative idea can benefit in both situations.

How to Foster Intrapreneurship Within an Organization

Fostering intrapreneurship within a healthcare organization closely parallels the concepts previously examined with regard to fostering innovation. Healthcare leaders can boost intrapreneurship by creating policies and an environment that cultivates innovation. There are several support tools in place from national healthcare organizations that help to support leaders to establish a culture of innovation. The American Nurses Association's (ANA) Strategic Plan for 2017 to 2020 has as Goal #2 nurse-focused innovation (2016):

> *Stimulate and disseminate innovation which increases recognition of the value of nursing and drives improvement in health and healthcare.*

The American Nurses Credentialing Center (ANCC) recognizes new knowledge, innovation, and improvements as one of the five major components necessary for Magnet recognition of a hospital (see www.nursingworld.org/organizational-programs/magnet/magnet-model).

To foster intrapreneurship, leadership can create an innovation committee in which team members can bring their innovation ideas forward for initial discussion and feedback. Ideas that merit further support and investigation can be followed by appropriate committee members and reported on each month.

Other activities to support intrapreneurship are:

- Innovation rounds
- Guest speakers
- Day or half-day innovation workshops
- Requests for ideas
- Informal idea pitch events
- Innovation newsletter/innovation column

CASE STUDY OF INTRAPRENEURSHIP WITHIN A HOSPITAL

Nurses in the pulmonary department of a Midwest hospital need a better method to follow up on asthmatic patients once they are discharged from the hospital. The hospital's readmission rates were high in this patient population, resulting in costs and Medicare penalties. To address the issue, the nursing team developed a method to provide extensive phone support to patients after they were discharged. Though this approach had never been taken before, it ended up being so successful that it was expanded to provide the same services to other hospitals nationwide. The nurses who developed the innovation negotiated with their own hospital administration for a percentage of the revenue generated from this specialty service. They ultimately became a service business within the hospital organization. This benefited both the hospital and the nurses providing the service. They continued to receive a salary and benefits under their hospital and, in addition, a percentage of the service fee charged to outside hospitals. Over a longer period, readmission rates at their hospital could be documented and a cost-saving model could be developed. The nursing staff was then able to utilize the data to negotiate better terms for their service.

CASE STUDY OF INTRAPRENEURSHIP WITHIN A MEDICAL DEVICE COMPANY

A hospital-based chemotherapy nurse changed jobs to work for a medical device company that manufactured implantable pumps for chemotherapy treatment. When the nurse saw the current product, based on her clinical experience, she realized there was an opportunity to use part of the existing product to create a new product, the first implantable vascular access device (VAD).

As a chemotherapy nurse, she dealt with the problem of finding adequate vascular access to give outpatient chemotherapy to patients. She saw an innovative opportunity to develop existing technology into another business opportunity for the company, but more important, she saw a way to help cancer patients undergoing chemotherapy. The result was a new product used for vascular access, which is now standard treatment for patients undergoing chemotherapy.

The Transition From Intrapreneurship to Entrepreneurship

A Personal Journey as a Nurse

Christine spent over 30 years working for both hospitals and medical device companies as an intrapreneur. She enjoyed working for small start-up device companies, which can be very risky. Many start-ups fail, not because the innovation was bad but for myriad other reasons—lack of sales, inadequate reimbursement, inappropriate management team, insufficient clinical data to support a new device and procedure/technique, and so on.

Christine realized that she actually liked taking risks and working on novel innovations, even though she could be out of a job in a short period of time. She was fortunate to have both her clinical expertise and her business/job experience when she needed to change jobs or find a new one. Having clinical nursing expertise made her unique within a nonhospital healthcare business. She had risen up the business ranks by sheer grit, determination, passion, and hard work, not because she had master's degree in business administration (MBA). Because she did not have an MBA, she did have to work harder than most people around her, but the advancement (financially and personally) was worth it. She believed that if you do have the chance and the interest to get an MBA, go for it. It probably would have made it easier to convince others that she was capable of running her own start-up medical device company, but by then she had no time to go to school and felt she had all the business experience she needed.

So after 20 years working for medical device start-ups, she was ready to create and run her own medical device company. She became aware of an interesting patent that was available for license from a university and took the plunge. She was able to convince the engineer and physician involved with the patent to join the company as co-founders, while Christine served as CEO. As she had been working for start-ups for 20 years, she knew she would have to "bootstrap" her company. *Bootstrapping* is a start-up term, which means that you use a variety of personal funds to get the company started and pay for the initial development until you can raise an angel investment or venture capital funding. Although she knew it would be difficult to raise funding for the company, it turned out to be harder than she could have ever imagined.

(continued)

(continued)

Despite the multitude of hurdles in front of her, she did, however, succeed, and sold the company to a private equity firm for a profit. She became a successful entrepreneur, but also came dangerously close to having her company fail due to the difficulty of raising the needed funds to keep it going. Entrepreneurship is exciting and challenging, but is not for the fainthearted. If you are ready to go out on your own and understand the financial risks, challenges, and *possible* rewards, then do so. Otherwise, keep your current job and continue to be a valuable intrapreneur for your current organization.

"If you can dream it ... you can do it." —Walt Disney

BUSINESS MODELS

Whether leading their teams as an intrapreneur or an entrepreneur, it is imperative for healthcare leaders to understand how companies make money. It is not only important for leaders to comprehend how their organization makes money, but also how vendors, competitors, and market leaders from other industries sustain their businesses. This knowledge can provide healthcare leaders with leverage when negotiating, insights on how they can differentiate their services, and the opportunity to develop new strategies to meet their community's needs.

How Companies Structure Themselves to Make Money

Les Wexner, founder of L brands, Victoria's Secret, and many other retail giants, is famous for his quote, "without a margin, there is no mission." This is one of the most important insights into any industry that wants to have an impact. Companies must develop a sustainable business model that allows them to make enough money to continue to provide their services. In business, *model* refers to an essential plan used to help organizations achieve their financial goals. Simply put, a business model is a company's plan on how it generates revenue and makes a profit; it is *how you make money.* Your job as a leader and innovator is to identify which model will serve you best with your business and with your customers.

As there are many different ways to make money, there are many different business models. Some of the most common models are:

- Service
- Software as a Service (SaaS)
- Franchise
- Manufacturer
- Direct sales
- Subscription
- Ecommerce

In healthcare, the most common business models are service, SaaS, and manufacturing. We'll dive into service and SaaS in this chapter, and tackle manufacturing in Chapter 24, Key Strategies for Moving From Research to Commercialization With Real-World Success Stories.

Business models also vary by who their customers are. To differentiate among these businesses, the terms *B2B, B2C, C2C,* and *C2B* are often used. In each of these acronyms, *B* stands for *business* and *C* stands for *consumer*. In a B2B model, businesses sell services products or other valuables to other businesses. An example of a B2B model is medical suppliers like McKesson selling their products to health systems. The B2C model is commonly seen in retail, when a business sells directly to a consumer. Any time you buy something at Target or Amazon or even at your local corner store, you are participating in a B2C model. The C2C model is less common, as it means consumers sell to consumers. Have you ever hosted a garage sale to sell your unused goods? If so, you've run a C2C retail business model for a very short period of time. Another type of business model is C2B, in which the consumer provides goods or services to businesses. This concept can be confusing to grasp, but is easily exemplified by an Internet blogger who sells advertising space on his or her webpage to companies. In my opinion, these four concepts are the most common methods used to reach customers as they can be combined with each other to capture revenue. An example of combined business models will be highlighted later in this chapter through a case study of NurseGrid.

You've likely interacted with just about every type of model as both a consumer and a healthcare professional. As you develop your entrepreneurial leadership skills, it is important to understand why certain businesses have adopted their chosen business model and how they leverage it for success.

▌ REAL-WORLD EXAMPLES OF HEALTH PROFESSIONALS AS BUSINESS LEADERS

Michelle Podlesni began her nursing career in a local hospital, never thinking she would be sitting in board rooms with customers that were Fortune 500 companies. From a nurse case manager to ultimately the CEO, she participated in three different SaaS company start-ups that generated multimillions of dollars in revenue. More important, her business prevented insurance fraud and abuse, saving billions of dollars for her customers. As she transitioned into full-time entrepreneur mode, she gained experience with the franchise-based business model and the subscription-based business model. Now with the advantage of hindsight, we can look back at Michelle's career to review three real-world examples of these business models (SaaS, franchise, and subscription), and examine their advantages and disadvantages through her experiences.

SaaS—Software as a Service-Based Business Model

Proprietary, customized, and innovative, SaaS businesses are typically the big winner business models with venture capitalists (VCs) and investment firms. The business creates and maintains software as a service in which the software is leased on a subscription basis allowing customers to focus on their core competencies and save money on server costs and in-house developers. An SaaS model can also leverage a subscription model, in which customers make recurring payments to the business in exchange for access to its services. Michelle spent her career working with the following companies to help them utilize variations of the SaaS model for success.

Crawford & Company

Michelle first learned about the workers compensation industry while working at Crawford & Company, the nation's largest third-party administrator (TPA). Worker's compensation costs are split between indemnity payments and Medical payments. Back in 1988, the TPA she worked with did not have automated support for its claims processors on medical billing. Claim processors had to manually apply paper-based volumes of fee-scheduled data.

Michelle came on board as a software product manager to act as the liaison between the medical director's proposed software and the programmers. She would explain to the programmers the outcome necessary in addition to the rules and regulations. For example, in New York, the fee schedule would pay radiology Curren Procedural Terminology (CPT) codes for up to two contiguous part body parts in an injury. This language was not familiar to programmers, but it was imperative for them to understand it in order to produce the desired outcome. Once completed, the software allowed for medical claim information to be processed. The enhanced value of medical claims processing created both a new revenue stream *and* profit center for the company.

General Care Review

Having a strong foundation in utilization review, Michelle was determined to start her own business providing these services in the Southeast. Her knowledge of case management as a nurse served as her unique-value proposition. She was able to recruit one of the executives from her previous employer to help her start the company who would supply the funding to get it started. Instead of building from scratch, they leased software that was available on the market and could hit the ground running. Within 12 months, the company had several national service centers.

As the company's client list grew, the payment to lease the software was nearing over $1 million per year, pulling much needed cash from the company. So they ended up negotiating with the software company to purchase its product. This would allow them to keep costs down in the long term, while being able to customize the product to better meet their needs. Within 3 years, the company had grown to $24 million in revenues and, in 1993, the company merged with General Rehabilitation Services and changed its name to Genex Services.

CompReview

Michelle's next position was as president of CompReview (CR), the software company she used in starting General Care Review. In 1995, CR generated revenues around $10 million. The company made money through two revenue streams: (a) licensing software (SaaS model) and (b) processing medical claims for clients (service model). In addition, CR allowed "white-label branding" of the software. This allowed clients to purchase a license for CR's software and it to make it appear as their own.

This ability to generate revenue using the two models most requested by their customers allowed for great growth. Within 3 years, CR employed nearly 300 people, was generating $40 million dollars in revenue, and captured over a third of the country's workers compensation market through licensing software and service center operations. CR was well positioned for acquisition and was acquired by HNC Software Inc., with a valuation of five times revenue.

Advantages of a SaaS-Based Business Model

Cost savings—These are significant savings that result from subscribing versus investing in onsite solutions, which typically have high upfront costs for installation, maintenance, upgrades, and an information technology (IT) infrastructure. With SaaS, you pay as you use. Most of the preceding examples involved a per bill, per line charge that was paid monthly. Contracts were at will annually with a 90-day notice of cancellation.

Accessibility—With an Internet connection work can be done anywhere, 24/7.

Scalability—SaaS software can scale easily to meet your company's growth and increasing demands. You can easily add more users and features when required. With in-house software, you would have to invest in additional software licenses and more server capacity.

Reliability—Upgrades occur on time and, in the case of the preceding examples, the changes to the fee schedules occurred so often that this proved a barrier for many competitors entering the market. Sites are monitored and supported 24/7.

Reduced risks—Customers are able to try the software before contracting the service. Data-backup servers and additional separate warehousing are available in case of emergencies. SaaS offers shorter deployment times and customized integration, guaranteed delivery, maintenance, and management of the IT services provided.

Customer retention—Value is high due to the lengthy contracting process, EDIs (electronic data interfaces), claims integrations, and implementation processes.

Profit margins—Profit margins tend to be higher as overhead is lower than in models that require hardware or large numbers of employees to deliver a service.

Disadvantages of a SaaS-Based Business Model

Lengthy customer acquisition—A typical licensing contract with corporate clients, such as Liberty Mutual, Marriott, and Walmart, ranges between 12 and 18 months. With service operations clients, the contract typically lasts 3 to 12 months.

Downtime—Outages can occur for any reason and, if you are using an Internet connection, it can go down, which means you cannot access the software application. SLAs (service license agreements) need to be thorough on both sides.

Security—Confidential company and customer data as well as business processes to a third-party provider needs to be addressed to ensure that only authorized people can view and edit sensitive areas. Health Insurance Portability and Accountability Act (HIPAA) regulations, encryption, and firewalls need to have the latest security measures.

Maximum control (most of the time)—The SaaS company owns, manages, and monitors the software, which means customers have minimal control over it. However, some clients and IT staff can become aggressive in testing the limits of the software.

Real-World Example of a SaaS Business Model

NurseGrid creates simplified nurse scheduling tools for healthcare facilities. Joe Novello, BSN/RN, is the CEO and founder of NurseGrid. In the text that follows he has answered some questions about how NurseGrid functions from a business perspective.

What Is Your Business Model?

NurseGrid's model is business to consumer to business (B2B2C). In this model, NurseGrid engages the end user with a "freemium" model (model is free, but add-on features cost money) and then layers on an SaaS model on top of the free experience.

By placing a free, value-added tool in the hands of end users, and then adding incremental value as the early adopters invite their colleagues to join (network effect), NurseGrid can move toward critical mass in the nursing market. With critical mass, NurseGrid is able to open conversations within targeted, well-saturated departments with the end goal of selling a monthly subscription to nurse leaders.

How Do You Apply It to Healthcare and Why Does It Work?

Selling into healthcare is difficult and cumbersome because of its long and often complex sales cycles. Historically, decisions are made top-down, either at the system or hospital level. The B2C2B model helps overcome some of the barriers to entry, which gives NurseGrid a competitive advantage over the larger incumbent solutions in the marketplace.

The premise of the go-to-market strategy is simple: Solve pain points for the end user by offering a mobile-first solution that the individual nurse loves to use, create a network effect whereby the end users get more value as they help recruit more nurses onto the system, use the product to attract and engage nurse managers, introduce NurseGrid Manager as a paid monthly subscription, prove your success (via return on investment [ROI] and other positive outcomes), introduce the results of the single department to the hospital executives with the goal of a house-wide rollout.

What Is Your Business Strategy (High Volume/Low Cost, High Cost With Differentiation, or Another)?

During the early years of NurseGrid, the strategy was twofold: Attract end users and create strong engagement, and implement a land-and-expand model whereby NurseGrid enters a single hospital department where positive outcomes can be demonstrated, documented, and delivered to the hospital C-suite.

How Do You Make Money?

NurseGrid has two main products that integrate seamlessly into one another: NurseGrid Mobile (launched first quarter of 2015) and NurseGrid Manager (launched first quarter of 2016). Both products have gained significant traction over the last several years. NurseGrid Mobile has been downloaded by more than 550,000 nurses and NurseGrid Manager is used by more than 500 nurse leaders.

NurseGrid Mobile is a free solution, acting as a loss leader that paves the way for NurseGrid Manager. NurseGrid Manager is a monthly subscription service with discounts for longer term agreements. In addition, NurseGrid has a menu of professional service add-ons that can be purchased at the discretion of the customer.

A *loss leader* is a product (in NurseGrid's Case, a software platform) that is sold below its cost or given away at no charge in hopes of attracting customers. Companies then hope to leverage the loss- leader product to get customers to purchase other products that, combined with the loss leader, allow the company to make a profit.

What Are the Benefits of This Type of Model Versus Other Models and Why Did You Choose It?

This model was chosen given the standard barriers to entry into healthcare technology. These include end user adoption failure, price sensitivity at the department level, lengthy sales cycles, and others. With NurseGrid's model, the solution has already proven to be successful at the end user level, can be deployed quickly with little friction and at an affordable rate that produces positive ROI rapidly, thereby allowing for rapid expansion throughout the entire hospital.

What Are Your Top Two Challenges?

The top two challenges for NurseGrid include:

1. Nurse managers as atypical buyers of healthcare technology. Although Nurse Managers are accustomed to budgeting and other types of purchases, historically they have not historically been the core decision makers for technology solution procurement. This creates a situation in which the NurseGrid sales team must walk the manager through the buying cycle.

2. There is a disconnect between nurse managers and C-suite hospital executives. The pain points that NurseGrid solves for are almost universally felt at the staff nurse and nurse manager levels. However, hospital C-suite executives are often shielded from the direct pain points and are often unaware of current workarounds used to overcome pain points unmet by incumbent solutions. Meanwhile, executives believe these incumbent solutions have the features and functionality to solve the pain points.

Why Doesn't Everyone Do It?

NurseGrid is not alone in the scheduling, communication, and staffing space. What is unique about NurseGrid is its go-to-market strategy. The competitive landscape includes large time-keeping solutions that have attempted to bolt on schedule management solutions, and hospital-specific scheduling solutions that deploy a traditional top-down model.

Franchise-Based Business Model

A *franchise* as defined by the Code of Federal Regulation (16 CFR 436.1) as: (a) "franchisor" (owner of the trademark) grants to franchisee (person or entity granted the right to use the trademark) the right to use the franchisor's trademark; (b) for a fee; (c) and franchisor exerts a "significant degree of control over the franchisee's method of operation," *or* "provides significant assistance in the franchisee's method of operation." A franchisor can expand and collect fees from others who want to purchase, own, and operate a franchised business system that is offered by the owner/entity and operates under its trademark(s), business systems, training, and ongoing support.

Franchise buyers will typically pay a substantial up front *initial franchise fee (IFF)* as well as ongoing royalties and other fees. Royalties usually are a percentage of each franchise owner's monthly gross revenue. These ongoing fees enable the franchisor to continuously improve the business systems and support the franchise community to help them grow their respective businesses.

Michelle's diversity as an entrepreneur also expands into experience with a franchise model. In 2002, corporate life and travel no longer appealed to her. She and her husband determined that that they wanted to have a business that would keep them home. In discussing this and looking at the trends in the healthcare marketplace, elder care services appeared to be the market to enter. They examined starting their own elder care business or purchasing a franchise of an established elder care company. After investigating senior care companies, they decided to buy a Comfort Keepers franchise for the territory where they were living in Ohio.

Michelle and her husband's franchise experience was very similar to the definition just outlined. They purchased an exclusive territory, which involved an up-front payment. They went to the corporate headquarters for training on their system. They didn't have to recreate the wheel. They put things in place, hired their first caregivers, and got their software ready. They paid a royalty to the franchisor each month that they felt was reasonable.

Michelle's background as a nurse was perfect for this new business. She and her husband built the company to include 70 caregivers who provided over 2,000 hours of service a week in their community. They hired an administrative staff and a professional employer organization (PEO) to handle employee payroll and insurance. They continued to grow their company for several years, but wanting to move back to the West Coast, they decided to put their franchise up for sale. Knowing all the Comfort Keepers franchise owners in the area, they leveraged their network and sold their franchise to an existing franchise owner in 2010.

Advantages of a Franchise-Based Business Model

Franchise owners receive help with:

Site selection: To gain optimal traffic with consideration of locations of competitive businesses

Training: To learn the business and proven operational methods

Grand-opening programs: To be able to jump start the business

National and regional advertising: To grow sales

Routine business operations: To maintain best practices for optimal efficiency

Access to bulk purchasing agreements: Offered by approved vendors to hold down operating expenses

Ongoing supervision and management support: Help is available if you run into problems or have questions

Disadvantages of a Franchise-Based Business Model

Control: Support from the home office is designed to take the guess work out of running a business, but for some entrepreneurs, this can be stifling. If you are looking for a business in which you want to apply your own personal touch and pricing, you have to make sure that the franchisor is willing to allow you that level of freedom.

Cost—It's not cheap to get a franchise up and running. The capital investment requirements for franchising vary widely depending on the industry.

Noncompete agreement—There is generally a significant period of time during which you are not permitted to have a competing business after you no longer own the franchise.

Real-World Example of Service-Based Business Model

Freelance Anesthesia is a traveling anesthesia practice that provides dentists and physicians more flexibility to conduct procedures within their own office space. Pamala Wilson, DNPA, CNRA, is the founder and CEO of Freelance Anesthesia. Here she has answered questions about how her company functions from a business perspective.

1. **What is your business model?** Freelance Anesthesia uses a B2B service model. We travel to dental facilities to provide pediatric, and sometimes adult, sedations in the dental office versus the patient having to go to the hospital just for behavior modification sedation. I would consider this company my own practice and the contracted providers (other certified registered nurse anesthetists [CRNAs]) receive 1099s, so they can have the beneficial write-offs that a contracted provider gets. They also have the flexibility to work for several groups if they desire and can set their own schedules. The benefit to the business is reduced costs for taxes and the additional benefits that an employee gets.

2. **How do you apply your service to healthcare and why does it work?** Essentially we provide a service that reduces the cost of services. The cost of anesthesia is often the same regardless of where we provide care (hospital operating room, surgical center, physician office, etc.). As an office-based anesthesia company that provides anesthesia services for medical and dental offices, we keep patients/insurers from paying facility fees for the hospital or surgery center for minimally invasive procedures done on relatively healthy patients. For example, state Medicaid programs save millions of dollars a year by not having to pay a facility fee when services are performed in the hospital.

   Physicians and dentists also benefit from our services because patients choose them to keep their out-of-pocket costs down, reimbursement is higher for some procedures conducted in the office setting, and they improve efficiency by seeing patients in between cases. Something that cannot be done during the procedure is performed in a hospital.

3. **What is your business strategy?** We offer cost-effective services requiring anesthesia outside normal institutional settings.

4. **How do you make money?** We bill directly to state Medicaid programs or collect from patients for their anesthesia services if they are private payers. We have started services in several other states. Depending on the state's dental regulations, we use a physician anesthesiologist or a CRNA. When we use CRNAs, we pay them 70% of the net revenue; when we use physician anesthesiologists, we act as a management service for them. We want to stay away from the fee-splitting and anti-kickback statutes when working with physician anesthesiologists. We charge physicians a daily fee for equipment leasing, for a proprietary trade secret sedation protocol, and for billing and back-office management services.

5. **What are the benefits of this type of model versus other models and why did you choose it?** Our business model allows the patient, provider, payer, and our contractors to all win. We chose it because there was a need to help at-risk populations, like the pediatric dental population, and this model allowed us the ability to serve this community.

6. **What are your top two challenges?**
   1. Our first challenge is that some state dental regulations don't allow certain anesthesia practitioners to provide anesthesia services in the dental office setting.
   2. Another challenge we face is getting the information regarding our services to doctors and dentists who would contract our services.
7. **Why doesn't everyone do it?** Most people don't want to spend the time, money, and deal with the risks incumbent in starting their own business. They just want to provide services and don't want to deal with the business side of things.

Subscription-Based Business Model

A *subscription model* is a revenue model in which the customer subscribes for a service; it is a recurring revenue model. The objective is to retain customers under a long-term contract and secure current revenues with repeat purchases of products and services. Companies operating online require the customer to sign up for automatic payment plans for a preset time frame. Subscription businesses are a favorite of entrepreneurs; its recurring nature is attractive to businesses as a stream of income and as a means for improving customer lifetime value. This model was pioneered by magazines and newsletters but has now pervaded nearly every industry. Think of Amazon Prime, Birchbox, StitchFix, Graze, and Netflix. This is the business model Michelle chose for her next company, when she acquired the National Nurses in Business Association (NNBA) in 2014.

Advantages of a Subscription-Based Business Model

Predictable income: Brand loyalty and a dependable consumer base are built, which are two key ingredients to a viable business. The overall value of each customer also tends to be higher. Therefore, the model reduces overall risk and makes for easier forecasting.

Good customer relationships: Companies have an extended time to build a relationship and receive feedback that allows them to learn what they value and further improve their offerings.

Word of mouth: In this social media-driven age, customers who love your product share it with friends and followers. Comments and reviews appear online in places like Facebook, LinkedIn, Amazon, and Twitter. Reviews and comments have fueled growth of the NNBA's membership and annual conference attendance.

Disadvantages of a Subscription-Based Business Model

Bigger budget needed for customer procurement: Because a subscription service is based on the idea of selling one idea, and getting that idea to stick on a month-to-month basis, the initial budget for reaching and procuring new customers can be somewhat larger than it would be with a more traditional business model.

Risk of cancellation: *Churn*, or cancellation, is one of the biggest risks of subscription service-based companies. Although it is true that there is some reliability of income when a customer signs up, what's going to keep the customer interested? More important, what's going to prevent the customer from cancelling when he or she decides the product is not worth the monthly fee? It is critically important to develop a good relationship with your customers and to make it easy for them to cancel the subscription. At the NNBA, we guarantee 100% satisfaction. Membership subscription is refunded immediately without any cancellation penalty. We maintain a 5-star reputation with the nurses in our community.

Difficulty maintaining value: This is a hurdle that subscription service business owners should anticipate. If your product gets old, or can be replaced by something cheaper and easier, the novelty will wear off. You need to provide new products and services. You need to be innovative in your marketing approaches. NNBA publishes a newsletter every 2 weeks with current and relevant articles, opportunities, new services, and programs. We have been consistent, never missing a 2-week publication schedule for over 4 years. You need to know how to shake things up and keep customers from moving on.

The Future of Business Models in the Healthcare Marketplace

Businesses fail when they don't keep up with changing market conditions. As leaders and innovators, you must be aware of socioeconomic changes, legislative changes, technologic changes, competitive changes, and customer changes. For example, leaders need to be aware of legislation that is being proposed. Medicare Rule 2019 IPPS (inpatient prospective payment system) will be published in the *Federal Register* and is then open for comment. This rule applies to about 3,300 acute care hospitals and 420 long-term care hospitals. It promises more price transparency for patients, reduced administrative burden on providers, and a greater emphasis on interoperability. There are multiple, innovative opportunities inside those 1,000 pages.

As Thomas Friedman (2005) states in *The World is Flat*, by *flat* he means connected. Exponential technical advances of the digital revolution make it possible to do business instantaneously with billions of people across the world. Over the next 5 years, we are going to see what has been taking place in retail begin to take place in the healthcare marketplace. You will start to see Priceline- and Ebay-like models used to auction off medical and surgical procedures. Is there any doubt when three corporate behemoths—Amazon, Berkshire Hathaway, and JPMorgan Chase—announced that they would form an independent healthcare company for their employees in the United States (Wingfield, Thomas, & Abelson, 2018)?

Many healthcare professionals, especially nurses, limit their potential influence and impact because of the internal conflict between altruism and self-interest. Jaana Woiceshyn's book, *How to Be Profitable and Moral* (2012), offers rational egoism to business leaders who want to maximize profits ethically. Nurses need to be at the table of the new players who want to effectively deal with inefficiencies throughout the cadre of providers, insurers, pharmaceutical companies, and IT systems. Most important, nurse leaders and innovators need to be agile, allowing for revenue models to change as the healthcare marketplace changes.

SOCIAL ENTREPRENEURSHIP

> *"It always seems impossible until it's done."* —Nelson Mandela

Social entrepreneurship is a relatively new term; however, the activity it describes is not and the phenomenon has been around for a long time. There have always been social entrepreneurs, though they may have been known by other terms. Before the term was coined, there were many entrepreneurs who worked for children's rights, women's empowerment, socioeconomic development, environmental issues, and more. Historically, three noteworthy social entrepreneurs are Robert Owen (1771–1858), the founder of the cooperative movement; Florence Nightingale (1820–1910), who founded the first nursing school and developed various modern nursing practices; and Clara Barton (1821–1912), founder of the American Red Cross.

Today, *social entrepreneurship* has been defined as the use of organizations and start-up companies to develop, fund, and implement solutions to social, cultural, or environmental issues that create societal value. The businesses differ from nonprofits as nonprofits must invest all profit back into the mission of the organization. Social enterprises have more freedom over how they can spend their profits and address their defined social objectives. Nonprofits also hold a 501(c)3 tax-exempt status from the Internal Revenue Service (IRS) in the United States. An example of a social enterprise is the shoe company TOMS. TOMS uses some of the profits generated by the sale of their products to "provide shoes, sight, water, safe birth and bullying prevention services to people in need" (TOMS, 2018).

In healthcare, many social enterprises have been formed to address issues that were not being previously met. These organizations require innovative approaches, the use of technology, and the entrepreneurial skill set of determination and hard work to succeed. Some of the most influential social entrepreneurship organizations operating today are descried in the text that follows.

Doctors Without Borders/Medecins Sans Frontieres

"An independent global movement, providing medical aid where it is needed most." —from Doctors Without Borders (https://www.doctorswithoutborders.org/)

This organization was informally started in 1968 with two doctors, two nurses, and two clinicians who went to Biafra (Southern Nigeria) to care for victims of war and starvation. It continues to operate today in 65 countries around the world during outbreaks of disease, war, and famine. It is one of the first organizations to respond to each outbreak of Ebola.

Heifer International

Heifer Intenational works with communities to end world hunger and poverty, empower women, and care for the Earth. It was started over 70 years ago by Dan West, a farmer from the Midwest. Heifer International works with communities to strengthen local economies by distributing animals and teaching families in need about agriculture to foster self-sufficeincy. Their value-based, holistic, and community-development approach focuses on increasing income and assets, food security and nutrition, and helping the environment.

CASE STUDY: THE MAKING OF A SOCIAL ENTREPRENEUR WITH SOCIAL MEDIA

On the evening of September 14, 2015, Jane Harvey Garner, an ER nurse in St. Louis, Missouri, was thinking about what she heard one of the commentators say on the popular talk show *The View* earlier that day. The commentator mocked the Miss America contestant, Miss Colorado,

Kelly Johnson, who was a nurse and who talked about her experience as a nurse for the talent component of the contest. She came out wearing hospital scrubs, wore a stethoscope around her neck, and talked about caring for patients. She is a real nurse. She was mocked by the commentators on *The View*, who asked, "Why is she wearing a doctor's stethoscope around her neck?"

This bothered Jane and later that night on her break at the hospital she created a Facebook page and tweeted out on #nursesunitepic.twitter.com, "Is any other nurse out there as angry as I am about those comments? Send me a picture of yourself wearing your stethoscope."

What happened next is history.

Within 5 minutes, she received 6,000 responses from nurses worldwide.

By noon the following day, her page had 260,000 members. It was the fastest growing Facebook page membership that Facebook had ever seen and it almost shut Facebook's system down with the traffic. Today **Show Me Your Stethoscope** (**SMYS**; smysofficial.com) has over 650,000 members and is the largest active online nursing community in the world.

Jane thought, "What am I going to do with this?" Luckily for nurses, she decided to use the power of social media to bring nursing issues and philanthropy to the forefront. Today, SMYS is using nurses' voices to address staffing issues and patient safety. In addition, SMYS's nurse-driven philanthropy is happening globally with healthcare missions to Ghana, actions to address the Flint water crisis, sponsorship of an Orlando shooting fund-raiser, and donations to the Bangladesh Asthma Fund. All started and supported by nurses.

"The power of one, if fearless and focused, is formidable,
but the power of many working together is better." —Gloria Macapagal Arroyo

🔑 KEY TAKEAWAY POINTS

- Healthcare providers are natural social entrepreneurs who have a long history of changing the world for the better.

- An intrapreneur is a leader who acts like an entrepreneur while working in a large organization.

- Healthcare businesses make money in a variety of different ways. Understanding how money is made in healthcare provides a leader with leverage to use when making key decisions and negotiations.

- Being an entrepreneur is challenging and is not the best path for everyone to take. However, entrepreneurial principles can be applied to almost any role/organization to help find success.

- The decision to become an intrapreneur or entrepreneur is individualized and should be made after much deliberation.

- It is possible to make global healthcare changes with the power of one. It is also possible to make these changes with a dedicated group.

REFERENCES

American Nurses Association. (2016). *ANA strategic plan 2017–2020*. Retrieved from https:// www.nursingworld.org/ana/about-ana/strategic-plan/

Code of Federal Regulations, 16 CFR 436.1 (2018).

Friedman, T. L. (2005). *The world is flat*. New York, NY: Farrar, Straus and Giroux.

Pinchot, G., III, & Pinchot, E. S. (1978). *Intra-corporate entrepreneurship* [White Paper]. *The Pinchot Perspective*. Retrieved from https://drive.google.com/file/d/0B6GgwqtG-DKcSlpsb GRBZkZYSlk/view

TOMS. (2018). Improving lives. Retrieved from https://www.toms.com/improving-lives

Wingfield, N., Thomas, K., & Abelson, R. (2018, January 30). Amazon, Berkshire Hathaway and JPMorgan team up to try to disrupt health care. *New York Times*. Retrieved from https://www.nytimes.com/2018/01/30/technology/amazon-berkshire-hathaway-jpmorgan -health-care.html

Woiceshyn, J. (2012). *How to be profitable and moral*. New York, NY: Hamilton Books.

Legal Considerations in Starting a Healthcare Business

Jonathon Vinocur

"There's lots of bad reasons to start a company. But there's only one good, legitimate reason, and I think you know what it is: It's to change the world." —Phil Libin, CEO of Evernote

LEARNING OBJECTIVE
- Obtain a high-level understanding of the preliminary legal considerations applicable to healthcare businesses.

INTRODUCTION

The purpose of this chapter is to identify the legal matters that should be considered when starting a healthcare business. Although certainly not the most important consideration in starting a business, certain legal issues might help you decide (if not dictate) whether or not it is even worthwhile to proceed beyond the idea phase. For example, if you have no appetite for completing and submitting forms, running a business that generates revenue by seeking and obtaining reimbursement from a government agency—which is a document-intensive process—might not be the right choice for you. To this end, we begin with a short section that very briefly explains how the laws work in the United States and then follow up with a short summary of certain regulatory schemes that apply to healthcare businesses, each of which is intended to help you determine the extent to which your healthcare business will be regulated and what the implications of those regulations will be on your business plan.

Once you have decided whether your path will be highly regulated, not at all regulated, or somewhere in between, we will summarize the legal issues most commonly encountered by healthcare businesses. When people (whether they label themselves as owners, principals, founders, partners, or something else) start a business, the most important (and most frequently repeated) exercise they undertake is the prioritization of their to-do list. Because there is never enough time in any day, week, or month to do everything that needs to be done, they are faced with constantly visiting and revisiting what comes next, not to mention their approach to determining which tasks should be prioritized over others. Our intent is that each section that follows provides a sufficiently high-level summary of the hurdles you might have to jump so that you can determine easily whether or not "now" (whenever that might be) is the right time to address the contemplated issue.

LAW SCHOOL 101

Statutory Law

The federal, state, county, and municipal governments all limit the actions taken by individuals and businesses every day. They do so by way of statutes (i.e., laws) that are typically approved by the vote of a legislative body (e.g., Congress) and approved by an executive (e.g., the president). Frequently, those statutes then allow a regulatory body to create rules and directives (i.e., regulations) that define the manner in which the statute is applied, interpreted, and/or enforced (among other things). Just by way of example, Congress passed a bill designed to control air pollution on a national level, which was signed into law by the president as the Clean Air Act. Thereafter, the Environmental Protection Agency (EPA) created and implemented regulations defining the maximum amounts of specific pollutants that industries are allowed to emit into the air, and what the penalty will be if those amounts are exceeded.

Common Law

When parties disagree with respect to how a statute, regulation, or other legal mandate should be interpreted, it can be further clarified when one of those parties sues the other and then a court issues an opinion with respect to the statute, regulation, or other legal mandate at issue. The aggregation of all of these judges' opinions is referred to as *common law*, which can be just as strong as, or stronger than, any statute. For example, the duty of confidentiality owed by a doctor or nurse to her patient is derived from common law. The common law is very important to litigators and may be important to you if you are deciding whether or not to sue someone, trying to figure out whether or not you are going to be sued, and/or trying to predict the outcome of a lawsuit in which you are involved or that may otherwise be meaningful to your business. Otherwise, it probably won't be of great concern to you from a business (nonclinical) perspective.

CHART THE REGULATORY LANDSCAPE BEFORE YOU GET STARTED

Before deciding whether or not to start your healthcare business, or as you determine what shape it should take and/or how it should expand, it is important to understand that some businesses are subjected to many laws and regulations, whereas others are subject to very few. Understanding the extent to which your business may be regulated will impact, among other things, the amount of capital your new business will require before it begins generating revenue (and until it is profitable), the amount of time it takes to start generating revenue, and the types of individuals and service providers you will need to progress with your business. For example, if your healthcare business will be developing a new medical device that uses electricity and transmits a patient's data to healthcare providers, you may be faced with obtaining approvals from, among others, the Food and Drug Administration (FDA), the Federal Communications Commission (FCC), and the Consumer Product Safety Commission (CPSC), and you will need to be sure that it complies with the Health Insurance Portability and Accountability Act (HIPAA). Alternatively, if your healthcare business will provide healthcare services to elderly patients in their homes, the business may need to obtain (and maintain) certain licenses with the state, county, or municipality where it operates and be sure that the individuals who are actually providing the services maintain their respective licenses (although the extent to which you help them obtain, maintain, and/or pay for these licenses is up to you).

Of course, none of this includes the costs related to forming the business or day-to-day legal matters, such as the preparation of contracts for use with customers and suppliers, employee disputes, investment and lending transactions, and so forth. As you can imagine, whether or not your healthcare business is subject to these various regulations can significantly inform your business plan or even result in your choosing not to proceed. In any event, it will be important to fully investigate these issues before deciding to start your new healthcare business and/or expand your current healthcare business.

CALL TO ACTION

Determine whether or not your venture and/or those working for it will be regulated, what regulatory schemes may apply, and how that will affect your growth objectives.

HOW YOUR ULTIMATE OBJECTIVE SHOULD INFORM LEGAL DECISION-MAKING

Like so many things, knowing where you are headed will help you chart the path forward, and this certainly applies when you are trying to figure out what legal decisions need to be made as you start and operate your business. In this section, we will address how your ultimate objectives for the business can be everything from instructive to determinative with respect to any number of legal matters.

High-Growth Ventures—Diligently Focused on Diligence

If you are starting your business with the intention of selling it someday, you will want to do whatever you can to increase its value as much as possible, so that you command as high of a selling price as possible. If you fail to do so, the extent of your return on your investment of all of the time and money you have spent will be the learning experience (the value of which, to be sure, should not be dismissed), but not a financial profit. However, if you are developing a medical device and you are able to prove its efficacy (among other things), or you have figured out how to sell a new electronic medical records add-on like hotcakes, your start-up's value can increase exponentially, which will bring you markedly closer to achieving your ultimate goal of selling the business.

Unless you are independently wealthy, you will need money from third parties—typically investors—to fund your value-creating progress. Before investors agree to invest their money, they complete a diligence process through which they evaluate a business's likelihood of significant growth. During this process, they will ask you innumerable questions about, and make unending requests regarding your product; how you define your target market; how you formed the business; how you acquired the intellectual property (IP; which will be discussed in more detail later in this chapter); and how you have grown the business. These potential investors will expect the answers to their product-market-fit questions to roll off your tongue, and they will expect you to have your entity's formation documents, IP assignment agreements, and confidentiality agreements at your fingertips. As you would imagine, this diligence process becomes only more comprehensive as the stakes are increased when a buyer comes knocking. Just by way of example, failing to have in place the proper documentation with the primary supplier of a certain device component could significantly decrease the price your potential buyer is willing to pay. Similarly, if the primary developer of your software still has not signed that IP assignment agreement you gave him when he started, this could delay the sale transaction's closing (or even require some additional payment to him before he will sign it).

When you are building your business to be sold, it will be critical to be sure that you have all of these boxes checked before seeking outside investment or proceeding with a sale process. These considerations should be part of your ordinary course and can have a significant impact on the ultimate value proposition you present to potential investors and buyers.

Considering the Development of a New Medical Device in the United States?

If so, the FDA requires that you either obtain premarket approval (known as *PMA*) or that you submit a premarket notification of your intent to market the device (frequently referred to as *510(k) pathway*).

The PMA process is significantly more involved and costly and requires lab testing and clinical trials with human participants (and sometimes many rounds of testing and trials). On the other hand, the 510(k) pathway requires far less testing and data and is, therefore, much faster and less expensive.

Whether your device will require PMA or can be shepherded through via the 510(k) pathway depends on how much harm the device could do once it is available for sale to the public. To be specific, the riskiest devices (i.e., those that are permanently implanted into a human body or that may be necessary to sustain life) require PMA. Low- and moderate-risk devices, such as dental floss and hearing aids, respectively, are examples of devices that can follow the 510(k) pathway.

To be sure, either process is wrought with pitfalls and cannot be taken lightly. However, if we take a look from 50,000 feet, it's actually quite logical—the greater the likelihood a malfunctioning product could cause a significant, adverse outcome, the more rigorous and thorough the approval process will be, whereas a product with a relatively low likelihood of causing harm can be sold after providing the FDA with notice.

Lifestyle Businesses—Doing What Makes Sense

If selling your business is not your ultimate goal, making sure that your legal house is in order becomes far less about proving to potential investors and buyers that you know your stuff than it is about making sure the business runs smoothly on a day-to-day basis. For example, if you have a business partner, you will want to agree on which decisions will be made by which partner, as well as how the money that goes into, and comes out of, the business will be allocated between you. On the other hand, although latex gloves and syringes might be absolutely critical for you to perform the services offered by your business, it is not necessary for you to have a 40-page contract assuring that your primary supplier will deliver, because there are many companies that sell these supplies and they can likely be purchased in smaller quantities in a pinch. Similarly, maybe a simple customer order form is all you need if the way you collect your fee is to take a portion of the payments patients make using the medical invoicing collection software platform you sell to doctors' offices. Because outsiders are rarely reviewing your business practices, it will be important that your approach to legal matters does not unnecessarily slow down your sales (or collections) or create unnecessary administrative burdens, and that it generally works for you and your business partners.

 CALL TO ACTION

Decide whether your new venture will be a "high-growth venture" or a "lifestyle business."

> *"When you find an idea that you just can't stop thinking about,*
> *that's probably a good one to pursue."* —Josh James, co-founder and
> CEO of Omniture, founder, and CEO of Domo

WHAT TO DO BEFORE YOU THINK THERE'S ANYTHING TO DO

Keep It to Yourself

IP is the legal term given to an intangible creation of the human mind, such as inventions, concepts, ideas, artistic works, logos, slogans, and the like. The law protects someone's IP from unauthorized use by others for a period of time. However, your ability to enforce certain IP rights starts to diminish the first time your idea enters the public domain (more on that later). There are exceptions to this diminution that help protect your IP (e.g., nondisclosure agreements and the like), and it does not apply to certain relationships (e.g., conversations with your lawyer). But telling your friend about your amazing new idea could start the clock running, and there's no way to turn back time. Similarly, no matter how close you are to that friend, he or she will be under no legal obligation to keep that amazing new idea a secret.

Toe the Line

Undoubtedly, all academic and research institutions (including universities, colleges, hospitals, labs, clinics, etc.) have policies in place that dictate the extent to which any IP that results from the efforts of their students, staff, faculty, and others using their facilities and/or resources is owned by the research institution (as opposed to the individual). These policies also almost always require the disclosure of this IP by the individual to the institution, after which the institution may choose to permit the individual to use the IP. Failing to comply with these disclosure policies can result in a significant diminution in value or even litigation (i.e., the institution sues the individual for IP misappropriation). For example, the founder of a high-growth venture who fails to comply with her or his university's disclosure policy will find it virtually impossible to raise capital, as no investor wants to invest in, and thus own, a part of a company that neither owns nor has permission to use the technology it is attempting to commercialize. Similarly, a court could decide that a lifestyle business that uses technology in which a research institution still has legal rights owes the institution a percentage of any profit generated using the underlying IP (i.e., royalties), or that such a business is prohibited from using the IP unless it secures a license to do so from the institution where it originated.

CALL TO ACTION

Determine whether or not you will need to make an internal disclosure with respect to the intellectual property you're planning to use for your business and/or enter into a license agreement to use it in your business.

Get on the Same Page

Of paramount importance should be to make sure you can do business with the other individuals with whom you are starting the business. This relationship will involve as much emotion as almost any other relationship you have. Plan to go away together first (to a weekend-long hack-a-thon) and then move in together (by jointly tackling a discrete project) before becoming legally joined (think—married!) by forming a company together.

CALL TO ACTION

Ask someone to serve as your hypothetical partner, let her or him pick what kind of business it will be (that way, she or he will think it's important) and then see how long it takes you to agree on (a) how the profit will be divided, (b) how the business's debts will be paid, (c) what happens if one of you can't contribute your fair share, (d) how things will be split if you add a third partner, (e) how you will decide when it's time to sell the business, and (f) how you will decide when it's time to shut down the business. Next, ask a second person to undertake the same process and see whether you reach agreement more quickly. If so (or if not), why?

CHOOSING A LAWYER

Much of what is discussed over the balance of this chapter is intended to allow you to know when the time is right to dig in on a given legal issue. That said, in many instances and for better or worse, you may find that you need the assistance of an attorney. Although you undoubtedly know not to ask the lawyer who prepared your will or handled your cousin's divorce for her or his advice on how to prepare your first licensing agreements, many attorneys hold themselves out as capable of performing a wide range of legal services as opposed to focusing on just one area of the law. To be sure, attorneys can (and should) help with respect to various and numerous matters throughout the lifecycle of a business. Some attorneys become integral parts of their clients' businesses. Others perform tasks on a purely transactional (i.e., discrete, project and/or noncontinuous) basis. Some lawyers have hourly rates that are less than $100, whereas others' are over $1,000. Although none of these attributes necessarily reflects how helpful (or not) an attorney could be to your business, the overarching goal of what follows is to provide you with a sufficient understanding of the issues to enable you to discuss them with an attorney if the time is right. Your being able to explain what is at issue to an attorney should allow him or her to identify what legal services you need, when you need (and do not need) those services, and how those services should be priced. When your lawyer hits all three of those nails squarely on the head, you know you have picked a winner.

 ## FORMING AN ENTITY

What Are Entities?

All state statutes allow individuals (among others) to form entities. For legal purposes, these entities are considered by the state to be parties that are legally distinct from their owners. This distinction is typically achieved by the filing of paperwork with the state that will result in an entity being legally formed. Once it is, the entity can obtain its own tax identification number (which is like its Social Security number and is called an *employer identification number [EIN]*), own property, sue and be sued, and otherwise act as any individual could act. Examples of entities are partnerships, limited liability companies, and corporations.

Conversely, when an individual merely has a "DBA" (which stands for *doing business as*), she or he might have the right to use a certain name to perform a service or sell a product, and to do so to the exclusion of others (or not—it's entirely dependent upon the applicable law). However, any action being taken by that business is really being taken by her or him as an individual, not as a separate entity. Similarly, even when an individual identifies his or her business as a sole proprietorship, no legal distinction is created between him or her and his or her business.

Why Do Entities Matter?

Entities give business partners a way to act together, as a single unit, with respect to the business and a mechanism to sort out how decisions will be made (including how any profits or losses will be allocated among them). Certain entities also protect the business partners from having to be responsible for liabilities incurred by the entity.

Which Entities Are Which?

Partnerships

Although states allow individuals to create different types of partnerships (general partnerships, limited partnerships, limited liability partnerships, etc.), the general purpose is to provide a framework according to which two or more individuals can agree to work together. Generally, and unless the partners enter into an agreement that says otherwise, they are all treated equally, each partner has the same rights and obligations as the others, and each partner can act with full authority on behalf of the business. For example, depending on the type of partnership that is formed, this means that if one partner signs a lease in the partnership's name, the other partners are responsible for paying the rent—and not just their respective percentages of the rent but rather the full rent payment each month. Although the partnership as an entity is not used frequently for businesses providing goods or services (so that one partner isn't on the hook when the other partner signs a bad lease), it is still frequently used by individuals who want to pool their money for investment purposes.

Corporations

States also allow individuals to form corporations, which is a form of entity that limits the stockholder's liability to the amount of capital he or she invests. That is, if you and a business partner form a corporation and each of you buys 10,000 shares for $1.00 each, and, after spending the $20,000, the business fails, neither you nor your partner can be held responsible for any other liabilities that the corporation may have incurred. This protection, however, can be lost if the corporation's stockholders fail to adhere to certain formalities set forth in the state's corporation law. For example, most state laws require that formal steps be taken so that a corporation's stockholders elect directors annually and that those directors elect the corporation's officers. These formalities require either a stockholder meeting to be held each year and board meetings to be held regularly, or that legal consent actions be prepared to document the stockholders' and directors' actions to comply with these formalities. In addition, a corporation's assets are to be kept separate and aside from those of its officers, directors, or stockholders. Thus, if stockholder meetings are not held annually, board meetings aren't held annually, and an individual comingles the corporation's assets with his own (e.g., deposits a check properly made out to the corporation into his personal account), a court could find that the individual is simply the corporation's "alter ego" and, as a result, the individual should be liable for the corporation's debts.

Limited Liability Companies

Limited liability companies mix attributes from partnership statutes and corporate statutes by allowing the business partners to reach agreement on things like how frequently the holders of shares (frequently called *members*) and the board will meet (or not at all) while at the same time limiting the liability of the members to only the capital they have contributed to the limited liability company. Generally, the members will be afforded this protection so long as the members make the filings the state requires to form the limited liability company, and they treat the limited liability company as separate and distinct from the members (e.g., no mixing bank accounts). In addition, the process for forming a limited liability company often is less burdensome than the process of forming a partnership or corporation. Table 20.1 summarizes a few of the more important distinctions among partnerships, corporations, and limited liability companies.

TABLE 20.1 **Important Differences Among Partnerships, Corporations, and Limited Liability Companies**

	Partnership	Corporation	Limited Liability Company
Ownership requirements	Two or more partners	One or more stockholders	One or more members
Form of equity	None (but can be included in the partnership agreement)	Stockholders hold shares of stock	Members hold interests (sometimes called *units*)
Formation document	None (but certain types of partnerships can be created with filings)	Certificate of incorporation	Certificate of formation
Typical governing document(s)	None (but partnerships can have partnership agreements)	Bylaws and stockholders' agreements	Operating agreement
Liability	None (but certain types of partnerships can provide for limited liability for some partners)	Limited to contributed capital	Limited to contributed capital
Owners	Partners	Stockholders	Members
Strategic decisions	Partners	Board of directors	Members (or the operating agreement can name a board of managers)
Management	Partners (unless the partnership agreement says otherwise)	Officers	Members (or the operating agreement can name managers or officers)

Employer Identification Number

After the entity is formed, an EIN, which is sometimes referred to as a *tax ID, taxpayer identification number,* or the like, should be obtained from the Internal Revenue Service (IRS). The EIN serves as the identification number the federal, state, and local taxing authorities will use to identify the business and is different from any discrete identifying number provided to it when it is formed at the state level (although that number can be required for certain state-specific functions, sometimes including those that are tax related). We discussed earlier the importance of keeping your business's assets separate from your personal assets. Although the easiest way to do this is to establish a bank account, banks require the business to have its own EIN before an account will be opened. In addition, even though the acronym *EIN* suggests that it would be applicable only to entities that are employers, it can be obtained before a business has employees and even if a business will not ever have any employees.

A Very Brief Word on Taxes

The benefits and detriments of various tax structures could fill volumes, but for these purposes, we look at just two alternatives. In short, after you decide which form of entity to use, you can then decide whether or not to ignore that entity for tax purposes. If you choose to ignore the entity for tax purposes, you will report its gains and losses on your personal tax returns. Conversely, if you choose not to ignore the entity for tax purposes, the entity will need to file its own tax returns as an entity. Some prefer the former approach under the assumption that the aggregate tax paid on the entity's profit is less when the entity is ignored. Others, however, prefer that the entity not be ignored so that decisions are being made without regard for any specific owner's personal tax situation.

CALL TO ACTION

Decide which entity, and which tax structure, is right for your new venture.

INTELLECTUAL PROPERTY

Property can be divided into stuff that is tangible (i.e., you can pick it up, sit on it, walk into it, etc.) and stuff that is not (e.g., your ideas, contacts, computer files, etc.). It stands to reason that a business can prove it owns tangible property with a receipt or, for example, a car's title. Likewise, you can lock up these assets or otherwise physically protect them from theft.

One form of intangible property, which is the subset that can be described as your thoughts and what's created from them, is particularly difficult to identify. This, of course, makes it very challenging to determine its ownership and, without laws, virtually impossible to protect. As a result, businesses use contracts, statutes, and the common law to protect their IP.

IP Assignments

When IP is valuable to a business, it can require any party with which it interacts (e.g., employees, independent contractors, service providers, suppliers, etc.) to assign that party's IP to the business. For example, if you hire a graphic designer to create your business's logo, the way you prevent that graphic designer from selling your logo to someone else is by requiring the designer to assign it to your business. In doing so, you are also staking your claim to ownership of the logo so that if someone else tries to use the same logo, you can prevent them from doing so.

Along these lines, requiring employees to assign to your entity their IP that relates to the business is quite typical. The best way to do this can depend on state law, but some employers do so by way of their employee handbooks, whereas others require separate IP assignment agreements to be signed before the employee starts work. Conversely, having a policy requiring disclosure (as addressed in the "Keep It to Yourself" section) is how businesses and other organizations collect (and then protect) their IP.

Statutory Protections—Copyrights, Trademarks, Patents, and Trade Secrets

The federal government and all states have enacted statutes that allow the owner of the IP to prevent another party from using it. The applicability of these laws can depend on a variety of things, including what form the IP takes, where it was used, and how it was used.

Copyrights

Copyright protection is generally used to protect books, articles, and songs. The United States Patent and Trademark Office (USPTO) has a process by which you can protect these works so that they cannot be plagiarized by others. Some businesses will copyright their marketing materials in an effort to prevent competitors from using similar verbiage and confusing the public into thinking the two businesses are the same. It used to be that technology companies would copyright software code so that others couldn't use it without approval. This rarely happens anymore given the pace at which software can be developed.

The common law (check out the "Common Law" section earlier in the chapter for a reminder of what this is!) can also provide copyright protection. This occurs when the state courts identify certain categories of content that they believe should be fundamentally protected even though they're not covered by the federal law. The level of protection provided by the common law will be dependent on the applicable law in the state where the material was used, is not generally seen as the best path to making sure others don't use your content, and can be costly because you will need to hire an attorney to help with this process.

Trademarks

Trademark protection is typically used for logos, special ways a business expresses its name, or even things like catchphrases. Like copyrights, the USPTO has a process by which you can protect these marks so that others cannot use them. You may decide to seek trademark protection of your logo right after starting your business, but it's important to remember that as you refine your logo or business's name, you will need to make an additional filing to protect the new or refined mark.

Unlike copyright protection under common law, common law trademark protection is generally stronger, as many states will provide the first party using a mark within a certain geographic area the continuing right to do so. In certain instances, these rights are further limited to the goods or services offered by the business. Put another way, if you have been using your logo in a certain city to offer home care services and another business that provides similar services starts using a logo that might be confused with yours, many state courts would prohibit the new business from doing so. Obtaining this level of enforcement can be costly, because it means you need to hire a lawyer. Plus, with similar new businesses starting in related fields every day, it is frequently difficult to prove when a mark was put into use and where.

Patents

Federal law allows the inventor of a process or thing to prevent others from using it by obtaining a patent when the process or thing is "new and useful." In short, you submit details about your invention and, if no one has done so previously, and its other requirements are met, the USPTO will issue a patent. There are a variety of different patents that can be obtained, but the vast majority are utility patents. After a utility patent is issued, the only parties who can produce and/or sell the patented invention are the inventor and those to whom she or he provides a legal right (usually via a license agreement). The patent application process can last for many years and be very expensive. An attorney's assistance is frequently required for this as well. Once the patent is issued, however, the inventor has a 20-year period during which he or she can exclusively use the invention.

Frequently, businesses will seek a provisional patent. Although the full patent application can require very specific drawings and details be provided, the provisional patent application allows for a minimal amount of information to be submitted to simply preserve a place in line. For 1 year after submitting a provisional patent application, the inventor can submit the full patent application as if it was submitted as of the date that the provisional patent application was made. This can be a useful tool in fast-growing fields and provide a new business a lower cost method of reserving its place in line. In addition, once the provisional patent application is submitted, the inventor can say it is "patent pending." Simply doing so can prove valuable and dissuade others from pursuing something similar.

As briefly alluded to earlier in the chapter, publicly disclosing your invention can result in the USPTO rejecting your claim. As mentioned previously, one of the requirements for approval of a patent application is that the invention must be "new." If it is determined that the invention has been publicly disclosed before the patent application was submitted, the USPTO may find that it is not "new" and reject the application. Using a confidentiality agreement can help in this regard as, once it is signed, disclosures made to the party signing it are not considered public disclosures. Finally, this limitation is another reason a business may submit a provisional patent application because once it is filed, the inventor can publicly discuss the invention.

Trade Secrets

Trade secrets, which are typically formulas, patterns, programs, methods, and so on that are used in business and provide the business an advantage, can be protected by state statutes and those states' common law. One of the most common examples of a trade secret would be a large soda manufacturer's recipe for making its soda. As a result, states' trade-secret laws protect trade secrets when others come into possession of them, although most states require that the business is taking steps to protect its trade secrets. When a third party comes into possession of another's trade secrets, courts can prohibit the third party from using the trade secrets and even require them to take steps to protect any further disclosure, which can be a costly outcome for the third party.

 CALL TO ACTION

Make a list of parties you expect to contribute IP to your business (and don't forget to include yourself!). Divide your IP among the copyright, trademark, patent, and trade-secret categories. After you do, try to decide when in your business's growth cycle will be the right time to begin the process of protecting each item of IP.

"In every success story, you will find someone who has made a courageous decision."
—Peter F. Drucker, management consultant, educator, and author

PEOPLE

Although you (or you and your partners) will be the initial contributor to your business, very few ventures grow without the contribution of others. These contributions can be made by employees, independent contractors, service providers, suppliers, mentors, advisors, and many others. However, each of these groups has different legal rights and, as a result, you will need to treat them accordingly.

Hiring Employees

Frequently, a business's decision whether to expand its team beyond the initial partners can be one of the biggest decisions it makes. Although this is not true solely for legal reasons, adding even one employee brings with it a variety of risk and potential for liabilities that were not previously present.

To help manage employees' expectations, many employers assemble a series of documents that they provide to new employees along with any forms required for payroll, benefits, or other purposes. These documents can include everything from an offer letter to an employee handbook and numerous others in between. The benefit of an offer letter that is delivered prior to the employee deciding whether or not to join the business is that it summarizes all of the employment-related particulars, including the employee's job title, wages, vacation days and other benefits, start date and reporting structure, among other things. In addition, some employers might request that employees sign an agreement that includes (a) IP assignment provisions (see the section on IP Assignments for more on this); (b) confidentiality provisions to ensure the business's proprietary information is not shared; (c) nonsolicitation provisions that prevent the employee, upon leaving the company, from hiring the business's employees or engaging with the business's customers or suppliers; and (d) noncompete provisions that prevent the employee from competing with the business if and when she departs. Similarly, some employers also use an employee handbook to outline the business's expectations with respect to, among other things, work hours, taking vacation time, expense reimbursements, nondiscrimination based on membership in a protected class (e.g., race, religion, gender, etc.), computer and Internet usage, public relations inquiries, use of controlled substances, carrying firearms, and the like.

Employee Benefits

To attract and retain employees and to create and preserve its culture, many businesses offer a variety of benefits to their employees. These benefits can include everything from a particularly employee-favorable vacation policy to performance-based bonuses to monthly parties celebrating employees' birthdays. Benefits provided to employees can have tax implications to the employee, which will be something to consider before rolling out any new offering. Along similar lines, many benefit plans, like health insurance plans, 401(k) plans and the like, also have so many legal requirements that most businesses work with an outside third party to provide these benefits to their employees. In considering what benefits to offer, businesses will frequently look to, and compare themselves with, the other organizations with which they might compete for employee talent. For example, if one home-health agency requires its aides to pay for their scrubs, another might reimburse them for this expense. Similarly, some healthcare providers give nurses paid time off to complete their continuing-education requirements, whereas others do so and also pay for the coursework.

If a portion of your business's employees will be licensed, it will also be important to consider how you will (a) confirm that their licenses are current and (b) ensure that they maintain their licenses. Although some businesses treat this as a box that must be checked by new employees, and thereafter annually by current employees, others may seize it as an opportunity to provide an added benefit by either paying for the license renewal or allowing the employee to take time off for any activities that might be necessary in this respect.

Employee-Related Laws

In addition to managing the individual's expectations with respect to her or him working with your business, as you add employees your business will also be required to comply with numerous federal laws like COBRA (Consolidated Omnibus Budget Reconciliation Act; which, among other things, requires an employer to make certain insurance benefits available after an individual's employment is terminated), FMLA (Family and Medical Leave Act; which, among other things, prohibits employers from replacing an employee who takes off time from work to attend to certain significant life events), OSHA (Occupational Safety and Health Administration; which, among other things, requires employers to maintain certain levels of workplace safety), and ERISA (Employee Retirement Income Security Act; which, among other things, controls the ins and outs of certain benefit plans like 401(k) plans, etc.). Although states, counties, and cities also have their own sets of employment-related laws, many of these legal requirements (whether at the federal, state, or local level) also have exceptions based on size (i.e., a business need not comply until it has reached a minimum threshold number of employees). This is not true of all employment-related laws but does help to alleviate the burden when a business is just starting out.

Employees Versus Independent Contractors

Many businesses do not externally (or even internally) distinguish between the individuals providing services as employees versus those doing so as independent contractors. This is an important distinction, however, so that neither your business nor your employees are burdened with unanticipated tax liabilities. Although its analysis includes a multipart test that primarily relies on the many courts' opinions in lawsuits related to this issue, it is generally a matter of control—if the business has control over when, where, and how the services are being provided and/or the payment for those services is being rendered, then it is likely that the individual needs to be classified and treated as an employee.

When a business has employees, it is responsible for (among other things) making various withholdings from the employee's wages. Because the types and amounts of withholdings change depending on the country, state, county, and/or city where the business and its employees are located, most businesses engage a payroll service provider to assist in determining what must be withheld from an employee's wages.

When a business's workers are independent contractors, there is no obligation on the business to make any withholdings, as the independent contractor is responsible for paying these amounts. Because many people have grown accustomed to their employers making income tax payments on their behalf by way of their regular withholdings, there are numerous instances where the tax ends up unpaid. When the taxing authority (frequently, the IRS) seeks payment, the independent contractor claims he was an employee in an attempt to shift the payment burden back to the business. This then results in the business being added to the lawsuit and a court deciding whether or not he or she was actually an employee or an independent contractor. Whether the court determines that there was an employment or an independent contractor relationship, whichever party is responsible for payment may also be required to pay penalties and interest on the amounts due.

Frequently, businesses attempt to use independent contractor agreements to avoid the confusion around whether an individual is an employee or an independent contractor. Although these agreements are not necessarily conclusive, they can sway a court in favor of determining that there is an independent contractor relationship. Moreover, not only do these agreements describe the work that is to be performed and the manner in which the business will pay for it, but can also include, among other things, (a) explicit language providing that the individual understands he or she is an independent contractor, (b) indemnification provisions requiring the individual to reimburse the business for its expenses in a matter contesting his status as an independent contractor and any other damages incurred by the business as a result of the individual's providing services to it, (c) IP assignment provisions, (d) confidentiality provisions to ensure the business's proprietary information is not shared, (e) nonsolicitation provisions that prevent the individual from hiring the business's employees or engaging with the business's customers or suppliers upon his departure, and (f) noncompete provisions that prevent the departing employee from performing services that are competitive to the business. If nothing else, these types of agreements serve to establish the ground rules for the work that the individual is going to provide and, if circumstances change, they can always be changed when the business and the individual agree to do so.

Terminating Employees

When considering the added costs and risks associated with hiring employees, businesses should not forget to consider the possibility that each employee may, someday, need to be terminated. Most states are "at-will" employment states, which means that employers can terminate employees for any reason whatsoever or no reason at all. However, there are federal laws that serve as exceptions to this rule and prevent many employers from discriminating against employees as a result of the employee's age, race, religion, gender, national origin, or disabilities (e.g., a business cannot terminate an employee because of his or her religion). In addition, many states have also enacted statutes that expand these exceptions to include marital status and sexual preference, among others. Plus, states also differ with respect to things like whether an employee must be paid for unused vacation days and, if payments are required, how those payments are to be calculated. Given the overlapping nature of these laws, and the fact that they change from state to state, terminating an employee can be difficult and costly.

In addition, states with unemployment compensation systems add to this decision-making process. Although these systems can vary greatly from state to state, the general notion is that the employer pays up front so that terminated employees can receive some amount of compensation until he or she finds new work. These systems will frequently allow employers to contest these unemployment payments if the individual's employment was terminated for cause (e.g., stealing from the cash register, etc.) and because their payments typically increase with the number of former employees they have seeking unemployment benefits, employers are motivated to contest unemployment claims brought by former employees terminated for cause.

🔑 KEY TAKEAWAY POINTS

Tackling the legal complexities of starting a business is a challenging endeavor even for those who are repeat entrepreneurs. So as you continue to engage with the legal aspects of owning a business, consider these key points:

- *Chart your path.* Deciding whether your business will be a high-growth venture or a lifestyle business will inform your business plan, ongoing operating plans, funding/revenue requirements, and hiring needs.

- *Adjust for regulatory requirements.* If the sale, manufacturing, or marketing of the business's products, or the delivery of your business's services, will be regulated by a federal, state, or local governmental agency, adjust your business or operating plan accordingly. If your business will not be subjected to significant regulatory requirements, consider yourself among the fortunate.

- *Protect yourself.* Establishing a corporation or limited liability company should limit your personal financial liability to the capital you contribute to the business. After forming the entity, obtain an EIN from the IRS. Once you have the EIN, open a bank account and run all of the revenue and expenses through it.

- *Achieve partner harmony.* Like oarsmen, if you and your partners are unable to row in the same direction, your business's growth will be limited (at best). Be sure that you are aligned with respect to (a) how the business's expenses and profits will be shared among you and your partners and (b) who is responsible for making which decisions, how many of you must agree when make major decisions, and what constitutes a major decision.

- *Protect the business's assets.* Intellectual property laws have been established to protect what is valuable to your business. Make sure you are doing what you can to protect the business's assets. At the same time, given the cost and time required, also be sure you are doing only what is necessary.

- *Consider the cost of people.* Although it may be difficult to achieve certain growth levels without adding resources, each incremental team member comes with added cost and potential liability, whether with respect to how he or she performs or in the event he or she needs to be terminated.

Building and Pitching Your Plan

Tim Raderstorf

"To achieve great things, two things are needed: a plan, and not quite enough time." —Leonard Bernstein

---

LEARNING OBJECTIVES

- Understand the importance of developing a (business) plan.
- Describe how to develop an individualized plan.
- Discuss the core components of business plans.
- Examine how to best communicate your plan to obtain buy-in.

INTRODUCTION

One of the more famous scenes from the movie *Apollo 13* occurs after the crew realizes that its air-filtration system is not be able to perform under unforeseen circumstances. The team had developed a meticulously precise plan that would allow for the ground crew to know exactly where the shuttle would be throughout its journey to the moon and back. But because of external forces (an explosion of an oxygen tank), the team was now forced to abandon its elaborate plan and rapidly innovate to save the lives of the three crew members on board. The crew members developed a solution to use an existing air filter, modifying it with the available supplies within the shuttle. Three days later, the flight crew safely returned to Earth. In all of the 12 previous Apollo missions, a meticulous plan had also been developed. And just as with the Apollo 13 mission, every plan needed to be adjusted at some point during each mission. The purpose of the plan was not to define exactly how every variable would play out. The purpose of the plan was to define what variables were most likely to occur, and how the team can adapt when less likely variables occur.

"If plan A doesn't work, the alphabet has 25 more letters – 204 if you're in Japan." —Claire Cook

We are going to explore the purpose of developing a (business) plan. *Business* is being placed in parentheses because many of you may never develop a plan to start a business, but as healthcare leaders you will very likely need to develop a plan for a new innovation within your organization. These entrepreneurial learning principles will help you whether you are serving as a healthcare leader in a large organization (those intrapreneurs we discussed in Chapter 19, Intrapreneurship, Business Models, and How Companies Make Money) or whether you are building a plan to execute as an entrepreneur. For those taking the entrepreneurial route, your plan will be helpful in obtaining funding from investors, a loan from your bank, or perhaps even recruit talent to join you as your business gets started. As an intrapreneur, you will be developing a plan to improve outcomes and obtain buy-in from key stakeholders.

The most important component of the plan is how well it can be communicated to those who have influence over its success. If you need to demonstrate how increasing staffing ratios on your unit would improve patient outcomes and/or increase the bottom line for your organization, then you need to find a way to obtain buy-in from key decision holders within your organization who can help you put your innovation into practice. This communication is often called *the pitch* in entrepreneurial circles (think *Shark Tank*). To help you hone your pitching skills, we also examine the best ways to communicate your plan to ensure that you receive the buy-in you need from key stakeholders.

DEVELOPING A (BUSINESS) PLAN

When developing a plan, reflect on the design-thinking principles outlined in Chapter 15, Design Thinking for Healthcare Leadership and Innovation. All plans should be validated by the end user prior to initiating the plan. For example, if you wanted to develop a new drug for individuals with elbow pain, you would first need to understand the desires of individuals with elbow pain. If they are able to purchase a cheap over-the-counter drug that already meets their needs, then developing a new drug that is just as effective or just as inexpensive would be futile, as it would be extremely challenging to get users to abandon their existing treatments for a product that achieves the same outcomes at the same cost. However, if you found that the existing drugs addressing elbow pain were all topical creams and users did not like having to apply the cream on a regular basis, then developing an oral tablet that achieved the same results could address the users' unmet needs. This the point when it's time to start developing a plan.

There are multiple ways to set up a (business) plan. The traditional approach takes anywhere from a few days to a few weeks to develop. The amount of time needed is often relative to the innovators' understanding of the market needs and their innovation's capabilities. Intuit, maker of small-business accounting software *QuickBooks* (n.d.) identifies these seven essential elements of the business plan:

1. Executive summary
2. Business description
3. Market analysis
4. Organization and management

5. Sales strategies

6. Funding requirements

7. Financial projections

Not to be outdone, *Forbes* magazine (2013) listed these 10 components as must-haves for your plan:

1. Executive summary

2. Mission or vision statement

3. Description of Your company (or for you intrapreneurs—a description of your innovation)

4. The scription of what makes Your company/innovation different from the status quo

5. Market analysis

6. Team

7. Marketing plan

8. A SWOT analysis (*s*trengths, *w*eaknesses, *o*pportunities, and *t*hreats)

9. Cash-flow statement

10. Revenue projections

The differences between these two lists are minimal. The take-home point here is the understanding that your business plan will need to be tweaked or modified irrespective of who your audience may be, and as your business/innovation evolves. This is a key component of *the pitch* and is writeed later in the chapter, but it is also important as you develop your business plan. As many of the principles outlined by these two business plan templates are likely foreign to most healthcare leaders, let's take some time to develop an understanding of each.

Executive Summary

An executive summary is an overview of your entire business plan. This summary serves as your elevator pitch for your business/innovation. Although it serves as the beginning of your business plan, write the executive summary last so that you have a full understanding of the full, final business plan and can identify what components of the plan would be most attractive to the intended audience. The value of the business/innovation should shine through in the executive summary.

Mission or Vision Statement

The mission or vision statement is an opportunity for the team to convey the inspiration behind the business/innovation. The most persuasive statements first explain *why* the team is doing something before it focusis on *how* or *what* the business/innovation is achieving. This focus on *why* evokes emotion from the audience and can persuade audience members to engage with your business/innovation. Mercy Health Ministry has perhaps one of the most compelling vision statements in healthcare today: *"We are the people of Mercy Health Ministry. Together, we are pioneering a new model of care. We will relentlessly pursue our goal to get health care right.*

Everywhere and every way that Mercy serves, we will deliver a transformative health experience." I'm sold, how about you?

Business Description

Although this element of the business plan may seem harder for intrapreneurs, the concepts are the same whether you are innovating or developing a business. Define your problem and solution (refer back to problem and solution statements in Chapter 20, Legal Considerations in Starting a Healthcare Business). If you are starting a business, this is where you outline also the structure of your business. Are you an LLC or C corp? Where are you located? In this section, you should also define your (business) model and identify any unfair advantages you may have over the existing market.

Market Analysis

A market analysis is your opportunity to evaluate your competition. When innovating, you always have competition. That competition may not be creating the same product as you, but the status quo is always competing against new innovations. Understand the size of your market. There are three distinctions of the market your business/solution can service (Figure 21.1): (a) TAM (total available market), this is self-explanatory; (b) SAM, service-available market, which is the market size that could be serviced by your business; SOM, service-obtainable market, this is the realistic market size your business can address.

Let's examine how these terms would apply for a nurse practitioner who is specializing in caring for patients with diabetes. For this nurse practitioner the TAM would be all patients with diabetes, or those who have risk factors of developing diabetes in the world. The SAM

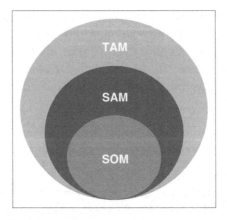

Figure 21.1 Three types of market sizes.

SAM, serviceable available market; SOM, serviceable obtainable market; TAM, total available market.

Source: Berry, T. (n.d). TAM, SAM, SOM, potential market. *Lean Business Planning*. Retrieved from https://leanplan.com/tam-sam-som-potential-market

would be all patients with diabetes or at risk for diabetes who are within a 3-hour drive from the nurse practitioner's office. The SOM could be further distinguished by patients within a 3-hour drive from the nurse practitioner's office with diabetes or at risk for diabetes who seek care from primary care providers within the nurse practitioner's healthcare network. Having a strong understanding of these three components allows leaders the ability to understand how much of the market share they currently hold, and how much realistic growth can be projected for the future.

Organization and Management (Team)

The Organization and management section is your opportunity to showcase why your team is the most likely collectively achieved the goals of your business. This is where you would highlight all key players and how their past experience will help lead your team to success.

Sales Strategies

Making money in a business is harder than most people think. This section allows the leadership team to showcase how much planning they have put into determining how their organization is going to make money. You will learn about business models later in the text. This is the section of the business plan in which you define what your business model will be and how you will leverage it to make money for your company/organization.

Funding Requirements (Ask)

This section is the most important aspect of your business plan and later you will find it is also the most important component of a pitch. Whether you call it *Funding Requirements* or *Needs Assessment*, this is your opportunity to ask for what your company will need to find success. Many times, this is an amount of dollars, but for those of you working in intrapreneurial settings, there may be many other types of resources that you can request to help aid in your success.

Financial Projections

The financial projections section is your opportunity to showcase how profitable your company or idea can become and in what timel frame. Often this is displayed by a profit and loss (P&L) sheet. A P&L sheet is a spreadsheet that showcases the amount of money coming in to the company and the amount of money being spent by the company. (An example of a P&L sheet is located in Chapter 24, Key Strategies for Moving From Research to Commercialization With Real-World Success Stories.) If you are starting a company, investors rarely expect that the company will actually make money in the first few years of business. One of the most common mistakes first-time entrepreneurs make is being overly optimistic with their financial projections. When completing this section, constantly evaluate **your assumptions and whether they are realistic.**

Marketing Plan

Projecting that you are going to be able to successfully attract customers is easy. Actually getting customers to use your services is extremely hard. This section of the business plan showcases *how* your company will find success attracting repeat customers through the use of a marketing plan. Marketing involves a skill set that not every person has, so this information should be created alongside the help of a marketing professional. After all, if you don't have customers, you won't have a business for very long.

SWOT Analysis

A SWOT (*s*trengths, *w*eaknesses, *o*pportunities, and *t*hreats) analysis is a tool that allows teams to effectively visualize and aggregate data that may impact their business or initiatives. Effective for entrepreneurship, a SWOT analysis is made up of a four-grid box (Figure 21.2), wherein each portion represents either the strengths, weaknesses, opportunities, or threats that impact the business or innovation. Teams are encouraged to list as many factors that impact each of the four boxes as possible. This exercise allows teams to both focus on what they are doing well and to be realistic about where they have room for improvement. It further provides an understanding of where they could further grow the business and how competition is impacting the business/innovation.

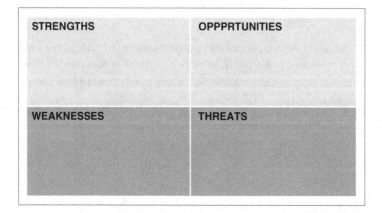

Figure 21.2 Strengths, weaknesses, opportunities, and threats analysis grid.

 CALL TO ACTION

Develop a SWOT analysis for your next project at work. Obtain input from key stakeholders and organizational leadership.

MAKING SENSE OF A BUSINESS PLAN

If all of this information overwhelms you, there are many tools that can help you rapidly develop a business plan. Two of the most highly recommended tools are the Lean Canvas and the Business Model Canvas (Exhibits 21.1 and 21.2). Both tools break down the complexities of the formal business plan into a one-page document that can be drafted (not completed as *your plan* is always evolving) in under an hour. Regardless of which canvas you choose to use, either can help you quickly identify the key players in initiating your innovation in business. Some people are partial to the Lean Canvas as it begins with a problem/solution statement. This may be easier for intrapreneurs to use when planning out their initiatives. Similarly, the Business Model Canvas focuses on the problem first by examining customer segments and then defines the solution through the value proposition. You can see from the side-by-side comparison that there are many similarities between each canvas type. A key variance between the two models is the three additional considerations included in the Lean Canvas.

Lean Canvas	Business Model Canvas
1. Problem	1. Key partners 8
2. Solution	2. Key activities 7
3. Unique value proposition	3. Value proposition 2
4. Unfair advantage	4. Customer relationships 3
5. Customer segments	5. Customer segments 1
6. Key metrics	6. Key resources 6
7. Channels	7. Channels 4
8. Cost structure	8. Cost structure 9
9. Revenue streams	9. Revenue streams 5

Note: Numbers following the Business Model Canvas elements are the recommended order to follow when filling out the template (i.e., start first with "Customer Segments," then consider "Value Proposition").

Additional Lean Canvas Considerations

1. Existing alternatives—How can customers address this problem without using your technology/innovation/service? How will customers address this problem in the future without using your technology/innovation/service?

2. High-level concept—This is your elevator pitch (more on that shortly), distilled into one brief sentence.

3. Early adopters—Who will be the first people to purchase your technology/innovations/service and serve as champions for your initiative?

These additional considerations provide further insight into factors that will impact your ability to find success.

EXHIBIT 21.1 The Lean Canvas

PROBLEM	SOLUTION	UNIQUE VALUE PROPOSITION	UNFAIR ADVANTAGE	CUSTOMER SEGMENTS
List your top 1–3 problems.	Outline a possible solution for each problem.	Single, clear, compelling message that states why you are different and worth paying attention.	Something that cannot easily be bought or copied.	List your target customers and users.
	KEY METRICS		**CHANNELS**	
	List the key numbers that tell you how your business is doing.	**HIGH-LEVEL CONCEPT**	List your path to customers (inbound or outbound).	
EXISTING ALTERNATIVES		List your X for Y analogy e.g. YouTube = Flickr for videos.		**EARLY ADOPTERS**
List how these problems are solved today.				List the characteristics of your ideal customers.

COST STRUCTURE	REVENUE STREAMS
List your fixed and variable costs.	List your sources of revenue.

Source: leanstack.com

EXHIBIT 21.2 The Business Model Canvas

The Business Model Canvas

Designed for: Designed by: Date: Version:

Key Partners

Who are our Key Partners?
Who are our key suppliers?
Which Key Resources are we acquiring from partners?
Which Key Activities do partners perform?

MOTIVATIONS FOR PARTNERSHIPS
Optimization and economy
Reduction of risk and uncertainty
Acquisition of particular resources and activities

Key Activities

What Key Activities do our Value Propositions require?
Our Distribution Channels?
Customer Relationships?
Revenue streams?

CATEGORIES
Production
Problem Solving
Platform/Network

Key Resources

What Key Resources do our Value Propositions require?
Our Distribution Channels? Customer Relationships?
Revenue Streams?

TYPES OF RESOURCES
Physical
Intellectual (brand patents, copyrights, data)
Human
Financial

Value Propositions

What value do we deliver to the customer?
Which one of our customer's problems are we helping to solve?
What bundles of products and services are we offering to each Customer Segment?
Which customer needs are we satisfying?

CHARACTERISTICS
Newness
Performance
Customization
"Getting the Job Done"
Design
Brand/Status
Price
Cost Reduction
Risk Reduction
Accessibility
Convenience/Usability

Customer Relationships

What type of relationship does each of our Customer Segments expect us to establish and maintain with them?
Which ones have we established?
How are they integrated with the rest of our business model?
How costly are they?

EXAMPLES
Personal assistance
Dedicated Personal Assistance
Self-Service
Automated Services
Communities
Co-creation

Channels

Through which Channels do our Customer Segments want to be reached?
How are we reaching them now?
How are our Channels integrated?
Which ones work best?
Which ones are most cost-efficient?
How are we integrating them with customer routines?

CHANNEL PHASES
1. Awareness
   How do we raise awareness about our company's products and services?
2. Evaluation
   How do we help customers evaluate our organization's Value Proposition?
3. Purchase
   How do we allow customers to purchase specific products and services?
4. Delivery
   How do we deliver a Value Proposition to customers?
5. After sales
   How do we provide post-purchase customer support?

Customer Segments

For whom are we creating value?
Who are our most important customers?

Mass Market
Niche Market
Segmented
Diversified
Multi-sided Platform

Cost Structure

What are the most important costs inherent in our business model?
Which Key Resources are most expensive?
Which Key Activities are most expensive?

IS YOUR BUSINESS MORE
Cost Driven (leanest cost structure, low price value proposition, maximum automation, extensive outsourcing)
Value Driven (focused on value creation, premium value proposition)

SAMPLE CHARACTERISTICS
Fixed Costs (salaries, rents, utilities)
Variable costs
Economies of scale
Economies of scope

Revenue Streams

For what value are our customers really willing to pay?
For what do they currently pay?
How are they currently paying?
How would they prefer to pay?
How much does each Revenue Stream contribute to overall revenues?

TYPES   FIXED PRICING
Asset sale   List Price
Usage fee   Product feature dependent
Subscription Fees   Customer segment dependent
Lending/Renting/Leasing   Volume dependent
Licensing
Brokerage fees   DYNAMIC PRICING
Advertising   Negotiation (bargaining)
               Yield Management
               Real-time-Market

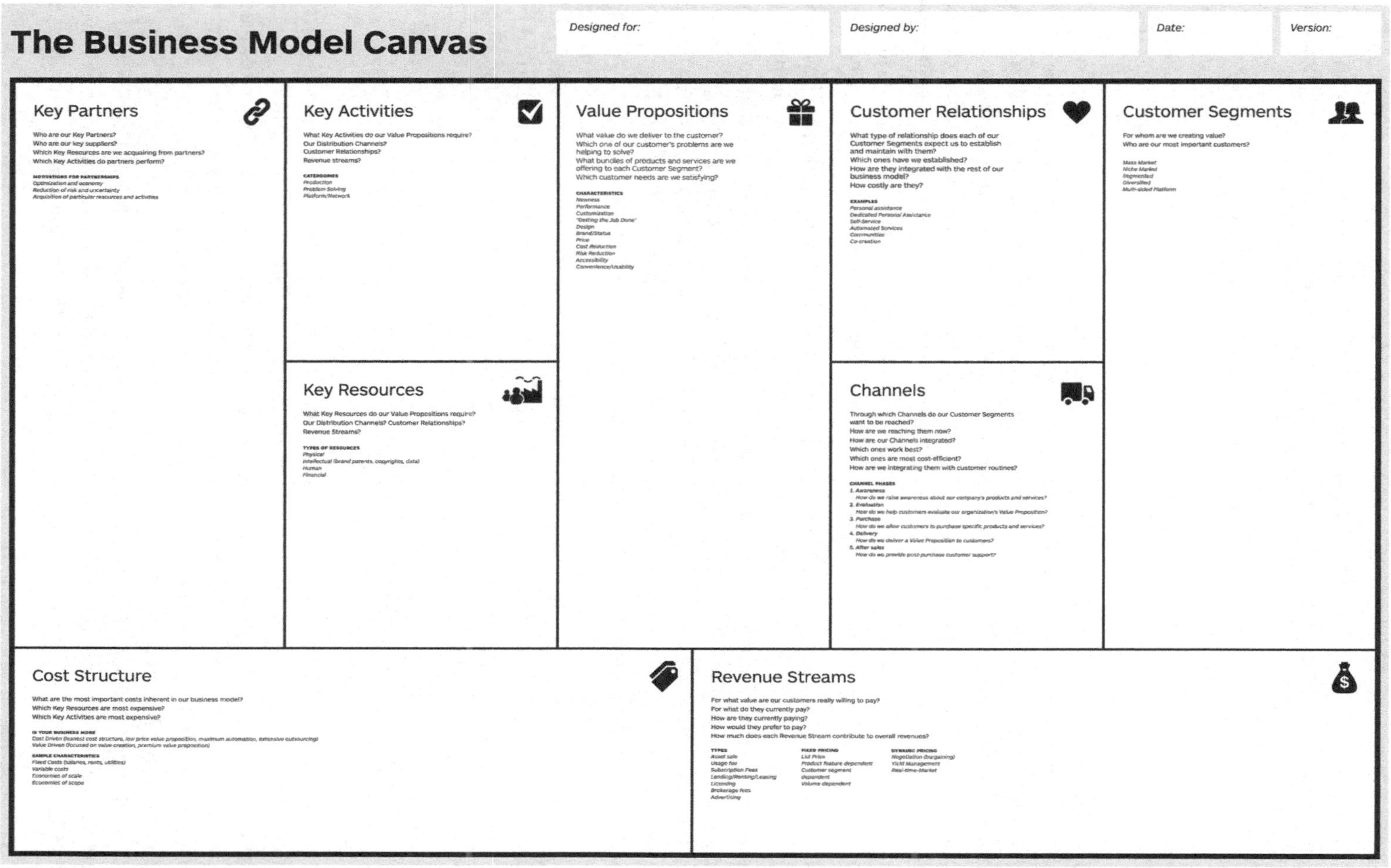

Source: strategyzer.com

Regardless of how long or accurate your plan ends up being, imagine how much better prepared you will be to tackle the variables that come your way when you have a firm understanding of these business-plan components. The beauty of the business plan is not in its execution, it is in the research, empathy, an understanding of your users' needs that is generated from developing a plan.

"Plans are nothing; planning is everything." —Dwight D. Eisenhower

THE PITCH

*SPOILER ALERT: You are about to learn the key component to all successful pitches. We dive deeply into how to properly construct and deliver a pitch in this section, yet there's one main component that separates successful pitches from unsuccessful pitches: **the person who delivers the pitch.** Whether the audience is the director of your unit, a potential customer, or potential investor in your company, the audience is looking for one thing from your pitch, a clear indication of your ability to solve the problem better than anyone else. If through your pitch you can project confidence in your ability to succeed, a willingness to incorporate feedback, and a determination to get the job done, your likelihood of obtaining the requested resources will skyrocket.*

Contrary to popular belief, coming up with the idea and developing a plan on how to implement your innovation are the easiest parts of the journey. The big challenge lies in putting your ideas into action. To put ideas into action, you are going to need something that many leaders often struggle to obtain: HELP. Although *help* is a four-letter word, it is also the cornerstone of success for entrepreneurial and intrapreneurial endeavors. Now it's time to let you in on a little secret, there's only one surefire way to receive help. You have to ask for it. Fortunately for leaders, help is often abundant and can be as easy to get as calling up a trusted colleague or leveraging your network. As an innovative leader, you will inevitably find yourself in a scenario in which you need to pitch your ideas to get the help/resources you need to be successful. The remainder of this chapter is dedicated to teaching you the core components of all great pitches, and how you can develop the skill set required to effectively pitch your ideas and obtain the help you need to find success.

How One Pitch Changed My Career—By Tim Raderstorf

In the spring of 2013, I found myself in front of the C-suite of my organization as I pitched them an idea I had for a software platform to improve patient outcomes. The C-suite team was complimentary of my pitch and encouraged me to seek support from other key leaders across the organization to obtain more buy-in. They said I must pitch my idea to the dean of the College of Nursing, Dr. Bernadette Melnyk, as she is an entrepreneurial leader who can help make these types of projects happen.

I had never met Dean Melnyk before, but heard her speak at an event earlier that year and was enthralled with her energy. A short time later, I found myself pitching my idea to Dr. Melnyk. After my pitch was completed, she expressed her full support for the idea.

(continued)

(continued)

I thought we would end on that note, but that's when things took a sudden turn that would change my life. Dr. Melnyk asked me whether I was faculty at the College of Nursing. Caught off guard, I told her I was unsure what she was asking. I was the quality manager in the emergency department. I didn't work at the college.

She replied that she understood what my current role was but wanted to know if I had an adjunct appointment at the college. When I told her I did not, she asked me whether I had a master's degree. After replying that I did, she said, "Congratulations, you're now faculty at the College of Nursing. I always look for people with a gleam in their eye and a fire in their belly. I see that in you and want you to join us as an adjunct faculty member."

A few months later, I started teaching online courses during the evenings for the College of Nursing, though I still maintained my day job as a quality manager. Within a year I would transition into a full-time faculty role at the college, and within 2 years I was named the first nurse to hold the title "craised innovation officer" in an academic setting. In truth, my career pivoted in a direction that I never imagined possible. That pitch didn't just bring me to a role as craised innovation officer; it also helped me turn that original idea into a healthcare information technology (IT) company. That pitch has helped me discover more about myself than I ever imagined. But the most amazing result of that pitch is the fact that I am writing this textbook to you today, sharing the evidence behind how innovation and entrepreneurship will make you a better leader. You never know where a pitch may lead you, but it can take you somewhere great. Step up to the plate. Seize your moment.

COMPONENTS OF GREAT PITCHES

Regardless of the setting and the structure of your pitch, first understand how to develop a pitch that compels your target audience to help provide you with the resources you need. Depending on the amount of time allotted for your pitch, you may not be able to incorporate all of these components of exceptional pitches included here into every pitch. These components should serve as the foundation for all of your pitches. After each pitch note what components resonated with your audience and explore how you can make adjustments for the future. Now let's explore eight essential components that will help you find success when pitching your idea/product/service.

Evoke Emotion Through Story

If you can only include one of these eight elements in your pitch, use "evoke emotion through story." In a world where facts and figures serve as the foundation for why a majority of decisions are made, an advantage lies within the excellent idea/product/service that also evokes emotion. Facts and figures are incredibly valuable, but in his well-known book *Actual Minds, Possible Words*, Jerome Bruner (1986) discovered that humans are up to 22 times more likely to remember stories than to remember just facts alone. Now that is a competitive advantage you can capitalize on!

The most effective way to evoke emotion is to use storytelling. Imagine that you are writing your pitch as a children's book. Like all stories, children's books have a beginning, middle, and end. The beginning defines the problem; there is great emphasis placed on understanding the entire breath of the problem. Then, focus is placed on the concise description of the solution (middle). The book culminates with the revelation or a recap of the emotional journey of the characters (end). In a pitch, the ending is a *summary and a request*. Also in children's books, more emotion is evoked through the use of pictures and body language than the actual words used to tell the story. Be sure to incorporate imagery as frequently as possible when telling your story.

Even though you are writing your pitch to mimic a children's book, still include complex details. The level of detail that you need to include in your storytelling is determined by the next essential component of pitches, *knowing your audience*.

CALL TO ACTION

Read a children's book and note how its structure compares to the structure of a pitch. Prepare your next work presentation based off the same model used in the children's book. Emphasize the use of pictures over words and seize the opportunity to evoke emotion.

Know Your Audience

When you find yourself in a situation in which you may want to pitch your idea, remember there must be two critical players and one critical element for the discussion to be a pitch. The critical players are the person pitching the idea and an audience. The critical element is that the audience must have access to the resources the person pitching the idea needs. If the audience does not have the resources needed or cannot connect the team to someone who has the resources needed by the person pitching the idea, this is not a pitch, it is a networking conversation. Networking conversations are incredibly valuable, but it is the duty of the individual who is pitching the idea to ensure that the audience contains individuals who have the potential to provide the resources needed for success.

If the audience is capable of providing you with the resources you need to find success, it is recommended that you tailor your pitch directly to the audience. Some audience members may be more likely to respond to pictures and graphs, whereas others appreciate learning more about how your idea/product/service works. If you are pitching your product to a world-class expert in the field, then you likely do not need to explain the scientific underpinnings of how your idea/service/solution works as he or she likely already has a strong understanding of those concepts. Instead, focus on explaining your unique value proposition (UVP) and how it positions your team for success.

To find success, seek out other individuals who have had discussions or pitched their ideas to your audience in the past. Ask these people what the audience responded to well and what they could have done to improve their pitch. Also be sure to conduct an Internet search on your audience to find ways to better connect with them. You may be able to uncover that they sit on a certain charitable board for which you have interest or there may be past connections within your network that could lead to a more personalized relationship with your audience.

Grab Attention

It is often said that the first 60 seconds of any interaction are the most important. This could not be more true for people pitching their ideas. Introductions and anecdotal stories are comfortable openings for most interactions, but often lack the ability to grab the attention of the audience. It is imperative for people pitching ideas to find a way to connect with the audience rapidly and grab its attention.

As an example, when delivering a workshop on "How to Pitch Ideas" at the Cleveland Clinic, Tim Raderstorf learned that his audience had an admiration for their hometown basketball star, LeBron James. Tim had a connection to LeBron James through his high school basketball career and decided to leverage that connection to grab the attention of the audience. He spoke to the audience about growing up with one of the greatest high school basketball players in Ohio's storied history. Never naming who that basketball player was, Tim went on to list the accolades of that player and posted a picture of Lebron James on the screen for the audience to see. Although the audience assumed Tim was talking about LeBron James, he was actually talking about Doug Penno. Doug was the young man who was guarding James in the picture on the screen (Figure 21.3). As Tim revealed his secret, he evoked laughter (emotion) from the audience, and had them hooked to be active participants for the remainder of his presentation.

Paint Your Unique Value Proposition

Your UVP is a clear and concise statement that highlights how you or your business is superior to all other solutions that attempt to solve the same problem. This is a message that should be conveyed often, so do not be afraid to repeat it a few times throughout your pitch. When developing your UVP, do not forget to consider your customers. Peter Thompson (2013) suggests that your value proposition should be composed around both your product and your customer. From the product side, consider the benefits, features, and experience. While from the customer side, understand your customers' wants, needs, and fears. A concise statement that addresses these six components will be your UVP.

Provide Enticing Solutions

Providing enticing solutions could also be called *understanding your customers' wants*. To effectively provide enticing solutions, you must have a clear understanding of the features that your target market most desires. With this understanding, you can tailor your product line as a tiered set of products or services that increase in features and create desire within your customer base. If you need a simple example of how to create enticing solutions, envision a 4-year-old at an ice cream parlor. For that 4-year-old, there are little to no options on the menu that would not result in euphoria. When creating a business or developing a new solution within an organization, strive to create a *menu* (metaphorically speaking) that would leave your customers ecstatic with any possible choice.

Show Results (or Evidence)

Showing results may be the most difficult aspect of the pitch because it can be very challenging to have results if you have not yet implemented your idea. If you are very early on in the

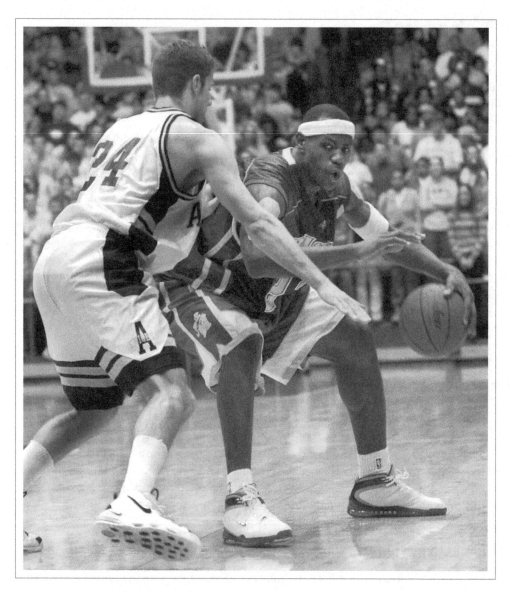

Figure 21.3 Doug Penno guarding LeBron James in 2003.
Source: Reuters/Brian Bergeron.

development of your company or idea, this is an opportunity to be creative with the way that you choose to show results. We have already thoroughly examined the impact and importance of using evidence-based practice in healthcare. If evidence exists for the potential impact of your business/innovation, leverage it now. You may also want to highlight the results that you or your team have been able to accomplish in the past. If you are further along in your implementation, use every opportunity you have to highlight the successes your team has achieved throughout your pitch.

Keep It Conversational

A pitch doesn't need to consist of one individual standing in front of others, preaching his or her message. And although that is a common delivery method of pitches, an opportunity is lost in this format. To truly evoke emotion through story and engage an audience, there must be a conversational nature to the pitch. Allow your audience to ask questions, and better yet, ask questions yourself. This will likely result in more time spent with your audience, and will showcase your ability to seek feedback and receive coaching.

Ask for What You Need

There's no way around it. Without a request, there is no pitch. All pitches contain a clear request that is individually tailored to the audience such that, if the request is granted, the person pitching the idea will obtain some benefit. Clearly stated, your pitch must contain a request for a resource you need to find success. Find your audience and start asking!

TYPES OF PITCHES

There are three main structures of pitches that are commonly used: (a) the elevator pitch, (b) the sales pitch, and (c) the venture pitch. The elevator pitch and the sales pitch are must-have tools in the healthcare leader's tool belt. As an entrepreneur, all three types of pictures are essential to finding success.

The Elevator Pitch

The name of the elevator pitch is itself an outstanding example of how words can evoke emotion and tell a story. The term *elevator pitch* describes a succinct explanation of your idea/product/service that is short enough to be delivered during a brief elevator ride (Kenton, 2017). With such a visual name like *elevator pitch*, one understands the meaning of the easily visualized term. By painting a picture through the usage of selected words, a story is told.

The Legend of Barnett Helzberg

As with many of the best legends, this is a combination of versions of the story told by Warren Buffett himself, to an often referenced, but rarely found *Harvard Business Review* article by Nick Wreden (2002). Although the exact details of this legend may be a little fuzzy, the lesson behind them is sound.

In 1994, Barnett Helzberg, Jr. was running his family's diamond business based out of Kansas City. A week after attending the Berkshire Hathaway shareholders meeting in Omaha, Nebraska, Helzberg was conducting business in New York City. While crossing the street, he

(continued)

(continued)

noticed a woman walking up to Warren Buffet, the famed billionaire and founder of Berkshire Hathaway. Helzberg had been contemplating opportunities to grow his business and decided that he was going to take a risk. After Mr. Buffett finished his conversation with the woman, Helzberg walked up to Mr. Buffet and with these 25 words, delivered *the most fruitful elevator pitch of all time.* "Hi, Mr. Buffett. I'm a shareholder in Berkshire Hathaway and a great admirer of yours. I believe that my company matches your criteria for investment."

Having heard this declaration many times before, Buffet replied, "Send me more details." Yet after receiving more details, Buffet concluded that Helzberg Diamonds did indeed meet his criteria for investment and Berkshire Hathaway purchased the company in 1995.

Now it is clear that Helzberg chose brevity over including some of the essential components of successful pitches included in this chapter. However, by indicating that his company did meet Buffet's criteria for investment, he was indicating that his company was open to an acquisition. Though he certainly could have been more clear with his request, Helzberg was tailoring his pitch to his audience, while also protecting the reputation of this company. (He didn't want to let everyone know his company was on the market.) Most important, Helzberg found himself in a serendipitous situation and had the intestinal fortitude to act on his good fortune. Great leaders surely take risks, but more important, they seize the moment when it is presented to them.

The Sales Pitch

Although you may believe that sales pitches are meant for individuals with greasy hair wearing leisure suits, it is very likely that as a healthcare leader you have delivered some type of sales pitch within the last month. A sales pitch does require money to exchange hands. In fact, in healthcare that's rarely the case. The common use of sales pitches in healthcare typically occurs in departmental meetings, C-suite boardroom, or even the cafeteria. Sales pitches can be formal or informal, and they differ from an elevator pitch in that they provide a greater depth of information regarding the idea/product/service. But just like the elevator pitch, they are conversations that contain a request in order to help the person pitching the idea find success.

The Venture Pitch

With the introduction of the television series *Shark Tank*, the venture pitch has become a common element in pop culture. A venture pitch typically contains much of the information that was outlined in the business plan section earlier in this chapter. Often delivered through PowerPoint slides over a 5- to 7-minute window, the venture pitch provides an entrepreneur or team of entrepreneurs the opportunity to showcase its confidence in its ability to succeed, a willingness to incorporate feedback, and a determination to get the job done while asking for the support needed to find success. If you are considering using venture capital for the advancement of your business, be sure to check with local start-up programs to determine the current protocol for pitching. Some organizations prefer a formal presentation. Others request that you send your *deck* (entrepreneurial speak for the slides from your presentation) in advance of the meeting, allowing for a question-and-answer session during the in-person meeting. Knowing your audience's preferences will increase your likelihood of success.

THE ROLE OF FEEDBACK IN SUCCESSFUL PITCHES

One of the most valuable benefits of pitching your ideas is the ability to receive feedback from key influencers within your target market. Oftentimes your audience is aware of market trends and can provide valuable insight that you may not be able to receive elsewhere. Fortunately for you, obtaining their feedback is a double win, as it also provides an outlet to showcase your coachability and ability to receive feedback. There is a fine line between sticking to your convictions as an entrepreneurial leader or innovator and leveraging the myriad advice and opinions you will inevitably receive from others. The successful leader demonstrates his or her listening skills and is able to be gracious for the time and effort the audience will put into providing feedback.

This can be a very challenging skill to master as oftentimes leaders are going to hear that their ideas are not worth pursuing or should be altered. After all, no one wants to hear that his or her baby is ugly, right? But one of the easiest ways to put this skill into practice is to have a prepared response that can be recited with grace when receiving feedback that takes you off guard:

> "Thank you for your feedback. We have yet to put the time into thoroughly examining your point. I will take that back to my team to explore how we could potentially make that happen."

Your actual response may sound different than that, but the lesson here is that your response needs to demonstrate two key factors:

1. You heard what the audience said about your product.
2. You value their opinion enough to discuss it with your team.

In demonstrating these two skills, you have the ability to showcase to even those who doubt your business/innovation that you have a desire to succeed, a willingness to incorporate feedback, and a determination to get the job done.

Record Yourself and Watch Your Performance

Practicing your pitch in front of a number of different professionals whom you can trust to be forthright with their feedback is a great way to polish your delivery. However, if you want to become an exceptional presenter, there is key step to take to improve this skill set. Dan Manges, founding chief technology officer (CTO) of Root Car Insurance *and* Braintree (yes that is an *and*. Look Dan up. You'll be pretty impressed with what this 32-year-old has accomplished), recently shared his secret to honing his pitching and presentation skills at a Starting Line event in May of 2018. At the event, Dan was asked by an audience member how he could speak for an hour without using the fillers "umm" or "uhh." Dan revealed that the secret to his success was the fact that he records his public-speaking endeavors and watches them afterward to observe his word choice and mannerisms. By understanding when and how he would exhibit a mannerism or make a word choice that he would like to change in the future, he was able to train himself to pause instead of exhibiting the unwanted behavior. Dan admitted that this pause sometimes feels like an eternity for him on stage, but it often is much shorter than he believes and it allows him the time to choose his words and mannerisms wisely. (A recording of Dan's interview can be found at www.go.osu.edu/startingline.)

📓 SUMMARY

Building a plan is a tedious task. Having the courage to follow through in convincing others to believe in your plan is all the more challenging. But now, you are armed with the skills to tackle these challenges head-on.

🔑 KEY TAKEAWAY POINTS

Plans are essential, but must remain fluid. The process of planning allows you to better understand your customers and their needs. As your level of understanding changes, so, too, should your plan. As World Heavy Weight Champion Mike Tyson once said, *"Everybody has a plan until they get hit."* Take your hits and change your plan accordingly.

- The Lean Canvas and the Business Model Canvas our simple tools that will help you quickly identify and understand the elements that will impact your likelihood of finding success.

- Pitching your ideas is nothing more than persuading an audience through storytelling.

- The five key elements of all great pitches are that you must (a) know your audience, (b) grab its attention; (c) paint your unique value proposition, (d) provide enticing solutions, and (e) ask for what you need—all while keeping it conversational.

- If through your pitch you can project confidence in your ability to succeed, a willingness to incorporate feedback, and a determination to get the job done, your likelihood of obtaining your requested resources will skyrocket.

REFERENCES

Berry, T. (n.d). TAM, SAM, SOM, potential market. *Lean Business Planning*. Retrieved from https://leanplan.com/tam-sam-som-potential-market/

Bruner, J. S. (1986). *Actual minds, possible worlds*. Cambridge, MA: Harvard University Press.

Hull, P. (2013). 10 essential business plan components. *Forbes*. Retrieved from https://www.forbes.com/sites/patrickhull/2013/02/21/10-essential-business-plan-components/#27c0f47d5bfa

Kenton, W. (2017, December 7). Elevator pitch. Retrieved from https://www.investopedia.com/terms/e/elevatorpitch.asp

QuickBooks. (n.d). 7 elements of a business plan. Retrieved from https://quickbooks.intuit.com/r/business-planning/7-elements-business-plan/

Thompson, P. J. (2013). Value proposition canvas template. Retrieved from https://www.peterjthomson.com/2013/11/value-proposition-canvas/

Wreden, N. (2002). How to make your case in 30 seconds or less. *Harvard Management Communication Letter*. Retrieved from https://hbr.org/product/how-to-make-your-case-in-30-seconds-or-less/C0201E-PDF-ENG

CHAPTER

22

Starting and Sustaining a Healthcare Business

Gary L. Sharpe

"If you want something you've never had, you must be willing to do something you've never done." —Anonymous

LEARNING OBJECTIVES

- Understand the role of creativity in generating innovation.
- Acknowledge the level of sacrifice required for entrepreneurial leadership.
- Apply principles to build a culture of innovation.
- Apply key learning from previous chapters to the journey of creating a healthcare business.

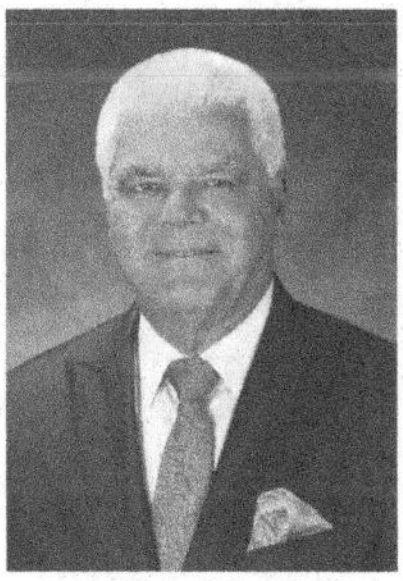

*Editor's note: This chapter is written in the first person in order to best capture **Gary Sharpe's** personal experience in starting his own healthcare business. Remember, the entrepreneurial journey is unique to each and every business. What works for Gary may be the exact opposite of what may work for your business. This chapter highlights what Gary has learned from over 40 years of innovating his business model, growing his business to over $100 million in annual sales, and employing over 320 dedicated workers. **Here's Gary.***

INTRODUCTION

How much are you willing to sacrifice?

Will you leverage all of your assets and work 80 or 90 hours per week for years? Will you persist for 10 or more years to achieve critical mass in sales, products, and the building space needed, all while never having enough cash or other resources? Thomas Edison once said,

"There is a way, find it." I have discovered that people are typically the most creative when they are the most constrained.

Needless to say, the struggle along our entrepreneurial journey was real. When our business was still very young, I visited a purchasing manager at a large hospital in Dayton, Ohio. At that time we were just a two-person shop, learning how to sell by direct mail and telemarketing. Wearing the many hats of the entrepreneur I was the CEO, and I was also our only traveling salesman. As I was sitting down, he said in a gruff manner, "What are you selling, Sharpe?" I have always had a problem with speaking before I think and before my derriere hit the seat, I blurted out, "What are you looking for you can't find?" The purchasing manager opened the center drawer of his desk and handed me a hand-written list on a piece of paper. I told him that I needed a week or 2, but I could take care of everything on the list.

Here's the catch, *I didn't have access to anything on that list.* I had to innovate and fast. I frantically found, made, or modified products to provide every product on the list. Two weeks later I shipped them, along with an invoice, to the attention of the "tough" purchasing manager.

The hospital paid the invoice in full without hesitation or negotiation, and I had an epiphany: *I should provide products no one else wanted to mess with.* Forty years later, we have $100 million in annual sales and 320 employees, but that does not mean it is not easy. It is a continuous struggle. Remember that saying, "If it is easy anyone can do it." You've heard throughout this book the importance of finding your niche. That concept is imperative to launching your own successful business venture or using entrepreneurial concepts within your organization to find success. Be different and find ways to solve your customers' problems. Think of it as taking away the customer's pain. In healthcare terms, provide palliative care, or better yet, a cure.

ENTREPRENEURSHIP AND MONETIZING INNOVATIONS

Entrepreneurship is an innovative process that joins and mobilizes the creation of something new to meet the needs of others through processes, products, and services. The pursuit of the market opportunity is the process in which entrepreneurship unfolds. Entrepreneurship is most commonly related to individuals; however, entrepreneurship emerges in a variety of settings, including small or large companies, nonprofit organizations, government entities, and sole proprietors. For the remainder of this chapter, I take you on an innovative journey describing how I started my company, Health Care Logistics, Inc. (HCL), by battling complexities, finding the customer's pain, and meeting the needs of the consumer.

When I was working for a pharmaceutical company after graduating from The Ohio State University, customers were asking for procedures and products they needed to convert their hospitals to provide unit-dose drug distribution and centralized intravenous (IV) admixtures. The pharmaceutical company selling the drugs invested in some of the product needs but not all of the small parts required. *Small parts* are defined as products that have only a small sales potential. I saw the opportunity in the fall of 1978 to build a company based on helping hospitals and nursing homes convert to unit-dose drug distribution systems and centralized IV admixture systems.

My wife, Connie, and I started HCL, Inc. in our home located near Circleville, Ohio, in 1978. Connie is a graduate of The College of Nursing at The Ohio State University and was working at the medical center in the thoracic surgery unit. Our spare bedroom served as the office and our garage was the warehouse and the factory. There was no heating or cooling in the garage (or insulation for that matter), and the first several winters were brutal trying to stay warm with just a kerosene heater. Air conditioning was provided in the summer by opening the garage door and using an electric fan.

We had about $1,000 in savings and I ripped my heart out by selling my beloved 1976 red Chevy Corvette for $7,600 to raise enough capital to help us launch the business. We also borrowed as much as any bank or financial institution would lend to us, including using as many credit cards as we could get to finance the business. It was a mighty struggle and absolutely could have ruined us financially. Looking back, I followed the steps I detail below to help me turn HCL into the company it is today. Some of these steps I mastered, others are still a work in process. I outline them here for you to serve as a guide, but know that every hospital, every business is different and adopting entrepreneurial principles is almost never done following a linear process.

FINANCING

Financing Your Invention

How much are you willing to risk? All of your savings and retirement accounts? Are you willing to get as many credit cards as you can and maximize the credit limits? Are you willing to get a second and third mortgage on your house? Are you willing to go to as many banks as you can to get loans? Are you willing to give up part ownership in your invention and business to private equity providers and venture capitalists? Are you willing to borrow from family and friends? If you are sales savvy and can convince people to see your point of view, you could also launch a Go Fund Me campaign online to raise capital for your business. Only you will know what fund-raising tactics you are comfortable with, and these are considerations you should thoroughly examine before launching your business.

You may be able to find a company that will invest in you, so it can add yours to its product line, but you will probably have to give up some ownership. Be aware that a business may buy your innovation and patents solely to remove it from the market and protect the sales of their existing product. If you take on partners, be sure to put in place a dissolution and breakup contract. Inevitably, one of the partners will want out or will want a bigger share of the ownership. Put an agreement in place in the beginning and it will save much stress and heartbreak and will reduce legal fees as well.

You Have an Idea for a Product or Service

There are multiple ways to structure the sale of an idea, and much of that depends on the buyer or seller's goals. But because this book is about you as an entrepreneur, we'll focus on the considerations from the seller's perspective. The seller must consider whether he or she wants to sell his or her innovation for a lump sum or license it for a royalty based on sales or a specific amount for a unit sold. The operative word here is *sell* and I will address that at the conclusion.

The entrepreneurs must also consider whether they want to make the product themselves or hire a contract manufacturer to produce it. If it is a product, should it be sold directly to the customer or through distribution, or both? If it is a process or service, should it be sold installed by the entrepreneur or through a distributor or a consulting firm? Do you want to give it away?

Remember that discussion in Chapter 20, Legal Considerations in Starting a Healthcare Business, on Food and Drug Administration (FDA) approval? That information may be the deciding factor on how your plans proceed if your product or process (software) requires an FDA 510(k). Getting a 510(k) designation is expensive and time-consuming and will require technical help. You can search the Internet for a consulting firm to help you. Also reach out to people you know in the medical product business and ask for recommendations on who they work with on FDA matters.

 ## LEGAL ISSUES

I know you have already read an entire chapter on legal considerations for healthcare entrepreneurs, but I want to share with you not only my legal experiences in starting a business but also those experiences in keeping that business flourishing for 40 years. As many of you work within healthcare settings, be sure to understand whether your employer has any legal claim to your innovation. Ask your human resources (HR) department and your employer for clarification. When you entered into employment, you may have signed away your rights to anything you invented while working at the company, even if you do it on your own time. It is important you clarify this with your employer now or when you take a new job.

Once you have made a decision on what you want to do with your innovation, you need to discuss it with business people you know and get legal advice on how to structure your business. You can get a business license and operate as a sole proprietor, set up a partnership, or establish a corporation. There are limited liability corporations (LLC), C corporations, subchapter S corporations, and others. You need to discuss this with a lawyer. There are pros and cons of every business structure and you need to understand the issues. You also have to think about liability insurance because we live in a litigious society. If you do not have a business structure that protects your personal assets, you could lose everything in a lawsuit or regulatory action. You should also consider liability insurance, which can get complicated and expensive. You can buy insurance to cover most things, such as product lawsuits, slips and falls, and other injuries at your place of business. If you start your own business, you will quickly discover how many situations for which you are liable—and you do not want to be surprised. Discuss this with your legal advisors and insurance providers. The more you educate yourself about liability, the better off you will be.

Patents

Another concern will be patenting your invention. You may think a patent will ensure a path for you to become rich and famous, but that is rarely the case. You need to know that getting a patent is expensive. If you are fortunate and if your invention is not complicated, it will only cost between $1,500 and $2,500. More likely, the cost to receive a patent will be many thousands of dollars. And receiving a patent is just the first step in a series of many more expensive steps.

If you make it through the first step and receive your patent(s) and build an inventory, the next (and hardest step of all) is to get customers to buy it (again, we'll discuss selling later in the chapter). But then after you start selling, several things happen. You find out others have copied your patented product and are selling against you. You or your lawyers send them a notice of infringement and they are to cease and desist their infringement. They may ignore you and continue the infringement. You begin legal action to stop them. To defend your patent, plan on spending $50,000 in legal fees and that is just the start. The infringer may file to overturn your patent and you will have legal fees again to defend your patent. Someone else may file a suit against you for saying you are infringing his or her patent(s), that his or her patent has precedence over yours. You may find yourself selling your inventions that are not patented and you get notice of infringement from someone who claims to have a patent that covers your product. You will have to defend your product, pay more legal fees, or cease and desist selling products you may have been selling for years. Sometimes your competitors will strategically prolong the process until you run out of money and can no longer fight back. It's brutal out there. Keep in mind patents generally last for 20 years, but there are ways to extend the life of a patent. Again, it's important to have a good lawyer at your disposal.

Several years ago, U.S. patent law changed from being based on the invention's discovery date to being based on the "first to file." There were several ways to legally document the discovery date. Even though someone else later patents your nonpatented invention, you could prevail by proving your discovery was made before the competitor filed for a patent. The language change brings the United States in line with international patent law. Now, even though you invented it first, your invention is now infringing on someone else's patent. You have to cease and desist with your product or defend it, which means more legal costs to you.

Another patent action that can put you out of business or hurt you financially occurs when a large company wants your product. It may offer to buy your patent(s) for a fair price or offer an absurdly low price. If you do not sell, this company can make your product, sell it illegally, and keep you tied up in court for years while you are forced to pay large legal fees. If this company wears you down with continuous legal action and causes you to spend even more in legal fees, you may be left with few choices and none will be satisfactory from your perspective. If, like me, you think this isn't fair, you are right. Fortunately, my parents and experience have taught me that life is not fair and you just have to deal with it. This discussion on patents is not meant to discourage you, but to make you aware of the challenges ahead of you and, I hope, prevent you from being blindsided in the world of business and commerce.

CUSTOMER DISCOVERY

The old saying, "Build a better mousetrap and the world will beat a path to your door" is not true. You have to find the customer who might want it and then sell it to that customer. Sometimes there are no customers for your invention or they are years away from realizing they have a need and want your product.

CALL TO ACTION

You may have this fantastic invention and your friends are impressed. They congratulate you and tell you it will be a huge success. Here's one way to test whether you are really onto something. Tell them it will be available soon and ask them how many they want at the price point you determine. If they say they will buy several at that price point, ask for a deposit now and the balance when you deliver the product. Suddenly, they are not all that interested in buying even with a money-back guarantee if you don't deliver. This is a brutal but proven test of the marketability of your invention.

THINK—QUESTION—DEFINE—INNOVATE—EVOLVE THE PRODUCT.

Listen to your customers, talk to them, question them, watch them work, get into their minds, then start the ideation process.

CUSTOMER ACQUISITION

Inventoritis

The dynamics surrounding your product change when you ask for money. Ask early for money-down orders and you quickly find out whether you have a viable product. This also helps you control your *inventoritis (the inflammation of one's ego, particularly inventors)*. You are in love with your invention and you are going to be rich. You know you will not need to search for customers because when the word gets out about your invention they will be lining up to buy it. *Inventoritis* will lead you astray. Trying to sell your product early will help keep this disease from hurting you financially and prevent ego destruction. I have had this disease and wish I had diagnosed it myself much earlier. Most inventors suffer greatly from *inventoritis*, so please keep this disease under control. A phenomenal book to read to learn more regarding inventoritis is called *Overcoming Inventoritis: The Silent Killer of Innovation* (Roosen & Nakagawa, 2008). Reading it assists you in learning the secrets of achieving better returns from your innovation investments.

DEVELOPING A TEAM

If you start a business, think about sales and marketing, finance and administration, production and logistics, and invent/innovate and develop. We'll dive deeply into sales, marketing, and finance soon (I know, the anticipation is killing you!), but first let's agree that you must have to have a plan to integrate all parts of your business. You will need computer systems, invoicing and collections systems, office space and an HR department to manage employees, and ways to manage regulatory compliance. You will need to develop in great depth your financial, accounting, computing, and HR needs with the goal of having fully integrated processes.

Next to consider is production and logistics. If you have a contract manufacturer making your product, you still have to manage purchase orders to the manufacturer, keep on top of quality and on-time delivery, as well as changes to the product and production problem workarounds. Do not simply issue a purchase order and think your work is done. It is not. You have to work closely with your suppliers to avoid problems, to find problems, and to know how to discover and fix them before they become serious and expensive. The concept of logistics is simple: right product, right quantity, right place at the right time. It also involves organizing a warehouse for your products, putting inventory away, keeping track of inventory and the picking-packing-shipping orders from inventory. The bigger your company becomes, the more complexity you will have to overcome and manage.

BUILDING CULTURE

Once you have thought through the details of your innovation, you need to build a team to make your dream (innovation—idea) a reality. The great innovators build creative and flexible teams. Find as many helpers as you can possessing many skills, such as experts in computer-aided design (CAD), 3-D printing, design, programming, manufacturing, as well as artists, engineers, and people who are interesting. Ask friends and friends of friends and coworkers whether they can refer you to people with various skills. Meet them and get to know them and what their quirks are. Many ideas come from personality quirks. Avoid putting labels on people and ideas because that limits the possibilities and ideas that can be generated. In a nonthreatening way, discover where they grew up, their education, and especially their hobbies. Sometimes people work to support their hobbies and they are usually creative team members that want to offer their expertise. Learn how to bring out the best in them and that comes from just talking and coaching them. Don't dictate or preach to them because that is a big turnoff. Ask questions, especially build a conversation around "what if" scenarios and magic will happen. As you and your team develop a sense of teamwork, keep their minds open to any and all ideas. Learn how to enhance their natural curiosity. Avoid negative comments because they are creativity killers. When you, a team member, or your team has a failure, celebrate it, discuss it, and learn from it. Let people fail and create an environment where your team is not afraid to fail. You will learn that many times those failures and what you learn becomes a new innovation or is a solution to a problem encountered later or on for another project.

A technique that I use is to devise an item or a product that I want made on a new machine I bought or a machine that I think we could be doing more with. I use this technique to get their eyes rolling and to see that look on their faces that suggest the old boy has finally gone around the bend. Then there is the "we can't do that phase," which is what I want because I can offer my ideas on how to achieve my new plan on that machine. Then they start saying it would be better to try this or that to do it, or to do a phase of the manufacturing on another machine then move it to the machine I want used. Then when they are really into it I say, "let me know when you have a prototype" and walk away. It is important to know when to butt out.

I had purchased a thermal laminator for use in our cabinets division. This machine fuses vinyl covering to particle board and expands the options for colors and textures that are not available commercially. It also lets us make cabinets and carts with rounded corners and complex curves. I got the look! Then I gave the cabinet team a picture of a cart with a modern design, including complex curves, a shelf, and a drawer. It was a perfect modern design for an EKG machine, other medical treatment devices, or for use in varied procedures in a treatment room or doctor's office. The team made one and the result was fabulous. One of the drawbacks of the work of the thermal laminator was that the back of the particle board was pale white and didn't look good. The shop floor manager took it upon himself to solve this problem. He did not seek permission; he just started working on it. One day I was walking through the cabinet department and the shop floor manager was working the thermal laminator and there was a pile of scrap on the floor about waist high. He had a look on his face that suggested he was in trouble. I asked what he was working on and he said he was trying to fuse vinyl to the back of the particle board. I asked how it was going, what problems he was having, and what he was going to do to be successful. I told him to keep working on it and let me know when he learned how to do it. About a week later he told me he solved the problem and we could now thermally laminate on the back of the boards. I asked him to explain the process and how he came up with the solution. He said it took him about 20 telephone calls to experts in the industry and he finally figured out how to do it. I thanked him for staying with the problem until he figured it out. The lesson is to let people tinker around and to celebrate their failures. This is how we learn.

In the label-printing department, I needed a small, easy-to-operate slitter/rewinder. There are no commercial machines on the market, so I knew we needed to make a machine ourselves to do what we wanted. I talked to one of our engineers about my idea on how to make one using a crank handle to pull the labels through and for a simple system to quickly change the cutter/slitter blades. He soon made one and it worked nicely. I had the slitter/rewinder operators working on the big and expensive slitter/rewinders try it and they loved it because it was easier to use and was just as fast as the expensive machines. One of the operators thought it should have an electric motor to pull the labels through instead of a hand crank, so he got a battery-powered electric drill from the maintenance shop and, with a flex shaft, connected the drill to the new tabletop slitter/rewinder and our new machine was even better. The team kept innovating and our new slitter/rewinder is now on its fifth generation and has a built-in electric motor with computerized controls.

Build a team, lead them, let them tinker. and celebrate their failures.

AUTHOR'S NOTE—Gary and his team put this ethos into practice. When conducting research for this book, we visited one of HCL's manufacturing locations. On October 29, 2 days before Halloween, members of Gary's team were dressed in Halloween costumes. Just another way that HCL celebrates its team members.

Inventing and innovating have been discussed, now you have to develop your product and your company. This requires a continuous effort because to survive and grow you should always work to make your innovations and business better. Innovate your business by finding new, better, and more efficient ways to do things. You must understand you will always be innovating and developing. There is an old Russian proverb: "When you are green you are growing, when you are not you rot." More money needs to come in than goes out. To keep growing and innovating new products and processes, invest earnings back into the business. Most overlook the power of DWYSYWD (do what you say you will do). A closing thought for you—and burn it into your thinking—is this: "May the problems you don't know about find you," accredited to Professor Tom Merrill, Xavier University, Center for Innovation. Learn to look for problems.

SCALING THE COMPANY

Scaling is a business term that refers to how a company can grow. As you work to bring your ideas to life, decide as early as possible whether your invention has commercial potential because the scope of your ideas could quickly morph into a mega project and potentially send it to an early grave. Once you have a narrow and well-defined creation, immediately shift your creative thinking to how it will be made if it is a physical product or how you will implement it if it is a process or service. Processes and procedures have to be detailed step by step. If you say, "here is a process or procedure" and just go do it, then your chances of success decrease. You have to explain it in detail, sell it, and walk people through the process. You have to train people on the process and follow up. Repeat this at regular intervals to drive the lesson home and encourage its adoption.

Gary Sharpe's Steps to Leading a Successful Business

I hope you have already started developing your personal way of thinking, generating ideas, inventing, and processing your innovation. Start thinking about a problem you want to solve or something that is troublesome to you and how you want to fix it.

> Think: "How can I do it better"?

> Remember: "Imagination is the ability to see what is already there."

> Do it "Now, you need to do it."

STEP 1: Develop a sales mind-set.

- Inventing, innovating, and manufacturing a product or service is the easy part. The hard part is selling the product or service.
- To create a business and have it grow requires a product or service that people will pay to acquire.

STEP 2: Continually foster ideation.

- Ideas come from thinking. Innovation and invention come from ideas.

STEP 3: Become an expert on how your company makes money.

- More money has to come in than goes out.

STEP 4: Do what you say you will do.

There are many books, courses, seminars, and publications on how to start a business, grow it, and make that business profitable. These offer a good starting point and you can learn some of the basics by reading them, but there are several caveats. Make sure the purveyors of these learning opportunities have done what they are teaching. *At some point during your entrepreneurship training (the sooner the better), you have to actually start a business built around your idea for a product or service.* It is important to think about a service as a process in which people perform physical or mental work for someone else. A service can be a process to do something more efficiently or a way to do something that has never been done before. Too often there is a focus on a product, but processes are just as important. Examples of items created through use of processes are software applications, a teaching system, or a "how-to" manual.

SALES AND MARKETING

Commit the following points to memory and think about them every day in different ways to develop your innovator's and salesperson's mind-set. Yes, you have to be a salesperson or your chances of succeeding are limited. Do not fear because selling is not what you probably think it is.

The word *sell* scares most people unless you are a natural-born salesperson. Nevertheless, you will have to do it. In the early stages, no one else will know as much about your invention/business and no one will have your passion.

📣 CALL TO ACTION

Think about your invention and write down all of its features and benefits. Define what your innovation will do to help your customer. Now write down who would benefit from your invention. If the beneficiary is a business, hospital, and so on, who are the decision makers? Pretend your mother is the beneficiary. How would you approach her and talk to her? It is pretty easy. "Hey, Mom, I have something you may be interested in." What will your invention do for your mother? How will she benefit? The main benefit is the product's unique selling proposition, often referred to as *USP* (not to be confused with the United States Pharmacopeia). Watch her facial expressions, listen to the tone of her voice, and listen to what she says. Then adjust your sales pitch. Sales pitches can seem cruel, but you have to master one not only to sell your invention but also to get financing, investors, suppliers, helpers, and so forth.

Marketing Leads to Sales

To fully develop your sales plan, you need a marketing plan. The difference between the two is that marketing is sales support. My definition of *marketing* drives marketing professionals crazy. They think it is demeaning. It is not. It is reality. A person has to get face to face with the customer and make the sale. Marketing will help you find potential customers and get their attention, but ultimately a person has to interact with real people who are customers. This may be done in person or on the phone. You may send a text or an email. You may connect through a web chat, at trade shows, or during public relations events your marketing team promotes.

If you have taken Marketing 101, you should be familiar with the four Ps: *product, price, promotion*, and *place*. The first three should be self-evident to you, but spend time thinking about them and put your thoughts into writing, then go back and think about them differently. Discuss them with your team or friends and create options to test your thoughts. *Place* is much more than the address of the potential customer. Think of it as how you will sell and distribute your invention: direct, multilevel marketing, wholesalers/distributors, or a combination of these.

Now, rethink your product in terms of:

CUSTOMER

SERVICE

MESSAGE

PRODUCT

Think about and write about who your *customer* is and envision this customer in as many ways as possible. Think about and write about what *service* your invention provides to the customer and how you will provide service to the customer when he or she uses your invention. Think and write about the *message* you want to convey to your customer. How will you convey this message? The Internet has made getting your message across easier and much less expensive than direct mail, personal selling, or journal advertising. Start writing a blog and set up podcasts; these tools will drive people to your website, where you can contact them and use your sales pitch.

PRODUCT, PRICE, PROMOTION, PLACE

There are four things our company measures on a continuous basis. Use Figure 22.1 to help you think more deeply and develop more sales and marketing options to try. I say "try" because you will constantly make changes as you get customer feedback and as you discover what is not working. Try. Fail. Adjust. Try again. Repeat this process and do it quickly and frequently.

Our company uses the matrix shown in Figure 22.2 to continuously reexamine how all of the elements of our products, services, and business are interrelated and must continuously evolve.

	Product	Price	Promotion	Place
Customer				
Service				
Message				
Product				

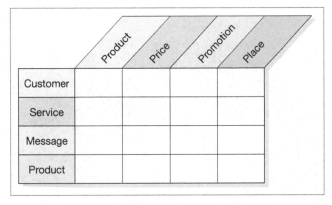

Figure 22.1 Matrix for developing sales and marketing options.

	Marketing	Administration	Logistics	Think	Imagination	Ideas
Sales						
Finance						
Production						
Invent						
Innovate						
Develop						

Figure 22.2 Matrix for examining the interrelatedness of products, services, and business.

Use Figure 22.2 to think about how an increase in sales will affect finance, inventory, production schedules, sales coordination, and so on. Teams should review Sales and Marketing, Finance and Administration, Product and Logistics, and Invent/Innovation and Develop matrices continuously. They all work together all the time. Optimizing these fields will be key to your success.

We've had our fair share of successes and failures over the last 40 years, so many that I could fill all of this book with lessons learned. But in the spirit of keeping this text a practical guide to success, I will showcase those lessons through a case study on one product that later evolved into an extensive product line by solving customer problems. Use this case as a template for innovating your product, process, or service as you launch your ventures.

CALL TO ACTION

Take a Rubik's cube and on it put a bunch of stickers with all different signs and symbols written on them to get your imagination going. The stickers should have all types of words pertaining to sales and marketing written on them. When you see the myriad combinations these stickers make, is amazing what starts coming to your mind!

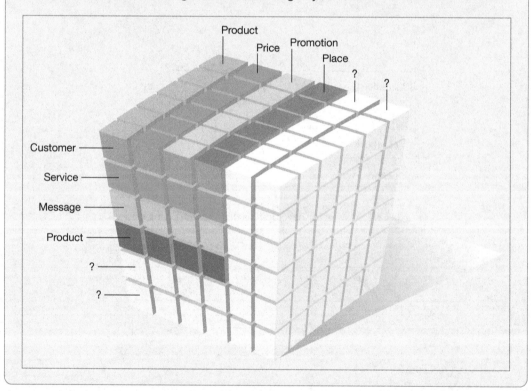

THE CASE OF THE MISSING TISSUE PLASMINOGEN ACTIVATOR AND STREPTOKINASE

When these clot busters hit the market, they were expensive and still are. They had to be refrigerated, accessible, and available for nursing staff without the usual delay that would occur if they were ordered from the hospital's central pharmacy. The problem was that they disappeared from the refrigerator and were not consistently restocked. This caused pain for my customers. To resolve my customer's pain, I had the idea to install a locking box onto one of the refrigerator shelves to prevent loss. At that time, the most common refrigerator shelves were made of wire, which was a design that I could leverage. I took a nicely sized tough plastic box from the warehouse and designed a stainless steel holder to fit the box that could be bolted onto the wire shelf. The slots in the top of the holder allowed it to be bolted onto any existing spacing within the wire shelf. The box holder was bolted in place with two stainless steel strips and stainless steel carriage bolts with locking nuts to prevent easy removal. At that time, I did not have my own metal fabrication shop, so I took the design or the holder to a local metal shop. They would make me 10 holders for $120 each. This would make the total cost of the product too expensive and people would not buy the locking box.

But then I remember a lesson on quantity pricing. I asked how much it would cost per holder if I bought 100 or more and they lowered the price to $20 each. After adding the lock, plastic bin, and packaging materials to the product, my cost was about $30 each. But I wasn't ready to order 100 of these without testing the market first, so I had them make me 10 holders at the $120 price. Unfortunately, I still had to sell the product as if it only cost me $30 to produce. I added a decent profit margin and launched the product and it was immediately successful. Everyone at the company thought I was crazy for selling a product for about $50 when it cost about $150. But spending $150 for the first 10 devices allowed us to determine whether it would sell and whether the price point was right. It did sell at the $50 price point and the rest is history; since 1997, we have sold almost 14,000 of the original design. We continued to add alternative designs and functionality as well as custom designs throughout the years. As of today, we have sold over 65,000 custom- locking refrigerator boxes as a result of continuing to innovate in order to meet the ever-changing needs of our customers.

As customer needs evolve, we develop products and services to take away the customer's pain. My company's innovation process is to listen to the customer and take away his or her pain. There is a caveat you need to be aware of. Steve Jobs said, "The customer does not know what they want until they see it," and I can attest that this is true. Jobs imagined and envisioned the iPhone in his mind and his team executed the idea. The iPhone is more than a physical product because of the software within it. Think about how the iPhone has evolved since it was conceived in one person's mind. You have to watch your customers work, relate and communicate with them, and read between the lines. Always imagine how you would like to do something and trust your gut. Using today's CAD software, you can design a product, create detailed pictures of the proposed solution, email it to the customer, and acquire feedback for possible modifications. When you get close enough, you can create a single prototype to take to the customer for further refinement. When the customer has it in his or her hands, it can be used in a real setting for further refinements. This reduces cost by eliminating a substantial amount of trial and error.

TAKEAWAYS FROM THIS CASE STUDY

The problem was clearly defined. Keep tissue plasminogen activator (TPA) and streptokinase from disappearing. Usually the question or problem is not so easily defined. Work hard on defining the problem and stating the question or questions about the problem as clearly as possible. State the problems and the questions in as many ways as you and your team can "imagine." This process gets your innovation started and speeds the prototyping process. But be mindful of scope and don't keep adding features. This usually slows development and sometimes kills innovation. Define narrow parameters and get your first iteration to market, then evolve it with customer feedback and improvements during the manufacturing process.

Think and use your imagination. In this case, I imagined a simple plastic box with a box holder that let the plastic box slide in and out. The box holder was adjustable to any wire shelving inside the refrigerator, was easy to install, and several lock options were available. Customers started using the box and began requesting different sizes, features, and better locks. Today, the product has evolved into many products that are standard and in stock for immediate shipment, as well as boxes that are customized to meet the customer's specifications. Many new features make their way into the standard stocked products. With continuous innovation the product keeps evolving. Along this continuum, new materials and manufacturing processes also are discovered and the product evolves even further.

Get the first "decent" iteration of the innovation to the market. Find out fast whether the market is going to buy the product. This also lets you test different price points.

CASE STUDY ON A PROCESS OR SERVICE

Sometimes hospital pharmacies have to package tablets, capsules, oral liquids, and topical agents in unit-dose packages because they are not available from a pharmaceutical manufacturer or a repackaging company. There are many products available to do this repackaging, but the problem (pain for the customer) is creating a label for the package containing the drug name, strength, expiration date, and lot number. Per regulations, everything packaged needs to be kept in a log with all the information on the label as well as how many were packaged, the date packaged, who did the packaging, and who verified the packaging and the logging.

Over the years we have offered several personal computer (PC) software programs with the capabilities required to make the labels. These programs evolved as needs changed and new technology emerged. The customer bought the program, which had to be installed on pharmacy computers. The installation could be problematic because of the hospital's technology department requirements and security protocols. Although the ease of use improved, over the years we all knew this process could still be done more easliy. We had several customer service representatives fully trained on installing, maintaining, updating, and troubleshooting this software. They also helped the customer set up their label templates and create a label database.

As more customers used the labeling software, two issues became prominent. Those working second and third shift were not adequately trained on the software program, which highlighted that the program was not as intuitive as it needed to be. Also, large hospitals and customers with multiple hospitals requested installation of the program on their networks, so all their pharmacies could use the software without having to perform constant updates to individual PCs. We knew this would be difficult because we would have to do programing for each hospital network and the maintenance would be never ending for us. If the multihospital groups had the same formulary in all their facilities and they made changes to that formulary, each computer had to be updated. This became a major point of pain for the customer and was time-consuming. It was time for our team to innovate.

The "pain" our customers needed removed and the innovations my company needed to make were as follows:

- Make the software intuitive and easy to use.

- Limit training to installing and using the program effectively while saving time for the customer and Health Care Logistics.

- Make it easier to create label templates that were not already available in the program.

- Find an easier way to keep the FDA National Drug Code (NDC) numbers' database current.

- Find an easier way to create and update multiple drug wholesaler product number databases specific to the hospital.

- Find an easier and faster way to create and maintain customer-specific databases.

- Find an easier and faster way to add and update printer drivers.

Our team started dreaming and innovating just as I wrote about at the beginning of this chapter. We wanted the new program to resemble an app similar to those found on smart devices. Simple enough to download onto your computer and to use to print unit-dose labels. The app needed to open on the home screen and to prompt the user to simply print labels. Once we had the vision, we had to incorporate these ideas and make them functional, so all of the problems (or as I like to say—*opportunities*) listed would be solved. Remember, find your customer's pain and innovate a solution for it.

Years ago we renamed our IT department the *Technical Services* department because it handles the business software, network, databases, telephone system, cloud computing, websites, security, and many other functions. This team stepped in and said they would start with a clean slate and incorporate all the features our customers desired into the new app. The end product was easy to use even if you are working the third shift and have no prior experience with the program.

Before the creation of this new program, we had to send the update on a CD or thumb drive to the customer, who would install it on his or her computers. Now our team handles all updates seamlessly for our clients. Since gohclabels.com (go online and check it out) was introduced, it has evolved with new features customers have requested, which is exactly what should happen. The product or service you have innovated should continuously evolve. With each iteration, it should keep getting better, last longer, become easier to use, and cost less.

The final question was *how do we price this software and get paid*? Charge an annual subscription fee? Charge by number of labels printed? Charge a one-time purchase fee? Charge a quarterly fee with submission of a quarterly invoice? Would we need a purchase order from the customer each time? How do we make it easy and affordable for the customer and for us? Finally, I made the decision to give the software away. It would be free to anyone who wanted to use it and we hoped these individuals would buy labels and unit-dose packaging supplies from us. This concept is often referred to as a *loss leader*. Remember that example from NurseGrid in the business models section (Chapter 19, Intrapreneurship, Business Models, and How Companies Make Money)? This loss leader has been a great success for our customers and my company!

CALL TO ACTION

Use an alternative setting where you can build out your ideas when you need to create. This "creative-thinking area" could be found at work or in your home. Getting your mind into that famous productivity zone is really fun and it continually gives substance to your ideas.

KEY TAKEAWAY POINTS

■ *Use your imagination to see what is already there*. Something you saw or have been doing caused you to have an idea for a product, process, or service that will be an improvement over what is available now or a way to do something better.

■ *Keep reworking your ideas, which comes from thinking*. Remember that thinking is the hardest job but you must train yourself to do it. Once you have your idea well defined, bring others into your project to help you bring your innovation into being. Use the power of other people and their skills to help you. This could be additional idea generation, CAD drawings, 3-D printing, computer programing, finance, manufacturing, and so on. When you are confronted with obstacles that are stopping your innovation from going forward and layers of complexity appear to be stopping you or slowing you down, find people with the proven skills to help you overcome them.

■ *Work hard to learn about the people working with you*. What are their personality quirks? Learn to avoid things that upset them and build on their strengths. Remember that you can't make an eagle out of a duck. Let eagles do what they do best and let ducks do what they do best. Now you are building a powerful team. You have to be the leader. Let people make mistakes. Celebrate mistakes and learn from them. Corporations and governments spend a lot of money trying to invent things. But it all boils down to individuals like yourself "tinkering" with ideas. From time to time the tinkering produces a viable innovation. Therefore, the more you "tinker," the more you learn and innovate.

NOW, GO INNOVATE.

DO IT. DO IT. DO IT.

NO EXCUSES—START NOW.

OH YES, HAVE FUN.

ADDITIONAL RESOURCES

Berkun, S. (2010). *The myths of innovation*. Sebastopol, CA: O'Reilly.

Descartes, R. (2009). *Discourse on method* and *Meditations on first philosophy* (4th ed., D. A. Cress, Trans.). Indianapolis, IN: Hackett Publishing. (Original work published 1637)

O'Sullivan, D., & Dooley, L. (2009). *Applying innovation*. Thousand Oaks, CA: Sage.

Sharpe, G. (2012). *Critical aspects of management.* Naples, FL: Sharpe Publishing.

Stewart, M. (2009). *The management myth: Why the experts keep getting it wrong.* New York, NY: W. W. Norton & Company.

Taleb, N. N. (2007). *The black swan: The impact of the highly improbable.* New York, NY: Random House.

Taleb, N. N. (2014). *Antifragile: Things that gain by disorder.* New York, NY: Random House.

REFERENCE

Roosen, P. P., & Nakagawa, T. (2008). *Overcoming inventoritis: The silent killer of innovation.* Cupertino, CA: Happy About.

Starting and Sustaining a Healthcare Practice

Candy Rinehart and John J. McNamara

"If you want something you've never had, you must be willing to do something you've never done." —Anonymous

LEARNING OBJECTIVES

- Understand the role of creativity in generating innovation.
- Acknowledge the level of sacrifice required for entrepreneurial leadership.
- Apply principles to build a culture of innovation.
- Apply key learning from previous chapters to the development of a healthcare business.

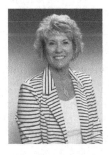

Editor's note: This chapter is written in the first person in order to best capture Dr. Candy Rinehart's and Dr. John McNamara's personal experiences in starting their own healthcare practices. Remember, the entrepreneurial journey is unique to each and every business. What worked for Candy and John may be the exact opposite of what may work for your business. This chapter highlights what they have learned from over 20 years of running their own private practices. Here's Candy and John.

INTRODUCTION

We were asked to provide a personal guide to launching and sustaining a healthcare practice, to share with you some of the insights we have gained along the way, and to really get you thinking about whether this an area of interest or a possibility in your career as a healthcare professional. We hope we will get you thinking and even doing some introspection and self-evaluation of your strengths, passions, and goals.

We thought that we should start our chapter with the personal stories of our journeys to become business owners and entrepreneurs in our chosen healthcare fields. We have different professions and have taken different routes to become business owners, but you will see that the passion to provide great healthcare is at the center of both of these journeys.

CANDY'S STORY

I am Candy Rinehart, and I am a family nurse practitioner. My original prelicensure nursing program was a BSN at a time when we were considered "book nurses." This was because we went to college for 2 years before we touched a patient. But soon, my nurse colleagues were going back to school to get that BSN. To be frank, I probably only went this route because my mother said I had to go to college and I knew I wanted to be in healthcare.

Thirteen years into my nursing career, I decided I should get a master's degree, but I was perplexed by what I should study. My choices were limited to administration or education tracks at the time, but coincidently (or was it meant to be?), during my second quarter of classes, the school of nursing announced that it was starting a nurse practitioner (NP) program. I was lucky enough to get accepted that first year and graduated just 6 months after the state of Ohio granted title recognition to NPs.

The NP role was so new in Ohio that at least a portion of each day I had to explain to patients and colleagues just what an NP's role entails. And no, I was not learning to be a "doctor" someday, as many people inquired. I just really wanted to be a great advanced practice nurse. I worked as an NP for two primary care practices for the first 8 years. The first practice promised to share monthly financial performance reports, but this never happened. After 4 years, I had become very concerned about their billing and financial practices and took a new position in a family practice across town. The next practice did share financial information and I was paid a bonus, quarterly, for a percentage of receipts earned over my base salary. This is where it really started to dawn on me that I could successfully generate enough income to start my own primary care practice, and, even more important, provide primary care, make employment decisions, and establish a caring work environment that I wanted to go to every day! I always joked that my motivation to start my own practice was that I finally had a say in how the phone was answered and how the receptionist greeted patients. These are important first impressions of you as the provider and of your business.

So, with the support of a loving husband, who throughout our marriage has teased that "you always have to have a project," and an attitude that I "could do it better myself," I held my nose and jumped. Starting my own practice was only possible because I had built a large following of great patients over the years that (I hoped) would follow me. A limited liability corporation (LLC) was formed (Remember that from Chapter 20, Legal Consideration in Starting a Healthcare Business?) and a practice site was selected. Initially, the practice employed one other NP and three full-time support staff.

Finally, the opening day arrived and the first patient came through the doors. The biggest surprise on our opening day was the large number of flowers and planters that were sent from our physician colleagues, primarily the specialists. There had been advertising and word-of-mouth promotion about the new family practice but it never occurred to me that there would be such an outpouring of support. In fact, one of the drivers for one of the florists announced, at around 4:00 p.m., that she thought we had "enough flowers" and that there was really no need to deliver any more the rest of the day. What a great way to start a new business and feel so supported.

In the first year or so, most days felt like I got in a covered wagon and went to the practice because there was so much pioneering to be done, especially in the world of reimbursement. NP practices were unheard of in Ohio at the time. The work that I had been doing for the past 8 years was primarily lumped with physician reimbursement. There were lots of meetings and negotiations with insurance companies and even a letter to the Board of Insurance and calls to state legislators when things were not going very smoothly. Little by little the barriers were chipped away. It was important not only for my practice, but for all NPs to be recognized professionally and financially for the work that was being done and the care that was being provided. I worked closely with our state trade organization, the Ohio Association of Advanced Practice Nurses, to be sure to include all reimbursement and practice concerns when working for change. Nurses have not historically been seen as business leaders, but we are. Nurses are also leaders in identifying where change needs to occur and possess the skills required to make those changes. All nurses have the responsibility to promote the image of nursing and to constantly inform the public of our important contributions to healthcare and population health.

For 10 years I practiced as a primary care provider and maintained a successful business. The practice was one of only four nurse-led practices in Ohio to be included in the state's House Bill 198, which provided an exceptional patient-centered medical home transformation project. We grew and maintained a reputation for providing exceptional primary care and excellent collaboration with specialists and other healthcare providers. This experience and reputation led to my next adventure ("project") with The Ohio State University College of Nursing, where (since 2014) I direct a nurse-led, interprofessional health center.

What were the biggest lessons that I learned from owning a healthcare practice? Building and maintaining a successful practice requires selecting a team of people who you know you can trust. It also requires the love and support of family, friends, colleagues, and the community. Above all it takes a desire to work hard to reach your goals and a true vision of what you want your practice to look like and how that practice will contribute to the community you serve.

JOHN'S STORY

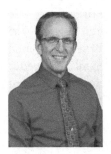

It is important to understand my background in order to better understand what influenced my decisions and motivated me to become an entrepreneur. My name is Dr. John McNamara. I am the fifth child in a family of 11 children: eight boys and three girls. As the father of three children, the thought of having eight more children is incomprehensible. However, growing up, I didn't sense the uniqueness of a large family since my friends all came from similar-sized families. It was a different time and different place. The important point is that, regardless of the family size, I was a middle child. Psychology courses have volumes written on the effects of birth order in a family and its impact on psychological development. I believe that the combination of my family size and my numerical birth order, impacted my development to be independent at a very young age. Money was not plentiful; so in order to acquire what I needed or wanted, I began working at a fairly young age. School for me was a requirement, not a love. In hindsight, a more serious approach to learning sure would have been more beneficial later in my career.

As I pondered what to do with my life after high school, I knew that going directly to college was not the right option for me at the time. I really lacked the motivation, focus, and goals that are required to be a successful college student. I knew I enjoyed working with people, so I accepted a job as a paraprofessional working with emotionally disturbed children in a middle school in the Bronx. My short tenure as a paraprofessional allowed me the rare opportunity, at a fairly young age, to experience helping others with special needs. I quickly discovered that I had an affinity for helping those with hearing impairments. I am not sure why I was attracted to that specialty, but at 17 years of age, I was fortunate enough to discover that I had found my true passion. Once I discovered that passion, learning became exciting and stimulating.

At the advice of a good friend, I entered college and pursued a degree in speech pathology to best prepare me for a degree in deaf education. During my studies in speech pathology, I was introduced to the field of audiology, the study of hearing disorders. I fell in love with audiology! I loved the mix of using sign language to communicate, the clinical aspect of diagnosing and treating hearing impairments, and especially taking advantage of the ongoing changes in technology that are involved in the rehabilitation process. My decision to pursue a master's degree in audiology rather than deaf education was one of many "forks in the road" that led me to ultimately own my own business.

I began my professional audiology career teaching communication to deaf students at the Model Secondary School for the Deaf (MSSD) at Gallaudet University and eventually moved to Rochester, NY, to teach and do clinical audiology work at the National Technical Institute for the Deaf (NTID). After a few years of teaching, I had an opportunity to move into private practice, and that began my business experience. Sometimes doors open for those who are looking. Choosing to move from a comfortable, secure, teaching position to a private practice environment was a frightening and daunting decision to make at the time, but it proved to be one of the best decisions I have ever made.

I was fortunate enough to work closely with the previous owners of the business I joined, and in doing so learned many skills that were never taught in my audiology program. Skills that included hands-on experience in marketing, financing, sales, repairing hearing aids, and the general management of a business. I combined these newly acquired skills with my audiology knowledge, a good work ethic, and some strong people skills, and felt confident that they would provide a strong enough base to allow me to successfully own and operate the business. So after 1 year I decided to purchase the practice from the owners. I wouldn't say it was a simple decision nor a simple path. There were and have been many sacrifices made over the course of 30 years. Fortunately though, I have had the support of my wife and children all along the way. I have been blessed with bright, hardworking, and passionate staff who have contributed immensely to the growth of the business. The joy received in seeing patients benefit from better hearing, the excitement felt when results and outcomes are positive, and the feeling gained from knowing I could improve others' lives by simply pursuing my vision, goals, and passions, far outweighs the challenges I've encountered and the sacrifices I've made.

 CALL TO ACTION

Create a list of opportunities you have been provided that help you believe that owning a healthcare practice is right for you. Then add to the list any potential reasons why owning a healthcare practice would not be right for you. When you think you are ready to own your own practice, first review this list with three practitioners who have started their own practices to obtain feedback.

FINANCIAL COMPETENCIES

The question that is probably asked the most by potential practice owners is "how much will it cost and where will I get the money?" We should also add "do you have the drive and personality to own a practice?" The bottom line is that there are financial competencies that must be attained prior to starting a business. If you do not have all or any of this knowledge and ability, then accomplish this first before taking the leap.

The American Organization of Nurse Executives (2015) identified and published the common core competency domains for healthcare leadership. Included within the business skills are the financial competencies. It is beyond the purpose of this chapter to teach and prepare you to be financially competent, but we will point out what competencies we feel are most important:

- Develop and manage an operating budget and long-term capital expenditure plan.
- Use business models for healthcare organizations and apply fundamental concepts of economics.
- Interpret financial statements.
- Manage financial resources.
- Ensure the use of accurate charging mechanisms.
- Educate you staff and providers on the financial implications of patient care decisions.
- Actively participate in negotiating and monitoring contract compliance (providers, billers, anyone you contract for services). Visit this webpage (www.e-mds.com/review-negotiate-monitor-managing-your-payor-contracts) for an example.

We admit this sounds overwhelming. In simpler terms, if you are able to create a business plan, include in the plan what you want to do and why, look at your financial resources, and can determine what the cost will be to see a patient, then you will be on your way. Just be sure to always pay attention. This is your baby and your constant love and attention will always be needed. No one will care as much about the business as you do.

HOW DO YOU KNOW WHETHER THIS IS RIGHT FOR YOU?

So you've done your research, gained the needed skills and competencies, weighed your options, reviewed your finances, and feel confident about venturing into your own business. Your excitement level and enthusiasm are high, but the list of "must dos" to start functioning as a business is very long. Where do you begin?

Let's start with **a name for your business**. This is a very important step in the planning process and is worth the extra time you take to make sure your name has meaning. Whether you are purchasing an existing practice or starting from scratch, there are many factors to consider.

If you are transitioning to ownership of an existing practice that has already established a patient base and has developed a reputation in the community, you'll have the option of changing the name and starting afresh, or continuing with the known business name (and not upsetting the cart). For ease of legal purposes and paperwork, the cost of modifying everything already in place, and keeping the security and familiarity with your existing patient population, maintaining the same business name might help the patient flow continue as is. However, this would be the ideal time to make changes to the name that you feel this would better reflect your vision and business goals. You might want to ask yourself: Does the existing practice have a good reputation or are you hoping to change its image? Does the name still reflect your brand identity and business philosophy?

If this is a practice start-up and you can pick any name you choose, make sure that the name includes words that tell the community what you do, so people don't have to wonder. Pick a name that you can live with forever and not have to change if you move to a different site. Questions that you might want to ask yourself are: How does the name look? Does the logo have appeal? Will it fit well with social media and potential modes of advertising? Is it unique? One very important question is: Does this business name already exist? You can search your state's business website to make sure your name is not already being used. Will you be able to use your business name online? You'll need to check to see whether the domain name (web address) is available. You can do this simply by searching online with the WHOIS database of domain names. Keep in mind that your domain name does not have to be the same name as your registered business name, but you'll probably want it to be somewhat similar. You can visit WHOIS at who.is to check for your desired domain name availability.

It is likely that at the same time you are coming up with a great name for your business, you are also looking for a **practice location**. This is not as simple as finding a nice building. "Location, location, location" is not just the real estate broker's mantra. Deciding where to locate your business is probably the single most important decision you will make. Without customers, patients, or clients entering your door, it will not matter how qualified you are, how much more you have to offer, or how good your customer service is, the business will ultimately fail. Any service-oriented business has to rely on a constant customer flow to generate revenue. The location of your business can significantly impact the amount of traffic coming through your door and eventually your ability to generate revenue.

To be successful, it makes the most sense to define what services you are going to provide and to explore where those services are needed and what the actual needs of the population are. It is also important to identify the present state of healthcare and business communities. If other practices have not been successful for that patient population, what do you have to offer that they did not?

When you have these things defined, you can start to look at the physical building itself. Once you find a location that will fit your needs, then look to see whether the rent/lease/purchase price fits into your budget. This is an important step in utilizing your negotiating skills. The amount of money saved on negotiating the "best deal" for where you set up shop is equivalent to receiving income from patients on a monthly basis. Don't forget to include any taxes that are required in your budget, too.

Here is a list of some questions to consider when making the selection of your practice location:

1. *Is the location appropriate and convenient for the patients you plan on serving?*

   Simply put, how easy is it to get to your office/business? Patients are twice as likely to choose a provider/business based on the convenience of its location, rather than the reported quality of its practice. When searching for suitable locations, consider the population you plan to serve.

- Walking distance from car into the office: Many seniors use walkers or canes, so an entrance that is close to the patient drop-off site is especially handy in the winter months.

- Ease of transportation, whether by car or metro: The office should be close to major highways or access points.

- Is there sufficient parking available? Is it free? Trying to find a parking spot in a crowded lot will elevate your patient's blood pressure and can lead to the demise of the business.

2. *Does the location reflect the population demographic you plan on serving?* If you plan on specializing in pediatrics, are the surrounding demographics represented by a community with young families? Or is it a mature community with many retirees that is better suited for someone wanting to specialize in adults or seniors?

3. *Is there potential space for expansion?* If your plan is to grow over the next 3 to 5 years, have you factored in either (a) the option to expand your existing space or (b) starting with more square footage than initially required with hopes of needing it in the future?

4. *Is there easy handicap accessibility?* The Americans with Disabilities Act (ADA) requirements are very specific about access and accommodations for persons with disabilities. You should familiarize yourself with these requirements to make sure the space you are considering is, or will be, within compliance. Any new build or modifications to an existing office should follow ADA requirements, but it's ultimately your responsibility to do so.

5. *What is the visibility of the signage?* Is your sign easily visible from the road or within your office building? The worst case scenario is losing a patient/client because this person couldn't find your office.

6. *Should you choose a downtown or suburban/rural location?* What region will draw more of your targeted patient population? Downtown locations are convenient for people passing by and allow for a street-level entrance, but the parking could be a challenge. In addition, consider whether or not there are people available in the downtown region to supply the workforce that will be needed.

When you settle upon a name and location, make sure you register the name with the state to protect it (see https://www.sba.gov/business-guide/launch-your-business/choose-your-business-name). This is an important step to make sure you secure your name online (domain) as well as register your name legally. You will want to check with your state and local agencies to see what their requirements are for business name registration, especially as this relates to healthcare providers. When your business name is registered, you'll be able to apply for a federal tax identification (ID) number (explained later).

Although there is in no particular order of priority, once you've settled on a business name, you'll want to decide **how your business will be structured**. We recognize that this topic was covered in Chapter 20, Legal Considerations in Starting a Healthcare Business, but wanted to provide you with the perspective of healthcare entrepreneurs who have put these legal principles into practice. Your choice of business structure has a direct impact on how you file your taxes as well as what your responsibility for personal liability is. There are several options for structuring a business, each with its own pros and cons. We strongly recommend discussing this with your attorney and accountant to determine what best fits your business model and current finances. Here are some basic options:

Sole proprietorship—This refers to one individual (or married couple) in business alone. This type of business is simple to structure, least expensive to set up, and has fewer tax and legal costs. However, the business owner is personally responsible for the liabilities incurred by the business. That means if your business gets sued, all of your assets are on the line. This is a very risky option for healthcare practices. Again, see the recommendation about discussing these options with your lawyer.

General partnership—This type of business model is composed of two or more partners who agree to contribute equally to the management, profits and losses of the business. Although this may seem appealing at first, simply because you're sharing your excitement, creativity, the prospect of being your own boss, as well as sharing the stress and responsibilities, you really need to give this option some deep consideration. Even the best of friendships and relationships deteriorate when trying to operate a business together. As with many relationships, when one partner feels he or she is contributing more to the business than the other partner, yet both still share equally in the profits, it can get ugly. This advice comes from personal experience. John spent his first 10 years with a partner, in an S-corp structure (structured so that profits/earnings/losses can be run through the individual shareholders before being taxed) before deciding to either dissolve the business or negotiate purchasing it from his partner. Fortunately, the latter prevailed. Candy also had a business partner (LLC) who decided to move out of state but wanted to remain a part owner. This caused a real rough patch for the business but was eventually resolved.

Corporation—A corporation has a more complex business structure that can be made up of a single individual, a partnership, or a group of people acting as a separate entity. The corporation setup has the same rights and privileges that an individual business would possess: that is, the ability to buy, sell, enter into contracts, or sue and be sued. There are generally two types of corporations, "S" and "C," with the major differences referring to how they are taxed. That's why having a great accountant vested in your best interest is so important. The greatest advantage to establishing your business as a corporation is that it provides limited liability to the owners (shareholders) with regard to business debts and actions. The disadvantage is the costs involved in starting a corporation, including the time and associated legal fees, as well as the ongoing costs associated with maintaining the corporation. John inherited an S-corporation structure, so it was a simple process to change the name of the shareholders and the ownership of the stocks. This worked to his benefit because of certain tax benefits that accompany an S-corp and not a C-corp, such as not having double taxation. If your finances are limited, choosing an S-corp or C-corp structure may not be the way to start. Always seek advice from your accountant and attorney.

Limited liability company (LLC)—This business structure is formed by one or more individuals and can be taxed much like a sole proprietorship or partnership. It is one of the most common choices in setting up new businesses because it shares many of the advantages and qualities of an S-corp or C-corp while allowing for more flexibility and a lot less paperwork and cost. Most important, it provides business owners with a much lower level of liability. The disadvantage is that because the tax is passed through personal income levels (self-employed), you may not enjoy some of the tax breaks that are permitted for corporations. Candy's business was an LLC. This business structure requires payment of quarterly taxes and what is left at the end of the year rolls back into the business. You have to be especially careful of your spending and be sure to pay yourself appropriately.

Professional limited liability company (PLLC)—If you are planning to form a business with other members of the same profession, you may want to consider forming a PLLC. A PLLC is very similar to an LLC in that it provides the same liability protection. However, it does not protect individual practitioners from malpractice claims against them. For this reason, malpractice insurance is essential. You should check with your state licensure requirements to see whether they permit your profession to form a PLLC.

Regardless of which structure you choose, if your business involves two or more owners, we strongly advise meeting with your attorney to put together a buy–sell agreement. A buy–sell agreement is set up between co-owners and details the process and provisions of a buyout if one of the owners dies, becomes unable to function and contribute to the business, or decides to leave. The contract can be written to detail the specific arrangements that partners agree upon in case something unexpected occurs. John's partner had a transient ischemic attack (TIA; mini stroke) 10 years into owning the business and was unable to return to work for over 6 months. The written agreement in the buy–sell contract stated that if one partner was unable to contribute to the business for more than 6 months, the other partner had the option of purchasing his portion. There was also a "right of first refusal" clause written into the contract, which simply means one of you has the first choice of buying the business at the other's asking price. In this instance, the buy–sell agreement made the process and transition simple and nonconfrontational. Another common option found in buy–sell contracts is an agreement to purchase life insurance policies on one another. The beneficiary of the policy is the surviving partner/s. The policy is often written so the death-benefit amount can be used as a viable funding option for the remaining owner/s. The selling price can be predetermined by establishing a set purchase price or using a formula to determine the price when needed. The surviving partner/s buy, and the heirs sell, the deceased owner's share in the business. It is a cost-effective means of purchasing the remaining portion of the business because it provides immediate availability of funds when death occurs. It also offers certain tax benefits to both the owner and surviving heirs because death benefits are generally tax free. In addition, it prevents any negotiating and haggling with family, heirs, or potential buyers during a difficult and stressful time. You'll want to ask your attorney to review many of the options available with buy–sell agreements.

GETTING RIGHT WITH THE TAX MAN AND GETTING PAID

Now that you have a business name and a business structure, what's next? You will want to **register your business** and become official (at least in the eyes of the Internal Revenue Service [IRS]). In order to operate a business, you need to obtain an employer identification number (EIN). This is the equivalent of a personal Social Security number, but for your business. You need an EIN to open bank accounts, pay local and federal taxes, secure business contracts, hire employees, and in almost any aspect of operating your business. Applying for an EIN is free and can be done online through the IRS website (www.IRS.gov).

Individuals who qualify as healthcare providers also need to obtain a National Provider Identifier (NPI) number. This is a unique number that allows healthcare partners (those who usually pay you) to identify you. It is required if you plan on working with any managed care plan, insurance companies, Medicare, or Medicaid. It is intended to provide efficiency throughout all healthcare systems as well as to reduce fraud. You can apply for an NPI number for free through the **National Plan and Provider Enumeration system website (https://nppes.cms.hhs.gov)**.

As we are on the topic of registering, licensing, and obtaining identifiers to work with insurance providers, this would be a good time to transition to the next task, which is **contracting with insurance providers**. Most healthcare providers need to bill for their services through third-party payers in order to survive. This includes Medicare, Medicaid, employers, insurance companies, or any combination of these payment sources. In order to work with these third-party companies, you need to be credentialed. It would be nice to say this is a simple, straightforward process, but it usually is not.

This process of credentialing usually involves having the **insurance companies** verify the provider's education, training, experience, competency, appropriate licensure, and malpractice insurance. Once you become a provider within the insurance company's network, you can begin to bill and be reimbursed for your services. Every insurance company you contract with has its own language, requirements, and levels of reimbursements. Some parts are negotiable and some parts follow strict requirements with no room for negotiating. Be very careful when reviewing and interpreting the language and provisions within these contracts. Once you are included in a network, you are agreeing to follow all its rules. You may want to consult with an attorney who specializes in health insurance contracts before singing any agreements. Although this may be costly in the beginning, it may save you time, money, and future headaches.

Many health insurance contracts and/or your own contracts with local affiliations may also require that you show proof of general business liability coverage. This coverage is designed to protect you from claims that can arise from your everyday business operations, such as someone getting hurt in your place of business, employees being injured while working, legal costs if you are sued, and replacement of equipment and property damage caused by fire or unforeseen occurrences. The amount of coverage and the options you choose depend on your type of business.

You will also want to set up a business bank account before you open your doors. A business bank account will separate your business money from your personal money. This makes it easier and simpler to track and manage your business cash flow. A checking account will allow you to write checks, use automatic teller machines (ATMs), deposit payments, and conduct business transactions. In addition, you should make sure your checking account has an overdraft line of credit. This allows you to withdraw an amount greater than the balance in your account without being penalized, or without bouncing checks due to insufficient funds. This feature gives your business some cash-flow flexibility.

A savings account (sometimes linked to a checking account) is usually set up to manage extra cash or provide a safety net for unexpected expenses. A savings account is a perfect place to deposit your 6-month cash "cushion" (recommended when opening a new business) because it can earn interest. Shop around to find the best rates on interest, services, and transaction fees, and keep in mind that many banks are willing to negotiate and reduce or remove many fees if you ask them to (from personal experience).

 CALL TO ACTION

Most healthcare programs have added business content to the curriculum but it has not been a focus. Healthcare is a business. What business education did you receive in your program?

YIKES! I HAVE A HEALTHCARE PRACTICE: WHAT DO I DO NEXT?

Pick a day to open and announce it publicly! There are so many ways to advertise now other than just using the newspapers and radio. Social media is an amazing source of advertising. If you have expertise in this area, great, but if not, there are lots of people who can help you with this.

We suggest you hang a sign. Don't skimp; make sure it is big and noticeable. Signage can make or break you. Place signs on the street, on entrance doors, anywhere they can be seen for directions and advertising. Before committing to the signage, however, check with local town or city requirements or limitations. Many towns have specific sign constraints and require approval through town boards before you can move forward. It took John 3 months to finally receive approval for signage from the town he moved his business to, so if he hadn't already been established with a database of patients, that would have been 3 months of limited business, which definitely would have been a showstopper.

You will need to start purchasing the items that contribute to your day-to-day business:

- IT support: You will need help with the Internet, phones, computers, fax, voicemail, and so on.
- Purchase an electronic health record (EHR) system that is user friendly and appropriate for your patient population. We highly suggest that you do not start with plans to keep paper charts then convert to an EHR, from personal experience, this is a nightmare.
- Make a spreadsheet of the supplies that you will need, both clinical and clerical. Contract with vendors to purchase these supplies. Don't be ill prepared to provide the care that you say you are going to provide (have you ever worked in a practice where there weren't enough supplies?). Put someone whom you trust in charge of ordering supplies and you can sign off on orders to oversee expenditures/control costs. You can increase your stock as you build your practice.

The most vital component of your business is getting paid for your services, so an essential step is to get credentialed with the payers you plan to bill for your services. You have to plan for at least 90 days to get *paneled* (the process of getting into the network of insurance companies) with Medicare, Medicaid, and most of the private payers. This process has been streamlined and the universal data sources are in one place. CAQH Proview (Council for Affordable Quality Healthcare, Inc.) collects self-reported provider data and streamlines credentialing by consolidating and standardizing primary source verification. This is essentially an online database that stores a provider's credentialing information that is often requested by various healthcare organizations. It eliminates duplicative paperwork by collecting your data using an electronic format and then sharing it with insurers. This way you only have to fill out and submit one application—you can eliminate the pain of filling out lengthy applications for every insurance provider you work with (www.caqh.org/about/about-caqh).

FINANCIAL SURVIVAL

How are you going to bill your services and follow up on the claims that are denied? There are medical billing companies that you can contract with for these services. The billing company should be familiar with the billable services that you provide.

If your services are not billable to third-party payers, establish a cash price and maybe even a payment system for your services and products. This again can be a lengthy process but in the end it can make the difference between success and failure. In the field of audiology, for example, many of the services are not covered by Medicare and insurance companies. John therefore had to establish options for patients to afford both his company's services and the products they were selling. He contracted with banks to provide long-term no-interest loans to patients and recently set up a lease program, so patients could afford to purchase hearing aids. Outline the costs for your services and products and clearly define those services that are covered by insurance and those that are not covered. Patients need to know what their financial responsibilities are before services are rendered.

How do you determine your hourly worth and what is your pricing strategy? Try putting together a monthly budget so you can look at short-term and long-term goals for the business. Our accountant told me most households and businesses fail to do this and we can sure understand why. It's tedious, but it's also critical for success. Look at your fixed expenses—for example, rent, insurance, salaries, lease equipment, insurance—and your variable expenses—for example, office and clinical supplies, credit card fees, hourly employee wages, cleaning services, utilities, advertising. If you are dealing with products, what are the costs of your goods? Is your purchase price for goods negotiable? Remember saving money up front is as good as making money on the sale. Analyze what your asking price will be, whether it's for a particular product or for your hourly service. Start by determining what the minimal baseline income you need to survive is. Then build up from there. The reason it's suggested that you have a financial cushion of 6 months is because you may need to supplement the "minimal" cash requirement to operate the business until the flow of your business is established. Review other similar businesses in your area to make sure your asking price is in a competitive range. Please see Exhibit 23.1 for a profit-and-loss (P&L) statement outlining how your revenue (amount of money made) minus your expenses (amount of money spent) determine the profitability of your business.

EXHIBIT 23.1 Example of a Simple Profit and Loss Spreadsheet

INCOME STATEMENT—Think Revenue/Expense	
P&L	
(Notice the number of income rows vs. the number of expense rows.)	
INCOME ACCOUNT	
Sales: (products, durable medical equipment....)	
Services: (diagnostics, counseling, follow-ups)	
Cash:	$9,628.00
Checks	
Insurance	$305,379.14
Patient	$79,408.50
Credit card	$64,589.20
TOTAL INCOME	$459,004.84

(*continued*)

EXHIBIT 23.1 Example of a Simple Profit and Loss Spreadsheet (*continued*)

EXPENSE ACCOUNT	
Advertising/Marketing	$12,367.00
Bank fees (including merchant service fees)	$1,570.00
Cost of goods	
Computer	$6,417.00
Continuing education	$1,400.00
Insurance	
Business/Workers compensation	$4,970.00
Health	$24,937.00
Janitorial	$2,200.00
Miscellaneous/other	$1,725.00
Payroll	$325,000.00
Postage/shipping	$2,389.00
Professional fees	
Accountant	$3,197.00
Attorney	$1,100.00
Rent	$25,300.00
Repairs/maintenance	$3,200.00
Retirement	
401(k)	$13,000.00
Pension	$—
Supplies	$1,950.00
Telephone	$9,443.00
Travel	
Meals and entertainment	$2,715.00
Convention/conference	$1,150.00
Lodging	$1,320.00
Flights	$3,800.00
TOTAL EXPENSES	$449,150.00
NET INCOME	
Total Income – Total Expenses =	$9,854.84
P&L, profit and loss.	

THE IMPORTANCE OF A GOOD TEAM

Staff appropriately and surround yourself with a team of people who want you to be successful. Remember, the person at the front desk is the face of your practice. When patients arrive at your facility for the first time, they should feel welcome. The waiting area should be clean, neat, and professional looking. Consider having coffee, water, and refreshments as well as current issues of magazines and reading material available, and offer free Wi-Fi. An inviting atmosphere shows that you've taken time and have pride in the services you offer. Equally important, if not the most important part of a patient's first visit, is the greeting he or she receives from your staff. Staff should exhibit a friendly, smiling, and positive impression at all times. Just look at the results of the classic Starbucks training given to all employees. A rude or agitated employee can offset any positive efforts you make to obtain a satisfied and happy patient experience. We have a policy that all grumpiness and complaining can be done in our back room away from patients. When we walk back out front, we're happy and smiling, regardless of our true internal feelings.

Start small and slowly increase your staffing as needed. You don't want to be paying people to sit around, or even worse, lay someone off after you have given him or her a job. Write good job descriptions, so the people you hire are aware of the responsibilities. Consider administering a personality profile test to potential new hires to determine whether their personalities match the needs of the job requirements. You can use the job descriptions to evaluate job performance. Someone needs to manage your staff and it will probably be you, at least in the beginning.

This can be difficult if you have worked for a company or institution that had these in place and you really never thought about how important they are. Make sure the policies, especially those related to staff (e.g., dress code), are enforceable.

Keep a constant eye on customer care. Remember, this is your baby and nobody loves your baby as much as you do. Make sure the staff and the care that is provided reflect the attitudes and goals that drove you to start a practice in the first place.

 CALL TO ACTION

If you were opening a business today, how would you publicize the grand opening? Develop a marketing plan for your grand-opening launch party!

FINAL WORDS OF WISDOM—LET'S HEAR THE PROS AND CONS

Well, to start with, owning a business is not for everyone. You are going to work harder than you ever have in the past. The hours may be longer, the workload heavier, the responsibilities greater. If you have a significant other, make sure your partner is on board before venturing forward. The demands on a significant other can be overwhelming at times—this person's support and belief in what you do are essential. Many challenges will come along the way but when you truly believe you are providing something special and that purpose is not only on paper, but also in your heart, then the business is bound to succeed. Remember how important passion is for the success of your business. Practice what you love and the success will follow. As previously mentioned, nobody loves the business like you do or is as willing to give up her or his free time for it. Sometimes it is hard to get paid for what you do, especially in the beginning. Be brave and stick to your plan. Just keep your eye on the prize. Having a practice that reflects your personal goals and ethical priorities emphasizing optimum patient care will provide you with inner success. We truly believe that maintaining this focus will lead you to financial success.

We hope that you have learned from and enjoyed us sharing our personal experiences and that if owning your own practice has been a personal goal, that we helped you make a final decision. Owning a practice is hard but very satisfying work. We believe that we have accomplished our practice ownership goals and achieved personal, professional, and financial success. We wish you the best in whatever direction your career path follows.

CALL TO ACTION

Interview at least two healthcare practice owners to learn more about their personal business experiences.

 KEY TAKEAWAY POINTS

■ Owning a business is not for everyone. You are going to work harder than you have ever worked in the past. The hours may be longer, the workload heavier, the responsibilities greater. If you have a significant other, make sure your partner is on board before you move forward. The demands on a significant other can be overwhelming at times—his or her support and belief in what you do are essential.

■ Many challenges will come along the way but when you truly believe you are providing something special and that your purpose is not only on paper, but in your heart, then your business is bound for success.

■ Remember how important passion is for the success of your business. Practice what you love and the success will follow.

■ Nobody loves the business like you do or is as willing to give up his or her free time for it.

■ Sometimes it is hard to get paid for what you do, especially in the beginning. Be brave and stick to your plan. Just keep your eye on the prize.

■ Having a practice that reflects your personal goals and ethical priorities and that emphasizes optimum patient care will provide you with inner success. We truly believe that maintaining this focus will lead you to financial success.

Key Strategies for Moving From Research to Commercialization With Real-World Success Stories

Caroline Crisafulli, Bernadette Mazurek Melnyk, Dianne Morrison-Beedy, and Mary Beth Happ

"When the going gets tough, put one foot in front of the other and just keep going. Don't give up." —Roy T. Bennett

LEARNING OBJECTIVES

- Define *commercialization*.
- Discuss one real-world success story that translated an evidence-based intervention into clinical practice.
- Describe the commercialization process.
- Identify the steps involved in translating research into the commercial market.
- Describe important considerations in forming a start-up company to disseminate an evidence-based intervention, technology, or product.

INTRODUCTION

Commercialization, or technology transfer, is a unique and exciting option used to increase the impact of one's research. Technology transfer can take many forms, which allows a wide range of flexibility in the level of involvement and engagement of the inventor. A technology may be licensed out to an established company or to an entity that will create a company around the technology, resulting in a start-up. If desired, the engagement of the inventor can be limited to essentially signing over the technology and letting someone else take over. A middle-ground option might be that the inventor remains a technical advisor or subject matter expert. The ultimate level of engagement on the continuum might be that the inventor decides to create and run a start-up company. By learning more about the process and becoming aware of the resources available, you can start to explore options in commercialization.

Commercialization is all about research and development, reiterative processes, proving hypotheses, arguing and defending, teaching, promoting, disclosing, responding to rejections, and the constant struggle against time and for adequate funding. The potential reward, particularly in terms of creating an impact in clinical practice or the community at large, is tremendous. The knowledge and satisfaction that something you created, designed, and developed is being used by others for the benefit of society is an exciting prospect.

WHAT IS COMMERCIALIZATION?

Commercialization, as defined by Merriam-Webster, is "(1) to manage on a business basis for profit or (2) to develop commerce in." The word *commercialization* may have a potentially negative connotation for some. Although making a profit may not be the primary object, it is a consideration and it is important to note that making a profit plays a significant role in the decision-making process of whether or not to pursue or invest in a technology. Simply speaking, for an idea or technology to be commercially viable, the product or service, ultimately, must be able to be created and sold at a profit. There are numerous factors that contribute to and drive that statement, these are described in further detail later in the chapter.

Not all significant scientific research is commercially viable. Not all good ideas are commercially viable for a variety of reasons. Commercialization is essentially a game with a certain set of rules and parameters, which is not unlike the program requirements of grants. If a particular idea is deemed "not commercially viable," it does not mean that it is a "bad" idea. Do not take a negative decision personally. The initial embodiment of an idea may not be commercially viable, but learning the commercialization process, essentially learning the "program requirements," will help you to incorporate a new perspective on how your research might be applied, translated, and transferred into the market.

CREATING OPPORTUNITIES FOR PERSONAL EMPOWERMENT (COPE)

One out of four to five children, teens, and college-age youth suffer from a mental health problem, such as depression and anxiety, yet less than 25% receive any treatment. Untreated depression is the leading cause of suicide, which is now the second leading cause of death in 10- to 34-year-olds (see www.nimh.nih.gov/health/statistics/suicide.shtml). If children and youth with depression and anxiety do receive treatment, it is often not the gold standard recommended cognitive behavioral therapy (CBT), mainly because of the severe shortage of mental health specialists across the country. Although the United States Preventive Services Task Force recommends screening all teens 12 to 18 years of age for depression (see www. www .uspreventiveservicestaskforce.org/Page/Document/UpdateSummaryFinal/depression-in-children-and-adolescents-screening), most providers across the United States do not screen for it because they do not have systems in place to manage depression. It is also typical for children and adolescents with mental health problems to wait 3 to 4 months for treatment. As a result of suffering from posttraumatic stress disorder and tremendous anxiety after witnessing my mother's sudden death from a hemorrhagic stroke that accompanied a sneeze when I was 15 years old and home alone with her, I became a nurse, then a pediatric nurse practitioner and psychiatric nurse practitioner, and a PhD-prepared researcher so that I could develop and test programs to improve mental health outcomes in children, teens, and parents.

I (Bernadette Mazurek Melnyk) began developing the Creating Opportunities for Personal Empowerment (COPE) program while practicing as a pediatric nurse practitioner in an in-patient child and adolescent psychiatric unit in Upstate New York. It was there that I recognized the huge need to teach children and teens suffering from mental health disorders cognitive behavioral skills and healthy lifestyle behaviors. I started to develop this program in the late 1980s and have conducted 16 intervention studies to support its positive effects in reducing anxiety, depression, stress, disruptive behaviors, overweight/obesity, and alcohol use, as well as in improving self-esteem, healthy lifestyle beliefs and behaviors, and academic performance (e.g., Hoying & Melnyk, 2016; Hoying, Melnyk, & Arcoleo, 2016; Kozlowski, Lusk, & Melnyk, 2015; Lusk & Melnyk, 2018; Melnyk, Kelly, & Lusk, 2014; Melnyk et al., 2013, 2015).

COPE offers a variety of evidence- and CBT-based manualized intervention programs with a goal to decrease anxiety and depression as well as increase healthy lifestyle behaviors in children, teens, and college-age youth. CBT is well established as the gold standard first-line evidence-based treatment for depression and anxiety, yet few children and youth receive it. By incorporating the key concepts of CBT into a manualized program that can be delivered by healthcare professionals other than mental health providers (e.g., pediatric nurse practitioners, family nurse practitioners, nurses, and social workers and teachers), substantially more children and youth who are affected by anxiety and depression can receive the evidence-based treatment they greatly need. Developmentally targeted versions of the COPE program are available for children 7 to 11 years old, adolescents from 12 through 17 years old, and young adults 18 to 24 years old.

CBT combines cognitive and behavioral interventions to produce changes in thinking, which then positively impact feelings and behavior, often referred to as the *thinking–feeling–behaving triangle*. It involves cognitive and emotional processing. Cognitive skills are taught and practiced. After the skill is learned, it is then used under conditions that trigger a negative thought or affective arousal. The goal of CBT is to help individuals turn negative thoughts into positive thoughts after an antecedent or activating event and to be more adaptive to their world by developing a coping template or schema. Until the development of the COPE programs, CBT had traditionally only been delivered by mental health providers, of whom there is a severe shortage, especially in rural areas throughout the United States.

COPE for children and adolescents with anxiety and depression consists of a seven-session brief manualized CBT-based program that is delivered in 25- to 30-minute sessions by a variety of healthcare providers in primary care, school settings, and community-based mental health clinics. The COPE Healthy Lifestyles TEEN (Thinking, Emotions, Exercise, and Nutrition) Program is a manualized 15-session CBT-based program that can be integrated into middle- and high-school educational curricula or delivered in small groups or individually to improve both physical and mental health outcomes in children and youth.

Table 24.1 presents the content and skills incorporated in the COPE 15-session program. The first seven sessions are delivered to children, teen, and college students with depression and anxiety.

TABLE 24.1 **Content of the COPE Sessions**

Session #	Session Content	Key Constructs From the Conceptual Model and COPE Intervention
1	Introduction of the COPE Healthy Lifestyles Pre-TEEN program and goals	Beginning introduction of CBSB
2	Healthy lifestyles and the thinking, feeling, behaving triangle	CBSB
3	Self-esteem, positive thinking/self-talk	CBSB
4	Goal setting, problem solving	CBSB
5	Stress and coping	CBSB
6	Emotion and behavior regulation	CBSB
7	Effective communication, personality and communication styles	CBSB
8	Barriers to goal progression and overcoming barriers. energy balance, ways to increase physical activity and associated benefits	CBSB and physical activity information
9	Heart rate, stretching, physical activity and its positive effects on mental and physical health	Physical activity information
10	Food groups and a healthy body, stoplight diet: eat red, yellow, and green	Nutrition information
11	Nutrients to build a healthy body, read labels, effects of media and advertising on food choices	Nutrition information
12	Portion sizes, "super-size," influence of feelings on eating	Nutrition information
13	Social eating, strategies for eating during parties, holidays, and vacations	Nutrition information
14	Snacks, eating out	Nutrition information
15	Integration of skills to develop a healthy lifestyle plan; Putting it all together	CBSB

CBSB, cognitive behavioral skills-building.
Note: Twenty minutes of physical activity are included in each session to build beliefs about engaging in regular physical activity.

The COPE programs offer evidence-based solutions that are now being delivered by a variety of healthcare providers, teachers, and counselors in primary care, community mental health clinics, and school settings in 43 states across the United States as well as in Canada, the United Kingdom, Australia, Lebanon, and South Africa. More than 11,000 children and youth have received treatment through the COPE programs. Healthcare providers who practice in primary care settings across the United States are receiving reimbursement for treatment using this program with the 99214 Current Procedural Terminology (CPT) code. The states implementing these programs are shown in bold type in Box 24.1.

COPE makes screening for depression feasible in primary care settings because this CBT-based program can be offered immediately to those children with elevated symptoms. Therefore, COPE

Box 24.1	States That Have Professionals Trained to Deliver COPE

Alabama | Alaska | Arizona | Arkansas | California | Colorado | Connecticut | Delaware | Florida | Georgia | Hawaii | Idaho | Illinois | Indiana | Iowa | Kansas | Kentucky | Louisiana | Maine | Maryland | Massachusetts | Michigan | Minnesota | Mississippi | Missouri | Montana | Nebraska | Nevada | New Hampshire | New Jersey | New Mexico | New York | North Carolina | North Dakota | Ohio | Oklahoma | Oregon | Pennsylvania | Rhode Island | South Carolina | South Dakota | Tennessee | Texas | Utah | Vermont | Virginia | Washington | West Virginia | Wisconsin | Wyoming

provides access to timely evidence-based treatment for children and teens who might not otherwise ever receive it. If not treated adequately the first time, depression has a reoccurrence rate of 60% to 70%. Being able to deliver an evidence-based program to both prevent and treat depression/anxiety by teaching children and youth cognitive behavioral skills that were once delivered only by mental health providers is an innovative solution to what is now a major public health epidemic.

Nationally, the most common and costly primary mental health diagnosis in children/teens is depression (44.1% of all mental health admissions; $1.33 billion/year). Healthcare providers across the United States are receiving reimbursement in primary care settings with the 99214 CPT code to deliver the seven-session COPE program (reimbursement, at $109 per session, totals $763 for seven sessions). For the 10,000 children/teens who have received COPE, the cost to the healthcare system for delivery of the program is $7.6 million. The average cost of a primary mental health hospitalization for a child/teen is $15,430 (Bardach et al., 2014). Using this cost number, if 10,000 children/teens were hospitalized for depression, it would cost the healthcare system $154.3 million. If hospitalization was prevented for the 10,000 children and teens who received the COPE seven-session program, the cost savings to the healthcare system would be $146.7 million. Conservatively, even if only 25% of 10,000 children/teens who did not receive COPE were hospitalized, the cost to the American healthcare system would be $38.6 million versus $1.9 million (the cost of delivering COPE to 2,500 children/teens), which would still be a savings of $36.7 million. These savings do not take into consideration the emotional hardship for the children/teens and families who experience a psychiatric hospitalization that could have been avoided through the use of the seven-session CBT-based COPE program.

The National Cancer Institute (NCI) has designated the COPE Healthy Lifestyles TEEN Program as a research-tested intervention program (RTIP) that is housed on the NCI website as an obesity control intervention program for adolescents (see https://rtips.cancer.gov/rtips/programDetails.do?programId=22686590). The NCI gave the COPE program its highest rating of 5 on a scale of 1 (low) to 5 (high) for its dissemination capability.

In the early years of my most recent university appointment, I sought the assistance of our technology commercialization office (TCO) as I was interested in developing a digital online version of the seven-session COPE program so that I could bring CBT help to any teen across the world who needed it. Key personnel from TCO directed me to launch a company and helped me to write a grant for small-business funding to digitalize the program. Although that grant was not funded, as soon as I launched the company that is named COPE2Thrive, LLC (www.cope2thrive.com) and hired someone to develop the website using my own personal funds, I started to receive multiple requests for the COPE programs. I also decided to personally invest in developers to create an online version of COPE for teens, which is currently available.

In addition, I took personal vacation days from my university job to develop online educational training for professionals who want to deliver the COPE program in their settings. I also hired a part-time employee to oversee the operations of the company because I currently do not have time to devote to the company and need to keep my role at the university totally separate to avoid any conflicts at work. In setting prices for my COPE programs, I had to conduct a careful analysis of expenses (e.g., part-time operations person, website, maintenance of the web platform for the online version of COPE, marketing/advertising, photocopying of the manuals, shipping) so as to be able to cover the costs of running the company and make sure I could keep the cost reasonable for healthcare providers, schools, and other entities wanting to implement the program and bring the desired COPE help and skills to children and youth. Recently, I worked out an agreement with my university to gift COPE to Ohio State for nonexclusive use so that we could deliver the program as a key strategy to prevent mental health disorders and to help our students across the university who are suffering from mild to moderate stress, anxiety, and depression. The program has been rebranded as MINDSTRONG for university use and is being delivered to both undergraduate and graduate health sciences students. If you are in an academic position at a university, seek the advice of your TCO and legal department when you seek to launch a company or if you have an existing company when taking a new position at a university. Legal affairs can assist you with learning about conflict policies and state ethics laws.

Based on several other clinical trials that I have conducted to support the positive outcomes of another COPE intervention program that I created to improve outcomes in hospitalized/critically ill children, premature infants, and their parents, I launched another start-up company in 2004, called COPE for HOPE, Inc. (www.copeforhope.com), with three other colleagues, which disseminates these COPE programs across the United States, the United Kingdom, and Switzerland. When launching a start-up company, seek legal guidance and consider very carefully whether you will be the sole owner of the company or have partners. Think through a partnership with specific terms and set up a legal agreement with any potential partners before launching the company to help avoid short- or long-term issues that might arise along your entrepreneurship journey. At the beginning of developing a program/product and testing it through research, think about its scalability and how you will disseminate the program/product if it is found to be efficacious through studies. Including hard "so what" outcomes in your research also will speed the translation of your evidence-based intervention into the real world (Melnyk & Morrison-Beedy, 2019). COPE for parents of preterm babies did not scale into real-world neonatal intensive care units (NICUs) until the findings from one of my National Institutes of Health (NIH)-funded studies showed a decrease in length of stay for the premature infants (Melnyk et al., 2006), which resulted in substantial healthcare savings (Melnyk & Feinstein, 2009). Developing scalable interventions that can make a real difference in improving people's lives and outcomes in real-world settings and mentoring others to do the same is a passion of mine. Research that gets grants funded and that is published will not automatically result in its being used in the real world. The research–translation time gap remains large, often lasting decades, so invest much time and thought into developing interventions that will be usable and easily scalable to real-world practice settings. The rewards of seeing your evidence-based interventions, products, or services used to transform health and lives are worth the many years of rejected grant applications and efforts to secure funds to develop and test your innovative ideas, so persist through all of the character-builders until your dreams come to fruition, and consult with others whose dreams have been realized and used in real-world settings.

◼ THE HEALTH IMPROVEMENT PROJECT FOR TEENS (HIPTeens)

Moving research through the translational continuum can be a slow-moving process; in fact, moving an evidence-based intervention from randomized controlled trial (RCT) testing to actual implementation in real-world settings takes, on average, 17 years (Balas & Boren, 2000; Melnyk & Morrison-Beedy, 2019). This time lag can be related to many different factors. For example, scientists who develop and test such interventions may lack the knowledge or skills to facilitate translational efforts. Certainly, in their busy roles in research and academia, these scientists also may lack the time, money, or needed resources to focus on translational aspects, and this may put the kibosh on such efforts. In truth, many researchers are thinking about next steps for scientific inquiry—"What is the next research study?" and "What is the next grant to focus on?" Naturally, translation from bench to bedside and into the community seems to drop off the slate of priorities. Yet, ultimately, if you ask researchers why they "do what they do," you will likely hear answers similar to this: "to make a difference in people's lives." To make this difference, we need to bring research full circle to translation into real-world practice settings and communities. This often requires changing hats—from scientist to business entrepreneur.

Here, I, Dianne Morrison-Beedy, tell my story of moving research to practice, of starting a business, of pushing out an evidence-based intervention (EBI) into the local, national, and global community. My story of moving an EBI to commercialization is likely different from others you may have read about or heard about because, in a nutshell, I was simply not ready to do so. Thus, I will provide you with a little insight into how I learned very quickly to, at the very least, get the ball rolling. In truth, my story of commercialization is probably one that demonstrates a lack of both planning and forward-thinking "what if" ideas and thoughts on how to capitalize on opportunities. I will tell you what happened when, as the saying goes, "the horse had already left the barn."

As a scientist and women's health nurse practitioner, I had a passion for improving the lives of young women and adolescent girls. After all, I had been one myself, and I knew those years were fraught with the challenges of navigating romance, sex, substances, relationships, and figuring out life. I knew that, clinically, these teens and young adults faced significant ongoing threats to their health and well-being because of high rates of HIV, sexually transmitted infections (STIs), and unplanned pregnancy. I also knew that, in my day-to-day clinical life, I saw clients over and over who were being tested for HIV, had been diagnosed with an STI, or thought they might be pregnant even though contraception and condoms were readily available. As I spent years working with these girls, I realized they might have some of the information they needed to be sexually healthy but lacked the motivation and skills to make and implement healthy choices.

Following years of qualitative and quantitative studies to develop and revise an intervention to reduce sexual risk in teens and young women (Morrison-Beedy, Carey, Cote-Arsenault, Seibold-Simpson, & Robinson, 2008; Morrison-Beedy, Carey, Feng, & Tu, 2008; Morrison-Beedy, Carey, Jones, & Crean, 2010; Morrison-Beedy, Carey, Kowalski, & Tu, 2005; Morrison-Beedy, Carey, Seibold-Simpson, Xia, & Tu, 2009), we ultimately completed a randomized controlled trial of nearly 800 girls, 15 to 19 years old, whom we followed for 1 year. Our brief, gender-specific intervention, The Health Improvement Project for Teens (HIPTeens), was provided in small groups to teens by trained facilitators and focused on providing sexual risk-reduction information, increasing the motivation to reduce sexual risk behaviors, and providing the skills needed to reduce risk. HIPTeens has a big focus on communication and negotiations skills, identifying triggers to risk behaviors, developing a future time perspective, and expanding behavior choices to include a wide array of healthy, safer choices along a continuum—in essence, a menu of options. We provided the intervention in four 2-hour sessions and added "booster" sessions at the 3- and 6-month follow-up visits. We recruited sexually active participants from a large urban area in western New York. These girls were predominantly Black, unmarried, non-Hispanic, impoverished, and 16.1 years old on average. We recruited through community-based agencies and other venues (e.g., dance clubs, after-school programs, and word of mouth) and successfully enrolled girls from across much of the area. Other methodologic and pilot details can be found here (e.g., Morrison-Beedy et al., 2010; Morrison-Beedy, Carey, Feng, et al., 2008; Seibold-Simpson & Morrison-Beedy, 2010).

Ultimately, the outcomes from the HIPTeens program were broad and long term. We significantly reduced the (1) total number of episodes of vaginal sex, (2) the number of episodes of unprotected vaginal sex, (3) the number of sex partners, and significantly increased sexual abstinence. In a subsample of approximately two thirds of participants on whom we obtained medical records, we significantly reduced pregnancy rates by 50%. More detailed information can be found in prior publications (e.g, Morrison-Beedy, 2012; Morrison-Beedy, Crean, Passmore, & Carey, 2013; Morrison-Beedy et al., 2012; Morrison-Beedy, Passmore, & Carey, 2013; Yinglin et al., 2012). Needless to say, we were thrilled to have had such an amazing impact, and that was about as far as we had thought about the intervention.

Following our published outcomes, we were contacted by the Centers for Disease Control and Prevention (CDC) for our data and more detailed information on our study and methodological details. We provided it, and did not think about it again until we were contacted by the CDC and were notified that HIPTeens was going to be included in the compendium of EBIs that were noted as efficacious in preventing HIV/STI. "Wonderful," we thought, "how nice!" We were also asked whether we could provide a phone number, in case anyone had any questions, and I promptly let them have mine. Similarly, the Department of Health and Human Services recognized HIPTeens as a teen pregnancy prevention EBI with strong evidence. Again, "How wonderful, and, yes, here is my cell number."

My phone started ringing, and ringing, and ringing. "Can you train us in HIPTeens?" "How much does HIPTeens cost?" "Do you have HIPTeens information on your website?" This is where I had to take a deep breath. Train people? Cost? Website? Yes, the horse was already out of the barn, but I desperately wanted to meet the needs of these agencies and nonprofits to provide girls with a sexual risk-reduction intervention that worked. So the clock was ticking, and I had to move quickly.

It was critical that I completed any work on HIPTeens outside of my professional job—considering conflict of interest and all. That meant taking vacation days or working only on weekends or late at night to get HIPTeens up and running as something that the community could use and implement in the real world. I filed the appropriate paperwork for a sole-owner limited liability company (LLC). I also paid for web domains to lock in my spot on the web so that ultimately I could build my website (see www.HIP4Change.com). One of the most important early decisions for me was determining that I would charge a fee to train people as HIPTeens facilitators, but that fee would cover the materials that would be needed to conduct the intervention (of course, including the costs of producing those materials). Since then, I have greatly expanded, improved, and added to the basic materials I first developed for the RCT

(Morrison-Beedy, 2018a, 2018b). This included developing and adding an online component to the face-to-face training for facilitators; filming video clips to be used for role plays; and developing a tailored intervention training manual and participant workbooks with professional graphics, business materials with professional logo, and a professional website.

Initially, I invested much of my personal vacation time and finances to get things started and conducted all the training myself. Over time, as I generated some (small) revenue from those early training sessions, I reinvested it into the business (HIP4Change, LLC: Health Improvement Programs for Behavioral Change) and hired contract workers to develop my webpage, graphic designers, and actors to "star" in my video clips. I took a course focusing on female entrepreneurship and the basics of starting a business. As time progressed and more clients came in, I continued to put any revenues into the business and to "up the ante" by adding two new people to my team, a contractor in social media and a graphics specialist.

Although HIPTeens is now being used in seven states and is in the process of being used internationally, we are still a fledgling business. I don't have enough time to devote to HIPTeens to grow the business as I should, so I know the real question is, how big do I want HIPTeens (and HIP4Change, LLC) to get? Determining that will require careful thought as to resources and expanding my very, very small team to push HIPTeens out and be able to meet demand. Keeping HIPTeens training and materials under my control was a critical decision that I made early on, when several companies expressed interest in buying HIPTeens. I have seen EBIs bought by companies that have been changed and altered and condensed so much that they do not resemble the original effective EBI; I wanted to avoid this issue, and so I still go across country to offer face-to-face training, still answer all the phone calls and requests for information, still do the voice-overs for the online training, and still send the thank you letters to clients. To me, those pieces are part of the personal touch that comes with HIPTeens at HIP4Change, LLC. Agencies work directly with the developer, namely, myself, who understands both the clinical and scientific aspects of this EBI down to the smallest details, who still has the same passion to make a difference in the lives of teens, and who is learning, step by step, what it takes to run a successful business.

THE SPEACS-2 PROGRAM: STUDY OF PATIENT–NURSE EFFECTIVENESS WITH ASSISTED COMMUNICATION STRATEGIES

A program of research to address the problem of communication disability among acute and critically ill patients led to the development, testing, and commercialization of an online communication training program and tool kit guided by an evidence-based clinical assessment and decision guide for choosing assistive communication strategies matched to the patient's functional abilities and preferences. The commercialization model used in this case exemplar is intended to promote dissemination and coherence of the program.

In preliminary work, our team observed that mechanically ventilated patients who were seriously ill and did not survive the hospitalization had periods during which they were communicative during the period of critical illness, even participating in communication about life-sustaining treatments, but received few tools or assistance to be able to communicate with family or clinical care providers (Happ, Swigart, Tate, Hoffman, & Arnold, 2007; Happ, Tuite, Dobbin, Divirgilio-Thomas, & Kitutu, 2004). The team also demonstrated that intubated, nonvocal mechanically ventilated patients and those following head and neck surgeries were able to use electronic, speech-generating devices (Happ, Roesch, & Garrett, 2004; Happ, Roesch, & Kagan, 2005). These studies and evidence from an integrative review of the literature (Happ, 2001) showed that although nonvocal patients were generally receptive to and appreciative of communication tools during serious illness, nurses lacked available tools and training in augmentative and alternative communication (AAC) techniques.

I (Mary Beth Happ) led an intervention study, funded by the National Institute of Child Health and Human Development (grant# 5R01-HD043988), to develop and test the effect of a multilevel communication intervention on nurse–patient communication performance (success, frequency, quality) and patient-reported communication ease with nonvocal patients in the ICU. Nurses received a 4-hour training program, decision aids, and low-tech communication materials developed in collaboration with co-investigator, Dr. Kathryn Garrett, a speech–language pathologist with expertise in AAC in the medical setting. In addition, one group received an additional 2-hour training session in AAC devices, speech-language pathologist consultation, and electronic AAC devices provided to qualifying intubated ICU patients.

Thirty nurses from two different ICUs and 89 nonvocal, intubated ICU patients who were awake and attempting to communicate participated in the study using a three-group sequential cohort design. The SPEACS (Study of Patient–nurse Effectiveness with Assisted Communication Strategies) communication interventions were associated with more successful communication exchanges about pain ($p = .03$; Happ et al., 2014). Patients receiving SPEACS interventions reported high levels of communication difficulty less often and utilized AAC techniques more often compared with those receiving usual care (Happ et al., 2014). Case exemplars illustrated the use and impact of the assessment protocol and AAC tools as guided by the speech-language pathologist (Radtke, Baumann, Garrett, & Happ, 2011). Overall, nurses evaluated the SPEACS communication training and AAC tools as helpful (Radtke, Tate, & Happ, 2012). They recommended unit-wide dissemination and implementation via an online training format (Radtke et al., 2012).

To translate the intervention for dissemination and implementation to nursing units, I condensed the SPEACS training program and prepared an online format of six, 10-minute online training modules (1-hour total), including video exemplars of desirable communication skills recorded from the original SPEACS study to reinforce content. SPEACS-2, a translational study funded by the Robert Wood Johnson Foundation Interdisciplinary Nursing Quality Research Initiative (INQRI), tested the impact of the online training course for nurses and low-tech communication tools program (SPEACS-2) on nursing care quality outcomes and on patient and family satisfaction with communication across six ICUs in two urban teaching hospitals. The study also tested nurses' knowledge, comfort, and satisfaction regarding communication with nonvocal ICU patients. SPEACS-2 utilized a web-based course, pocket reference guides, instructional manual, "low-tech" communication materials, and bedside communication rounds led by a speech–language pathologist to train ICU nurses on communication techniques for use with nonvocal patients (Happ et al., 2010; Happ, Sereika, et al., 2015).

The SPEACS-2 program was implemented across the six specialty ICUs using a stepped wedge approach with implementation order randomly assigned over eight quarters (2 years). More than 84% of eligible nurses participated (323 of 384). Nurses' communication knowledge ($p < .001$) and satisfaction and comfort communicating with nonvocal patients ($p < .001$) increased significantly after participating in the SPEACS-2 program (Happ, Sereika, et al., 2015).

More speech–language pathology consultations were initiated for communication in the ICUs after SPEACS-2 implementation. The electronic records of 1,440 mechanically ventilated patients (30 patients/ICU/quarter) were evaluated for nursing care quality outcomes (pain ratings, days in heavy sedation, physical restraint use, pressure ulcers, unplanned extubations). Nursing care quality outcomes remained unchanged after program implementation. This study also demonstrated that more than 50% of mechanically ventilated ICU patients screened for inclusion in the study met basic criteria for communication interventions, for example, being awake, alert, and responsive to verbal communication from clinicians for at least one 12-hour nursing shift (Happ, Seaman, et al., 2015)—an indicator of the potential unmet need.

Focus group debriefing with nurse participants revealed unit-based barriers to full program implementation and adherence at the bedside, such as problems with online training access, lack of protected time for training, and deep-seated attitudes about patient communication and practice change (Tate, Devido, Thompson, Barnato, & Happ, 2012; Tate, Happ, Sereika, George, & Barnato, 2014). Because communication is a set of learned, habituated behaviors, new communication approaches require deliberate, intentional change. SPEACS program consultations reinforce the importance of super users or communication champions, role modeling by experts such as speech-language therapists, simulated practice opportunities, decision aids and/or reminders, and the ready availability of communication tools for use at the bedside.

To package the online program for wider dissemination and implementation, it was refined using an updated format, professional narration, and high-fidelity video recordings of patient actors to simulate the communication skill exemplars, adding attainment of a required posttest score of 7/10 items correct (70%) for course completion to obtain credit for one continuing-education unit and using an improved delivery platform through The Ohio State University College of Nursing e-learning platform. The individual user cost is intentionally minimal and includes access to downloadable PDF files of communication tools (e.g., communication boards, tip sheets, clinical assessment and decision pathway, resources). The developers also structured in reduced rates for institutions to promote unit-based implementation and provide phone consultation emphasizing lessons learned from the SPEACS-2 implementation.

To date, the SPEACS-2 program has been implemented in hospitals and primarily critical care units in 10 cities across the United States, Canada, and Ireland. At the Hospital of the University of Pennsylvania (Philadelphia, PA), a group of clinical nurse specialists collaborated with the director of nursing research to evaluate the impact of implementing the SPEACS-2 program on nonvocal patients in five ICUs using the Plan–Do–Study–Act quality-improvement methodology with a pre-and posttest design (Trotta, Polomano, Hermann, & Happ, 2019). Nurses ($n = 385$) across five ICUs were trained in SPEACS-2, and 354 awake, nonvocal, mechanically ventilated patients (18–95 years of age) were evaluated over three 2-week periods; one preintervention and two postintervention intervals. Of the patients who completed the ECS ($n = 204$), scores improved significantly ($p = .027$) from baseline (mean 25.86 ± 12.2, $n = 71$) to postintervention period 2 (21.22 ± 12.2, $n = 63$). Nurses' use of communication techniques and communication plans of care increased incrementally across the posttraining periods (Trotta et al., 2019).

Difficulties encountered in the commercialization of the SPEACS-2 innovation are the attempts by interested constituents to circumvent registration and requests for free downloads or use of parts of the program rather than the whole. This raises concerns about intellectual property and derivatives as well as issues about potential degradation of content and impact of the selective use or alteration of program components. Although modifications and improvements are necessary and inevitable, SPEACS-2 partnerships and collaborations for such improvements would be a preferable route.

An additional dissemination pathway for the SPEACS-2 program is nursing education curricula at the undergraduate and graduate levels and for faculty teaching future clinicians. To that end, a team of clinical educators, led by Dr. Judith Tate, has developed an undergraduate module placed in the sophomore Health Care Communication course at The Ohio State University College of Nursing that includes completing the SPEACS-2 online program, additional reading and a lecture on the evidence supporting the intervention, and a simulation laboratory with case applications of the SPEACS-2 clinical assessment and decision aid. Thus far, approximately 900 undergraduate students and faculty have received SPEACS-2 training with positive comments about the program and exemplars of application of the skills on follow-up surveys. Dr. Tate recently obtained a university instructional grant to expand the program to the graduate entry (accelerated) and RN-to-BSN programs and to construct a curriculum implementation workbook for case study method instruction and other guides.

RESOURCES WITHIN A UNIVERSITY

The technology transfer office (TTO) is a customer service organization that assists members of a university in all aspects of the commercialization process, including activities such as pursuing intellectual property protection, obtaining funding for proof-of-concept work, completing initial market analysis, identifying potential business leads, and facilitating corporate engagement. All technology transfer activities in a university go through the TTO. Get to know the individuals in the TTO early on and view them as part of your team. The inventor is the technical subject matter expert, and the TTO is the team that drives and guides the process. Although the inventor does not need to have expertise in patent law or market strategy or in negotiating licenses, and so on, having an understanding of the process is empowering.

ADDITIONAL RESOURCES

For scientists and researchers who are interested in learning more about entrepreneurship and starting a business involving National Science Foundation (NSF)-funded research, the NSF Innovation Corps, or I-Corps, offers an immersive 7-week program that prepares scientists and engineers to extend their focus beyond the university laboratory and accelerates the economic and societal benefits of NSF-funded, basic research projects that are ready to move toward commercialization. The National Center for Advancing Translational Sciences (NCATS), part of the NIH, also offers various programs and webinars concerning small-business resources.

RESOURCES IN THE COMMUNITY

If your idea or technology is developed outside of the auspices of a university, look into complementary and extended programs and resources offered by technology and business incubators and innovation labs, such as Rev1 Labs in Columbus, Ohio. In addition to some funding mechanisms, discussed later, the Small Business Administration (SBA) is an excellent resource when developing a business plan and starting a business. These programs dovetail with the efforts of the TTO, providing a continuum of resources and education about entrepreneurship, small-business creation, and development.

THE TECHNOLOGY TRANSFER PROCESS

Disclosure

Typically, any technology developed at a university utilizing university resources, be it space, equipment, or personnel, is governed by the invention, patent, and copyright policies of the university and needs to be disclosed to the TTO.

The best way to start the transfer process is to contact your TTO and find out how to engage with it. Each TTO has its own specific process and set of procedures, but the overall process will be similar. The first formal step, typically, is to file an *invention disclosure form,* which is an internal document. In many cases, it is a simple online form that enables the inventor to give an overview of his or her idea or technology. Filing this form officially starts the conversation between you and the TTO. The idea or technology does not have to be fully developed, nor does the problem have to be fully solved. This is just the start; it is a very dynamic process. Err on the side of contacting the TTO too early. If it is too "early," they can help formulate appropriate next steps.

On receipt of your invention disclosure form, a licensing manager will follow up to learn more about your research and ask more detailed questions based on your invention disclosure form. Typically, a licensing manager will have an advanced degree or extensive industry experience in a related field and will be technically versed, not only to understand your research, but also to ask probing questions to help with patent applications, envision additional commercial applications and potential industrial partners or business leads. Regularly communicate with and update the licensing manager on any new discoveries and/or disclosure plans.

There are many types of disclosures, including published papers, poster sessions, conferences, TED talks, basically anything that informs another party about your research. The invention disclosure in and of itself does NOT offer any legal protection of your intellectual property. Since it is an internal document, it is not a public disclosure and is protected by the university.

In terms of intellectual property, ensure your ideas are sufficiently protected before you do any type of public disclosure. The TTO can help manage the timing issues. As long as the TTO knows what the disclosure plans and timing are, they will be able to file the appropriate applications with the United States Patent and Trademark Office (USPTO). It is never too early to contact the TTO. However, it can be too late if certain disclosures or other activities have already been undertaken. The earlier the TTO is engaged, the more assistance and guidance they can provide. Once a disclosure has been made to the TTO, they will start a formal evaluation process assessing the intellectual property and market potential to make a decision about how to proceed.

INTELLECTUAL PROPERTY PROTECTION

Intellectual property (IP) refers to your idea, invention, or a process you created. The IP is the asset that a company is purchasing the right to utilize in the form of a **license**. IP may be the only actual asset of a start-up. A *patent* is the formal protection of IP; this is what legally prevents other companies and competitors from doing what you are proposing to do. For licensing or attracting investments and/or an acquisition, you must have comprehensive IP protection. You can imagine that an investor or acquirer would be very reluctant to spend money on a company with technology that another company could utilize or replicate unimpeded.

The first step in protecting your *IP* is talking to your TTO. You do not have to be an expert at patent law, but the more you understand about the patent process, the more confident you will feel about the whole commercialization process. The TTO team will review your invention disclosure and research the current patent landscape to look for any existing patents or any other *prior art*, which is any previous public disclosure of the same or similar technology that would challenge the originality of the proposed patent. For a technology to be patented, it must meet the definition of an invention by fulfilling three requirements: (1) it should be *novel* (2) it should be *useful*, and (3) it should be *nonobvious*. These terms have clear legal definitions in patent law.

There are three patent categories: utility, design, and plant. A *utility patent* is the typical patent you think of, defined as the customary type of patent issued to any novel, non-obvious, and useful machine, article of manufacture, composition of matter or process. A *design patent* is legal protection granted to the ornamental design of a functional item. *Plant patents* are patents granted to new varieties of asexually reproduced plants (www.uspto.gov).

There are two types of patent applications: provisional and nonprovisional. *Provisional patent* applications are frequently filed initially, as they are relatively quick and inexpensive. The provisional patent is essentially a placeholder. It is not reviewed or examined by the patent office and does not result in issued patents. It does establish a U.S. *priority date*. If two or more patents are ultimately filed with the same invention, the invention with the earliest filing date has priority and receives the protection.

After a provisional patent is filed, the inventor has 12 months to file a *nonprovisional patent* application, sometimes referred to as a *full patent* application. A provisional patent is automatically abandoned after 12 months if a corresponding nonprovisional patent application is not filed. This 12-month period is used strategically by the TTO and the inventor. The TTO uses this time to further assess the commercial viability of the technology. The TTO allocates its financial recourses on the basis of those technologies that have a high patent potential and also a high commercialization potential, so the TTO will use this time to thoroughly review and assess the patent landscape to make an informed decision about whether to file a nonprovisional patent application. This 12-month period is also used by the inventor to demonstrate and prove as much as possible the value of the invention in the research before the more detailed and involved nonprovisional patent application is filed. Nonetheless, any future discoveries can always be added after a nonprovisional patent application is filed in a continuation application or separate filing, depending on the additional discovery. The goal is to protect as much as possible the first filing, but invention, by its very nature, is a dynamic process. The ideal strong *IP portfolio* will contain multiple patents expanding the reach of the original patent.

A nonprovisional patent application is very detailed, including technical drawings and fully fleshed out claims. The drafting and filing of a nonprovisional patent application are time-consuming and cost around $25,000 to $35,000 for the application and legal fees. A nonprovisional patent application comprises an abstract, background, description, figures, claims, and summary. The **claims** define and delineate the boundaries of what is actually protected by the patent. The nonprovisional patent application is reviewed by patent examiners. It takes anywhere between 18 months and 3 years for the patent office to communicate back to the inventor about the initial evaluation of the patent claims. These communications are called *office actions*.

The patent office will evaluate and render an assessment of each claim individually. There are three types of office actions: (1) rejection, (2) objection, or (3) allowance. A **rejection** is based on an assessment of the claim's not meeting the standard of novel, nonobvious, or useful. An **objection** is typically more of a minor point of clarification. An **allowance** is an official recognition of the validity of the claim based on novelty, nonobviousness, and usefulness. The most common action is, of course, a rejection, but this is not the end of the line. The inventor and team have 90 days to respond to the office action and supply additional information or clarification in support of each claim. The patent office may reject or allow none, some, or all of the claims. This entire process may take between 3 and 10 years for a patent to finally be issued. During this process, nonprovisional patent applications are **published** and searchable on the United States Patent and Trademark Office (USPTO) website 18 months after filing. A published patent is NOT the same as an issued patent and offers no legal protection.

Another question, particularly in a university setting, pertains to inventorship. Per U.S. patent law, an *inventor* must contribute to the conception of the idea or subject matter. This differs from who might be listed in a corresponding publication, where everyone involved may be listed. Who the actual inventors are is also important with respect to ownership in technology transfer. The TTO will be able to help determine who should be considered an inventor because this affects issues such as royalties and equity, a subject that will be discussed later.

Copyrights and trademarks are another form of protectable property. A **copyright** grants the exclusive right to reproduce, publish, sell, or distribute the matter and form of something, such as literary, musical, or artistic work. A **trademark** is a device, such as a word or symbol, pointing distinctly to the origin or ownership of merchandise to which it is applied and legally reserved for the exclusive use of the owner as maker or seller. For instance, an educational program that is developed with proprietary content may be copyrighted to prevent reproduction without the author's consent. The name of the program could be trademarked.

MARKET ANALYSIS

The other major analysis the TTO will undertake on receipt of an invention disclosure is an initial **market analysis**. The market analysis assesses the commercial potential of the technology, including identification of the target market, specifically the volume and value of the target market, the market need, the current competition, barriers to entry, and regulatory requirements. All of these factors affect the commercial viability of a product or service.

On a high level for the **target market,** you need to define who the potential customer is, how many of them there are, and how much they will use. Determining the potential volume and value of the target market gives the **total addressable market.** The total addressable market is a revenue figure that investors look for when considering an investment. The greater the total addressable market, the greater the commercial potential. The **market need** is addressed by identifying the benefit that the product or service will render and some initial sense of whether potential customers really need this product or service and whether customers are willing to pay for it. Thorough validation of the market need will be addressed later. Assessment of the **competition** deals with the question of whether anyone else is addressing this issue currently, and, if so, who it is and with what products. **Barriers to entry** are things that may make it harder to gain market entry and traction. Examples in healthcare include brand recognition, which may govern hospital access, enrollment in purchasing organizations, and contract approval. **Regulatory** hurdles include approval by regulatory bodies such as the FDA and CE marking.

 ## TTO DECISION

The TTO bases its decision on how to proceed by assessing commercial viability. The risks involved in the pursuit of commercialization are assessed; these are the same risks an investor or potential acquirer would also review.

Risk in a commercial setting is the possibility of failure or lack of success. There are a few broad categories of risk that the TTO will take into consideration:

Technical risk: Does the technology actually work?
Patentability: Can the IP be protected?
Regulatory risk: Will the technology be approved by the appropriate regulatory body?
Market risk: Is the product wanted, and are consumers willing to pay for it? Is the market large enough to create an acceptable profit?

An additional risk that plays a larger part for start-ups is:

Execution: Can all of the preceding considerations be resolved or decided before the funding runs out?

Certainly, there are many additional risks, but these are the high-level categories and represent milestones that correspond with valuation and commercial viability. The value of the technology is inversely proportional to the amount of risk remaining. So the more risk you can mitigate or eliminate before a financial transaction, the more the technology will be worth.

As part of this evaluation, the TTO may generate a **due diligence report,** which will summarize the findings regarding the patent landscape and market potential. On the basis of this information, a decision will be taken on how the office will proceed. Often the decision is predicated on the completion of additional testing or research. If there is IP potential, the TTO may proceed with the provisional patent giving the inventor and team another 12 months to further refine and develop the research.

The due diligence report or assessment is quite valuable in assisting the inventor in viewing the research through a commercial lens. Even if the TTO's initial decision is that the technology most likely cannot be protected or the market segment is not large enough to support the pursuit of the expense of a nonprovisional patent, there are very many things to learn from the process: Perhaps the technology can be adapted to another market or emerge in a different embodiment. Perhaps additional unmet needs may be uncovered by investigating other products in the market. Just the process of viewing research from a commercial perspective and application is valuable. If the decision is favorable to both the patent landscape as well as the potential market, the next step is to focus on mitigating the first risk on the list: technical risk.

 ## PROOF OF CONCEPT

Proof of concept is a critical milestone in mitigating technical risk. The proof of concept is a compelling demonstration that the technology or product works. It shows that the technology or product is no longer theoretical and enables an investor to envision extrapolating it to a commercial product. The TTO team can facilitate this process by helping define what a corporate partner or investor would find compelling or would need to see to make a decision. What needs to be demonstrated or proved to elicit the right reaction from an investor or partner? Engage with resources that have commercial experience early on, not only for market assessment and strategy, but also in terms of assisting with validation tests that may be helpful or applicable to the pursuit of IP protection or regulatory clearance.

Many things need to happen in parallel for commercialization of a technology or product. As development continues and a proof of concept is being designed, it is beneficial to engage with resources or mentors who have commercial experience. Regularly communicate with the licensing manager as patent claims are being developed. Engage with potential *stakeholders* or any entity who will be in contact with or affected by the product. This process of engaging with stakeholders is frequently referred to as the *voice of the customer*.

STAKEHOLDER ENGAGEMENT

To ensure that the product is actually what the end user wants, engage early and regularly with stakeholders. This feedback and information is also compelling for investors and potential corporate partners.

Identify all stakeholders. The entity that purchases the product may be different than the end user. Having an understanding of the market and product life cycle early in the development process can save a lot of time, money, and heartache in the end. No matter how much you think you know the space, there will always be things that you did not predict. This process of stakeholder engagement also assists with the **product definition**.

For instance, with a surgical device, the end user may be the surgeon, but attributes of the product, such as packaging, storage requirements, and sterilization, may affect many other individuals such as the first assist, the scrub tech, the circulator, or sterile processing. In a hospital setting, purchasing involves a completely different set of stakeholders. The surgeon may want the product, but purchasing and a value analysis committee have to approve and order it.

Understand who all the stakeholders are, their interests, constraints, and the process. In addition to determining who the customer is and what the customer wants, what is the product? What, specifically, will the customer be purchasing? Is it a piece of capital, software, a service, a program, or a disposable, or perhaps a combination of a few of these products or services? Exactly what the product or service will be drives the revenue model or specifically answers the question of how you are going to make money and how much money you will make over what period of time.

FUNDING

A significant challenge for university technology transfer is the transition from the research stage to what might be considered a functional and compelling proof of concept. Funding mechanisms that enable dedicated resources to be focused on creating that proof of concept are very valuable to the process. These are grants or awards specifically designated for development and validation of a proof of concept and generate an impetus to get the project done instead of the project's being relegated to one's spare time.

Creating a funding continuum or bridging the gap between basic science and research and traditional funding associated with start-ups and the commercialization process enables technologies to be further developed and validated internally within the university. This effectively assists in de-risking the technology or product to an extent before it is either licensed to an industry partner or start-up. The further along the development continuum a technology is, the more valuable it is with respect to a license agreement. With respect to start-up companies, the further along the continuum and the more risk that is mitigated, the greater the likelihood that the company will succeed.

There are specific funding opportunities available in conjunction with the SBA such as small business technology transfer (STTR) and the small business innovation research (SBIR). SBIR and STTR programs are funded by federal agencies with extramural research and development budgets, such as the NSF, Department of Health and Human Services (HHS), and Department of Defense (DOD). The STTR is a grant program for small businesses available in collaboration with nonprofit research institutions. STTR's objective is to bridge the gap between performance of basic science and commercialization of resulting innovations. Other SBA programs are the SBIR, and federal and state technology partnerships (FAST). These programs are designed to assist small businesses to engage in federal research and development that has the potential for commercialization (www.sba.gov).

TRANSFER OF TECHNOLOGY

The actual transfer of technology can take a few different forms, depending on the type and stage of development of the technology. In general, technology is licensed to another entity; either an existing company or a start-up company is created. *Licenses* are legal agreements authorizing a company to utilize or commercialize the technology. Milestones are usually attached to the license as a mechanism to ensure that the licensing entity is putting forth a good-faith effort to actually develop, utilize, and/or market the technology and not just "shelve" it. If milestones are not met, the TTO has the prerogative to call back the technology and license it to another entity. Licenses usually include an upfront fee, a royalty rate, and delineation of equity. In addition to the license agreement between the university and the licensing entity, there is another agreement between the university and the inventor that delineates how the royalties and equity are distributed among the inventor(s), college, and university.

In the initial discussions between a prospective licensing entity and the TTO, the licensing entity may request an *option*, which is a temporary hold. For some monetary consideration, the TTO may grant an option to a prospective licensing entity while the entity does its own due diligence to determine whether it wants to proceed with a license. The option will be granted for a limited period, perhaps 3 to 6 months, and during that time the TTO agrees not to actively pursue other licensees. During this time, the potential licensee with the option has no right to commercialize the technology until the technology has been formally licensed.

Another common technology transfer mechanism is a **collaborative development agreement** with an industry partner. In this case, both the university and the industry partner participate in development. The agreement clearly delineates the rights and responsibilities of each party. These terms are dependent on the type of technology and its stage of development.

CONSIDERATIONS IN FORMING A START-UP COMPANY

For some, exploring technology transfer and commercialization through the TTO may be just the start. The idea of continuing to be intimately involved with the development and commercialization of the technology, product, or service may be very appealing. The desire to control the direction and grow the idea into a full-fledged company may be very attractive. A start-up, based on a new technology or product, is a very exciting and extremely demanding undertaking, full of risks and unknowns but with tremendous potential. A start-up requires leadership that possesses tenacity, flexibility, imagination, and effective communication skills.

The goal of this section is not to give you a step-by-step guide on how to create a successful start-up; a number of excellent resources are available that go into great detail on best practices and recommendations for creating an effective start-up such as the I-Corps program mentioned earlier. There are online resources and books, such as *Disciplined Entrepreneurship*, the *Business Model Canvas*, and the *Lean Start Up* Model, that give very detailed step-by-step guides and recommendations. The goal of this section is to provide a generalized overview of the process to understand how many of the activities interact and overlap, to understand what investors are looking for in an opportunity, and, this is important, to give you some foundational guidelines on best practices to avoid some of the most common pitfalls. In a start-up company, all of the risks mentioned earlier become less theoretical and more real. The overarching risk in a start-up is **execution risk**. Execution is existential for a start-up. Will the company be able to create the product and get customers to buy it reliably for more than it costs to make it *before* the company runs out of money? That is the ultimate question.

EXECUTION

The Team

How do you mitigate *execution risk*? The single most important driving factor in execution is the *team*. Surround yourself with a team that shares the same vision, goals, and belief system you do. Embrace diversity within the team. Team members with different and complementary perspectives, skill sets, and life experiences can aid with creative problem solving and develop effective solutions. In a start-up, have people on whom you can count, who work very well together, and are as passionate and invested as you are in the project. This is also very good for moral support and resiliency. For these reasons, the team is frequently a deciding factor for investors. Investors evaluate whether the team has the subject matter experience, passion, and skills to execute the plan.

The Market

Mitigating **market risk** is a very large component of successful execution. The initial market assessment may be based predominantly on third-party data, such as reports on market size, projected market growth, research regarding current competitors and products, and some initial feedback from potential end users. Extensive **primary research** must be undertaken early and often in the development and commercialization process. This primary research involves numerous interviews with potential end users and other stakeholders, ideally, in person. This input validates the need for the product and the actual **product definition**. It is not uncommon for researchers and clinicians and any type of subject matter expert to be somewhat biased and myopic about their technology or product. You are heavily invested in this technology and are eager for it to be successful, but also remain open minded and unbiased when interviewing potential end users. The purpose of these interviews is discovery, not confirmation of previous assumptions. You want to listen to the end-users' descriptions of the problem and learn what they are currently doing. Are they using another product? If so, what do they like and dislike about that product? This first-hand experience and input will allow you to validate what the pain points are and best determine how you can solve any unmet need or needs. New questions may come up, and so may additional pain points and unmet needs. Primary research requires persistence, the ability to get people to talk, and then to remain open minded and to really listen. Solicit end-user interaction at the beginning to develop the initial product and throughout the development process, and as actual customers start to use the product to confirm whether the product is meeting the customer's needs. Stakeholder engagement becomes critical again when any product modifications are considered. Re-engaging with end users after you have made an improvement or iteration based on their input is a powerful tool for generating goodwill and enthusiasm and encouraging their interest in continuing to help. The importance of continuous stakeholder engagement cannot be overstated.

> One of the biggest and costliest mistakes that is made in product development is launching a product prematurely without adequate stakeholder feedback.

As a last note on primary research and end-user engagement, it is very valuable in a start-up in which the inventor is still involved, for the inventor to interact with end users. That does not mean the inventor has to or should do all the primary research, as that requires a certain skill set, but for the inventor to directly interact with end users and hear their input, even if it is not what you wanted to hear, sometimes *especially* if it is not what you wanted to hear, can facilitate problem solving, increase creativity, and improve the ultimate probability of success.

In addition to continual engagement with stakeholders or customers, a very **focused market strategy** must be developed. Start-ups are constantly balancing time and money. Efficiency is paramount. By systematically developing a clearly defined **target market**, that is, determining who is most likely to recognize and benefit from the technology and most likely to purchase the product, the odds of success increase. It is very tempting to try to please everyone and go after a very large market from the outset. Focusing on one clearly defined **market segment** and executing effectively in that segment greatly increases the odds of long-term success. This focus enables you to allocate your time and resources more effectively. The ultimate goal is to have paying customers who reorder.

 CALL TO ACTION

Who is the target market for your product or service?
What specific questions would you ask stakeholders about your product or service?

TIMELINES AND MILESTONES

Time to market will take several years for regulated products, such as medical devices. Many processes happen in parallel and reiteratively. To give an example of a path or road map, the following is a high-level overview of steps and major milestones for a medical device once a product is defined. Development follows a methodical and incremental progression. The goal is to try to add value with every step.

Functional prototype: Having a physical prototype to demonstrate the capability of the technology for end-user engagement as well as for use in presentations is necessary for potential investors. Being able to see and experience how a product works is much more powerful than talking about it and showing pictures and diagrams. Actually seeing the technology work animates the opportunity. A prototype is typically a "one-off" that is individually made, perhaps not even to scale and with little or no form factor, or what you might expect to see in a final product. The first of these iterations would be used and demonstrated on the bench in a lab. Ultimately, a functional prototype might be used in an animal lab.

Final prototype: This is the first embodiment that could be used with human patients. If required, it would be sterile or sterilizable, biocompatible, and incorporates human ergonomic factors. This is the embodiment that can or will be used when appropriate regulatory clearance is achieved.

Regulatory clearance: Regulatory clearance requires planning, strategy, and a significant amount of time. Depending on the technology, you may be able to start trials or use under institutional review board (**IRB**) approval while waiting for U.S. Food and Drug Administration (FDA) clearance. The complexity of the product and the potential risk or injury associated with the device affect the duration of the approval process. Something low-risk like bandages or exam gloves may require no formal approval or clearance. Something with a higher safety risk like an infusion pump may require a premarket notification based on a **predicate device**, a substantially similar device that has already been approved. Successful clearance of this type comes in the form of a **510(k) certification.** This process can take 90 days to 18 months. The most complex and highest safety risk items, such as a pacemaker, may require a **premarket approval (PMA)**, which requires a scientific review to ensure patient safety. This process could take years depending on the studies required. The risk, in addition to how long it takes, is that the device or product may never get approved. If that happens, it cannot be sold or used in patients. Achieving regulatory clearance is a significant milestone that allows you now to legally market and use your product.

First time in human. The first time the product is used with a human patient is another significant milestone. At this point, there are actual end users using the product in the setting for which it was designed. Data and feedback obtained from this point forward are even more meaningful. The product is no longer hypothetical; it is being used by real people in real situations.

Initial/soft launch. Launch your product in a very controlled fashion with limited variables so as to be able to focus on the function of the product and on how the end user uses the product. Often, this is with "friendlies" or end users who you already know and who will be amenable to trying and retrying the product, as well as being patient and understanding about the process. Listen to them and be agile. No matter how well you planned, no matter how many failure-mode analyses or focus groups were conducted, there will be all kinds of things that were not predicted once other people interact with and use the product. Listen, learn, implement, and repeat.

Market entry. Once the initial glitches and challenges are sorted out and addressed, the product is launched in a broader market. This is the official market entry with regular customers with whom you don't have a preexisting relationship. Again, engage with the end user, gather feedback, and make adjustments as necessary.

First order and first reorder. Quite a few free trials may be done to secure the first paid order. When the first actual purchase order comes in, it is a real milestone. You have now officially entered the market. The financial types in your organization may delay celebrating until the actual payment for that order comes in. It is especially exciting when customers start to reorder, indicating that the product worked and the customers like it and want to use it again.

Market adoption. When customers start reordering your product on a regular and reliable basis, you are entering the market-adoption phase. This is a very important inflection point. Reordering customers indicate satisfaction with the product, confirming utility and value. This is a critical milestone for obtaining the funding to move to the next level. At this point, an investor or acquirer is able to start extrapolating growth and revenue.

FUNDING

Commercialization funding is different from research funding. Although typical research funding comes in the form of grants from federal and state sources for basic science, research, and testing, most commercialization funding comes from private investors, such as individuals, angel investors, or venture capitalists. These investors receive **equity**, or a percentage of ownership in the company in return for the funds invested. Commercialization funding is used to develop the technology or product and grow the company. It is **dilutive** funding, that is, as additional funds are raised, the equity, or ownership, of the inventor and management decreases as additional equity is granted to the incoming investors.

Raising capital is a never-ending endeavor in a start-up and occupies a significant portion of a CEO's time. Start-ups will typically go through multiple rounds of investment, each associated with the level of maturity of the company as determined by the milestones achieved and the associated value of the company. Private sector funding can come from a variety of sources, such as angel investors, venture capital, and private equity. **Angel investors** may include individuals, such as family and friends of the investor, or may be an organization of individuals investing their own money early in the process. The purpose and intent of angel investors is to help entrepreneurs take their first steps. Venture capital is the next step. **Venture capitalists (VC)** invest in businesses that they feel will not only be commercially viable, but also create a certain return on their investment (ROI). Before VCs invest, they will undertake a formal and lengthy appraisal process, called *due diligence.* VCs are essentially investing other people's money. VCs have their own investors, called *limited partners.* VCs are investing money specifically to make money. It's not that angel investors don't want or hope to make money on their investment, but they focus on helping entrepreneurs get started. Venture capitalists typically invest at a more mature stage of the business than angels do, but some VC firms do specialize in early stages. The stages of funding have a variety of names that loosely correlate with levels of business maturity. These funding stages include terms you may have heard, such as *preseed/seed, validation, series A, series B,* and *series C.*

Different funds are appropriate at different times in the life cycle. The early funds may have descriptive names such as *preseed, seed, concept,* or *validation funds.* These are typically smaller investments, and the investors accept and expect a higher degree of risk. These early rounds fit into series A funding. **Series A** funding is designed to further develop and refine the product. The intent of **series B** funding is to build the company. Series B typically occurs when venture capital funding comes in. This is a larger amount of money designated to build the company once the product and the market are validated. This may include hiring more people and investing in manufacturing. **Series C** funding is designated to scale the company. Series C funding represents a large investment to expand the company to maximize its market presence.

CONCLUSIONS

The bottom line is that you need to do your homework well before commercializing your research to ensure its success. Take the time to work through the process, and consult with others who have been successful in this endeavor to ensure successful translation of your research into the real world.

KEY TAKEAWAY POINTS

- *Get the conversation started.* Contact your TTO, even if you think it is too early and you are not ready. Your initial idea may not be commercially viable, but that does not mean it is a bad idea. In fact, it may mean it is a great idea but that someone else has already pursued it. It may be that it needs to be tweaked and redirected, or it may just not have a sufficiently large commercial potential for the TTO to allocate resources. One way or another, do not take this personally. It is an educational process, and no matter what, you will learn something, and learning ignites additional creative thoughts and imagined solutions and opens doors and possibilities to increase the impact of your work and research. The TTO team is an excellent resource to help get started, set milestones, and establish timelines.

- *Develop a strong team.* Whether you are pursuing commercialization within a university or decide to spin out a technology or product in a start-up company, having an engaged team, with complementary experience and perspectives, will increase the chances of success. Talk with other inventors and develop a network of resources.

- *Involve stakeholders early on and frequently.* Knowing your target market and maintaining regular interaction with them will keep you aligned with the market needs. Customer needs may change over time; you have to be aware and poised to respond. The only way to understand the market needs and to keep up is to continually interact with your end users.

- *Stay focused.* Plan carefully, and focus on executing effectively in your target market. Efficient use of time and resources is paramount.

CALL TO ACTION

Meet with the TTO. Make an appointment to go to the TTO, meet with a licensing manager, and learn about the services the TTO provides and the process for engagement.

Market research. Start researching on your own what the market looks like. How big is it? What other products are in it? Discuss the market for your idea with the TTO. It will have an analyst do some initial searches to help you further understand the space.

Intellectual property. Be sure to share your disclosure plans with the TTO when you talk to a TTO representative. Discuss with this person what kinds of things you can and cannot protect. Look at an actual patent and read the claims. Again, the TTO will have analysts to assist you and can gather other patents in this space to review and help you to think through how your idea differs.

Network. Find other colleagues and near peers who are pursuing or have pursued commercialization of their technologies. The TTO may be able to help identify other inventive colleagues and may even host events for exactly that purpose. Take advantage of those encounters and ask candid questions as they relate to you, perhaps regarding how the process fits in with the other inventors' career paths, families, or other goals. Also, network with colleagues from complementary disciplines (e.g., engineering, design, nursing, medicine, and social work). This may provide additional technical perspective and expertise.

Develop and practice your "pitch." Get comfortable promoting yourself, your idea, and why it is needed. Practice really does help. Practice with TTO staff, colleagues, and your people in your network.

REFERENCES

Balas, E. A., & Boren, S. A. (2000). *Yearbook of medical informatics: Managing clinical knowledge for health care improvement* (pp. 65–70). Stuttgart, Germany: Schattauer Verlagsgesellschaft.

Bardach, N. S., Coker, T. R., Zima, B. T., Murphy, J. M., Knapp, P., Richardson, L. P., … Mangione-Smith, R. (2014). Common and costly hospitalizations for pediatric mental health disorders. *Pediatrics, 133*(4), 602–609. doi:10.1542/peds.2013-3165

Happ, M. B. (2001). Communicating with mechanically ventilated patients: State of the science. *AACN Clinical Issues, 12*(2), 247–258.

Happ, M. B., Baumann, B. M., Sawicki, J., Tate, J. A., George, E. L., & Barnato, A. E. (2010). SPEACS-2: Intensive care unit "communication rounds" with speech language pathology. *Geriatric Nursing, 31*(3), 170–177. doi:10.1016/j.gerinurse.2010.03.004

Happ, M. B., Garrett, K. L., Tate, J. A., Divirgilio, D., Houze, M. P., Demirci, J. R., … Sereika, S. M. (2014). Effect of a multi-level intervention on nurse-patient communication in the intensive care unit: Results of the SPEACS trial. *Heart and Lung, 43*(2), 89–98. doi:10.1016/j.hrtlng.2013.11.010

Happ, M. B., Roesch, T. K., & Garrett, K. (2004). Electronic voice-output communication aids for temporarily nonspeaking patients in a medical intensive care unit: A feasibility study. *Heart and Lung, 33*(2), 92–101. doi:10.1016/j.hrtlng.2003.12.005

Happ, M. B., Roesch, T., & Kagan, S. H. (2005). Patient communication following head and neck cancer surgery: A pilot study using electronic speech generating devices. *Oncology Nursing Forum, 32*(6), 1179–1187. doi:10.1188/05.ONF.1179-1187

Happ, M. B., Seaman, J. B., Nilsen, M. L., Sciulli, A., Tate, J. A., Saul, M., & Barnato, A. E. (2015). The number of mechanically ventilated ICU patients meeting communication criteria. *Heart and Lung, 44*(1), 45–49. doi:10.1016/j.hrtlng.2014.08.010

Happ, M. B., Sereika, S. M., Houze, M. P., Seaman, J. B., Tate, J. A., Nilsen, M. L., … Barnato, A. E. (2015). Quality of care and resource use among mechanically ventilated patients before and after and intervention to assist nurse-nonvocal patient communication. *Heart and Lung, 44*(5), 408–415. doi:10.1016/j.hrtlng.2015.07.001

Happ, M. B., Swigart, V. A., Tate, J. A., Hoffman, L. A., & Arnold, R. M. (2007). Patient involvement in health-related decisions during prolonged critical illness. *Research in Nursing and Health, 30*(4), 361–372. doi:10.1002/nur.20197

Happ, M. B., Tuite, P., Dobbin, K., DiVirgilio-Thomas, D., & Kitutu, J. (2004). Communication ability, method and content among non-surviving patients treated with mechanical ventilation in the intensive care unit. *American Journal of Critical Care, 13*(3), 210–220.

Hoying, J., & Melnyk, B. M. (2016). COPE: A pilot study with urban-dwelling minority sixth grade youth to improve physical activity and mental health outcomes. *Journal of School Nursing, 32*(5), 347–356. doi:10.1177/1059840516635713

Hoying, J., Melnyk, B. M., & Arcoleo, K. (2016). Effects of the COPE cognitive behavioral skills building TEEN program on the healthy lifestyle behaviors and mental health of Appalachian early adolescents. *Journal of Pediatric Health Care, 30*(1), 65–72. doi:10.1016/j.pedhc.2015.02.005

Kozlowski, J., Lusk, P., & Melnyk, B. M. (2015). Pediatric nurse practitioner management of child anxiety in the rural primary care clinic with the evidence-based COPE. *Journal of Pediatric Health Care, 29*(3), 274–282. doi:10.1016/j.pedhc.2015.01.009

Lusk, P., & Melnyk, B. M. (2019). Decreasing depression and anxiety in college youth using the Creating Opportunities for Personal Empowerment Program (COPE). *Journal of the American Psychiatric Nurses Association, 25*(2), 89–98. doi:10.1177/1078390318779205

Melnyk, B. M., & Feinstein, N. F. (2009). Reducing hospital expenditures with the COPE (Creating Opportunities for Parent Empowerment) program for parents and premature infants: An analysis of direct healthcare neonatal intensive care unit costs and savings. *Nursing Administration Quarterly, 33*(1), 32–27. doi:10.1097/01.NAQ.0000343346.47795.13

Melnyk, B. M., Feinstein, N. F., Alpert-Gillis, L., Fairbanks, E., Crean, H. F., Sinkin, R., … Gross, S. J. (2006). Reducing premature infants' length of stay and improving parents' mental health outcomes with the COPE NICU program: A randomized clinical trial. *Pediatrics, 118*(5), 1414–1427.

Melnyk, B. M., Jacobson, D., Kelly, S., Belyea, M., Shaibi, G., Small, L., … Marsiglia, F. F. (2013). Promoting healthy lifestyles in high school adolescents: A randomized controlled trial. *American Journal of Preventive Medicine, 45*(4), 407–415. doi:10.1016/j.amepre.2013.05.013

Melnyk, B. M., Jacobson, D., Kelly, S. A., Belyea, M. J., Shaibi, G. Q., Small, L., ... Marsiglia, F. F. (2015). Twelve-month effects of the COPE healthy lifestyles TEEN program on overweight and depression in high school adolescents. *Journal of School Health, 85*(12), 861–870. doi:10.1111/josh.12342

Melnyk, B. M., Kelly, S., & Lusk, P. (2014). Outcomes and feasibility of a manualized cognitive-behavioral skills building intervention: Group COPE for depressed and anxious adolescents in school settings. *Journal of Child and Adolescent Psychiatric Nursing, 27*(1), 3–13. doi:10.1111/jcap.12058

Melnyk, B. M., & Morrison-Beedy, D. (Eds.). (2019). *Intervention research and evidence-based quality improvement: Designing, conducting, analyzing and funding, a practical guide for success* (2nd ed.). New York, NY: Springer Publishing Company.

Morrison-Beedy, D. (2012). Communication strategies to facilitate difficult conversations about sexual risk in adolescent girls. *Journal of Clinical Outcomes Management, 19*(2), 69–74.

Morrison-Beedy, D. (2018a, October). *EBI to practice: Whose business is translational science?* Paper presented at American Academy of Nursing 2018 Conference. Oral Presentation, Washington, DC.

Morrison-Beedy, D. (2018b, June). *Whose business is translational science? Moving an evidence-based intervention into practice.* Paper presented at Faculty of Health & Social Care's 7th annual postgraduate research conference: Health & Social Care: Whose business is it? Keynote address, University of Chester, England.

Morrison-Beedy, D., Carey, M. P., Cote-Arsenault, D., Seibold-Simpson, S., & Robinson, K. A. (2008). Understanding sexual abstinence in urban adolescent girls. *Journal of Obstetrical, Gynecological, and Neonatal Nursing, 37*(2), 185–195. doi:10.1111/j.1552-6909.2008.00217.x

Morrison-Beedy, D., Carey, M. P., Feng, C., & Tu, X. M. (2008). Predicting sexual risk behaviors among adolescent young women using a prospective diary method. *Research in Nursing and Health, 31*(4), 329–340. doi:10.1002/nur.20263

Morrison-Beedy, D., Carey, M. P., Jones, S., & Crean, H. (2010). Determinants of adolescent female attendance at an HIV risk reduction program. *Journal of Nurses in AIDS Care, 21*(2), 153–161. doi:10.1016/j.jana.2009.11.002

Morrison-Beedy, D., Carey, M. P., Kowalski, J., & Tu, X. (2005). Group-based HIV risk reduction intervention for adolescent girls: Evidence of feasibility and efficacy. *Research in Nursing and Health, 28*(1), 3–15. doi:10.1002/nur.20056

Morrison-Beedy, D., Carey, M. P., Seibold-Simpson, S., Xia, Y., & Tu, X. (2009). Preliminary efficacy of a comprehensive HIV prevention intervention for abstinent adolescent girls: Pilot study findings. *Research in Nursing and Health, 32*(6), 569–581. doi:10.1002/nur.20357

Morrison-Beedy, D., Crean, H., Passmore, D., & Carey, M. (2013). Risk reduction strategies used by urban adolescent girls in an HIV prevention trial. *Current HIV Research, 11*(7), 559–569. doi:10.2174/1570162X12666140129110129

Morrison-Beedy, D., Jones, S., Xia, Y., Tu, X., Crean, H., & Carey, M. (2012). Reducing sexual risk behavior in adolescent girls: Results from a randomized controlled trial. *Journal of Adolescent Health, 52*(3), 314–321. doi:10.1016/j.jadohealth.2012.07.005

Morrison-Beedy, D., Passmore, D., & Carey, M. (2013). Exit interviews from adolescent girls who participated in a sexual risk-reduction intervention: Implications for community-based, health education promotion for adolescents. *Journal of Midwifery and Women's Health, 58*(3), 313–320. doi:10.1111/jmwh.12043

Radtke, J. V., Baumann, B. M., Garrett, K. L., & Happ, M. B. (2011). Listening to the voiceless patient: Case reports in assisted communication in the ICU. *Journal of Palliative Care Medicine, 14*(6), 791–795. doi:10.1089/jpm.2010.0313

Radtke, J. V., Tate, J. A., & Happ, M. B. (2012). Nurses perceptions of communication training in the ICU. *Intensive and Critical Care Nursing, 28*(1), 16–25. doi:10.1016/j.iccn.2011.11.005

Seibold-Simpson, S., & Morrison-Beedy, D. (2010). Avoiding early study attrition in adolescent girls: Impact of recruitment contextual factors. *Western Journal of Nursing Research, 32*(6), 761–778. doi:10.1177/0193945909360198

Tate, J. A., Devido, J., Thompson, D., Barnato, A. E., & Happ, M. B. (2012, September). *Taking the time to communicate: Characteristics of nurse workgroup engagement vs disengagement in the SPEACS-2 program.* Council for the Advancement of Nursing Science 2012 State of the Science Congress, Washington, DC.

Tate, J. A., Happ, M. B., Sereika, S. M., George, E., & Barnato, A. E. (2014, September). *SPEACS-2 program: Measuring and monitoring implementation.* CANS 2014 State of the Science Congress on Nursing Research, Washington, DC.

Trotta, R., Polomano, R., Hermann, R., & Happ, M. B. (2019). Feasibility study to improve non-vocal critical care patients' ease of communication using a modified SPEACS-2 program. *Journal of Healthcare Quality.* doi:10.1097/JHQ.0000000000000163

Yinglin, X., Morrison-Beedy, D., Jingming, M., Changyong, F., Cross, W., & Tu, X. M. (2012). Modeling HIV risk reduction intervention: The zero-inflated poisson regression models [Special issue]. *AIDS Research and Treatment, 37*(5), 367–375. doi:10.1155/2012/593569

Leveraging Social Media and Marketing for Personal Branding and Business Influence

Betsy Sewell, Dianne Morrison-Beedy, Linsey Grove, and Vibeke Westh

"You've got to get your team to not only understand your company brand, but also to understand their personal brand."—Amber Hurdle

LEARNING OBJECTIVES

- Identify the advantages and disadvantages of social media use as a leader.
- Describe the elements that comprise a personal brand.
- Define the basic steps to follow to create a digital presence.
- Determine ways to use social media and other digital platforms for the benefit of your organization.
- Identify strategies to partner with organizational teams to support goals.

INTRODUCTION

As a leader, a critical part of your role is to effectively communicate information to your organization, community, competitors, clients, and supporters. The collective of online communication options can help you to be successful in your messaging. The truth is, you will need to integrate all these options in your communication strategy to "get the most bang for your buck." Social media can help you to rapidly respond, communicate, and push out messages to a variety of audiences. If you are wondering why you would choose social media versus more traditional forms of communication, you might ask yourself these questions. Would you like to educate the public about issues related to your organization? Or would you like to influence politicians to see your side of the story? Or do you have a cause you are deeply committed to and you want to rally the troops to take up this cause? Maybe you are trying to get some good public relations (PR) and want the media to know about a new initiative your organization has undertaken? Perhaps you want to cheer your team on and make sure it is recognized for all its hard work and innovative ideas? If you answered yes to any of these questions, then using social media is an approach you want to include in your messaging.

As a leader you can leverage social media to assist you to encourage conversations and knowledge sharing in your organization among your colleagues and others with whom you are trying to develop a relationship and engage your customers or organizational members to help to create a brand and increase brand loyalty. However, there are both productive and, unfortunately, nonproductive ways to use social media, so we will discuss some of the perils and pitfalls as well at positive aspects of its use. It is important to understand uses of the various platforms in social media and how to leverage them to your advantage to connect with the audience you are trying to target. A savvy leader uses social media to analyze what's out there in his or her industry so she or he can stay one step ahead when it comes to decision-making for the organization. It allows you to keep track of emerging trends, innovations, and what's happening with the competition. Social media allows you to take a fresher, more up-to-date approach to getting your message out than you would achieve just by posting on your website alone.

"Tweet me, SnapChat me, text me, email me . . . just don't forget me. Use this need people have to connect to make change in the world." —Dianne Morrison-Beedy

CALL TO ACTION
Create an inventory of the social media accounts used in both your personal and professional lives.

As a leader in today's world, understanding and leveraging personal branding also is critical to the success of both you and your organization. Employees want to feel a sense of belonging—and trust—with the leaders and companies for whom they work. They want to feel as though they have a voice in the organization, and that their opinion matters and is valued—no matter their position in the organizational chart. As such, leaders need to find a way to connect with *all* employees on both a personal and professional level, across a multitude of channels.

Personal branding not only helps you, as a leader, connect with employees; it also drives external support from industry leaders, clients or potential clients, the community, the press, and other influencers. Consider the following reasons for creating a high-profile personal brand:

1. You want to influence change in your industry or the community.
2. You want to educate others about issues related to your organization.
3. You want employees—or future employees—to embrace the culture of your organization.
4. You want to amplify business initiatives, celebrate wins, and communicate positive messages to a wide audience.

THE FOUNDATION: PLANNING YOUR PERSONAL BRAND

The logical first step to developing your personal brand is to identify what you want to stand for as an individual. Determine the values that you want to exude, the personality that you want to project, and how much of your personal life you feel comfortable sharing with the world.

Next, you need to consider how your personal brand reflects on your organization. Are there controversial topics that you or your company might want you to avoid? What about the use of off-color humor or tactless language? As a leader of an organization, your personal brand is intrinsically linked to the company's reputation. It is your responsibility to ensure outsiders see that as a positive connection.

Consider all of the settings in which people may judge your character:

- A business or personal meeting, with opportunity for individual interaction
- A large presentation to the company or a community organization
- Attendance and participation at an event
- Sharing content online, via email or other channels
- Participating in conversations, both online and offline
- Simple interactions, such as waiting in the cafeteria line or sharing an elevator
- Any situation involving other people

By taking the time in advance to define your values and your desired perception, you create guidelines that you can easily apply when considering how and when to engage in a variety of topics or conversations. These guidelines will help you create a successful personal brand that reflects positively on your organization.

 CALL TO ACTION

Jeff Bezos, founder and CEO of Amazon, said, "Branding is what people say about you when you are not in the room." What do you want people to say? Take time to define aspirational goals and set clear guidelines for your personal brand.

CREATING INFLUENCE: DEVELOP A CONTENT STRATEGY

Once you identify your North Star and set guidelines for yourself, you're ready to develop an action plan to establish your personal brand. You don't need to create a full-blown content marketing strategy, but you should follow the same basic principles to create a simple plan. This helps to ensure that you focus your efforts in the right areas. Use these steps to help formulate your plan:

1. Define your goals and KPIs (key performance indicators).
2. Understand your audience.
3. Plan your content.

4. Create a distribution plan.
5. Start building community.

Your content plan should focus on your digital presence, rather than your offline behavior (though you should always ensure alignment between your online and offline personas). After all, Internet use among adults is nearly ubiquitous (Pew Research Center, 2018a) and seven in 10 Americans use some form of social media (Pew Research Center, 2018b). Take a look at each planning step in more detail to determine the best course of action.

1. **Define your goals and KPIs.**

   What do you want to achieve? How will you measure success? For example, if you wish to engage with your digital audience, you might track the number of comments on your posts. If you want to generate awareness about a particular subject, you could track the number of individuals who share your posts.

2. **Understand your audience.**

   How does your audience prefer to receive information? What online channels do they use? What are their interests? Take the time to do the research; knowing these details about your audience will help you to plan where—and what—to share. Not sure where to begin? Start by asking your colleagues and employees about their own digital habits.

3. **Plan your content.**

   What type of information do you want to share? Are there certain topics that you want to focus on or avoid? Do these topics align with your desired audience's interests? This last question is extremely important. To capture and grow a following, your content must resonate and even inspire your audience.

   Joe Pulizzi, founder of the Content Marketing Institute, popularized the 4-1-1 rule for content. That is, "for every self-serving tweet [or post], you should retweet one relevant tweet and share four pieces of relevant content written by others." The fastest way to lose an audience is to consistently share a barrage of advertisements or other self-serving content. Your audience expects to receive some value by following you—make sure you give it to them!

4. **Create a distribution plan.**

   Identify the channels that you want to focus on. How do these channels complement each other and reach different segments of your audience? These channels might include social media platforms, but also consider company-sanctioned internal communications platforms, e-newsletters, blog contributions, and even industry-specific online forums or communities like AllNurses.com or Nurse.com. Refer back to your audience research and identify which channels your desired followers use most often. You should also consider the *way* that users leverage each channel and what type of content is appropriate. For example, if you wish to disseminate an industry-specific, thought-leadership piece, you might choose LinkedIn or a specific online forum rather than Snapchat.

   "Content is fire, social media is gasoline." —Jay Baer

Let's take a closer look at social media channels, specifically, as those audiences and uses tend to vary more (Table 25.1).

TABLE 25.1 **Percentage of U.S. Adults Who Use Each Social Media Platform**

	Facebook	Instagram	LinkedIn	Twitter	Pinterest	YouTube	Snapchat
Total (%)	68	35	25	24	29	73	27
Men (%)	62	30	25	23	16	75	23
Women (%)	74	39	25	24	41	72	31
Ages (%)							
18–29	81	64	29	40	34	91	68
30–49	78	40	33	27	34	85	26
50–64	65	21	24	19	26	68	10
65+	41	10	9	8	16	40	3
Education (%)							
High school or less	60	29	9	18	18	65	24
Some college	71	36	22	25	32	74	31
College graduate	77	42	50	32	40	85	26

Source: Reproduced with permission from Pew Research Center. (2018). Social media fact sheet. Retrieved from https://www.pewinternet.org/fact-sheet/social-media

5. **Start building community.**

   When all is said and done, a good plan is only effective when executed well. More than anything, focus on engaging your audience in an authentic way. As a leader, leverage social media or other digital channels to encourage conversations and knowledge sharing, engage your customers or industry colleagues, understand your community, or simply build rapport with influencers whom you admire. Take the time to ask questions, provide thoughtful answers to questions, share interesting content that others post, and provide public kudos to employees or others who do amazing work. Make sure to include your organization's internal communication platform as part of your effort—by interacting with employees at all levels, you help to build trust and support from inside the walls, which often carries over to external-facing channels. As you continue to engage, you'll slowly begin to build a solid digital community over time.

🎥 REAL-WORLD EXAMPLE: KATIE DUKE, ACNP-BC

As a cardiology nurse practitioner in New York City, Katie Duke was featured on several hit documentaries. According to Duke's website, katiedukeonline.com, she leverages her exposure from television to fill the female healthcare and nursing professional void in the media. Duke created a platform to reach "her followers with powerful health promotion messages that embody the experiences of real-life lessons, women's empowerment, and positivity." In addition, she hosts the *Duke It Up* mentoring and networking event series and is a key contributor to *Scrubs Magazine*, the nation's number one lifestyle publication for nurses. Duke boasts nearly 103,000 Instagram followers, 25,000 followers on Twitter, and over 30,000 followers on Facebook—in addition to the audience she reaches via her blog. She takes the time to write about a variety of topics across her platforms, and engages with her followers on a regular basis.

Katie Duke
March 12 at 9:11 PM · ⚙

One of the best parts of being on #NYMed on ABC News was that I was able to portray my profession in a real, relatable manner.

There are many days where we leave work and feel defeated, where we leave feeling frustrated, where we leave feeling very burnt out.
We experience every human emotion on the spectrum in every shift. We deal with death, we deal with loss.

We are not robots.

We are not capable of "turning off" our human side, but we are capable of staying focused in times where duty calls: resuscitating the father & husband who was pulled out of a cab in cardiac arrest while his wife stands in the corner of the room, nourishing a neglected infant who has suffered the worst forms of child abuse, caring for a patient who has just murdered two children, holding a woman's hand as she experiences her 3rd miscarriage.

Duty calls in many forms. But we are not immune to feeling defeated and we are not immune to feeling loss.

We each take it home with us in different ways, and that's ok. We each have our coping mechanisms and if it wasn't for those, we wouldn't be able to do the amazing work we do everyday.

I salute all healthcare providers, and thank you for the work you do, but more so, thank you for your emotional strength and grit.

Tag someone who needs to hear this message and let them know that feeling emotion is ok!

Source: Reproduced with permission from Katie Duke. Retrieved from https://www.facebook.com/pg/thekatieduke/posts/?ref=page_internal)

 KATIE DUKE

ABOUT   SPONSORSHIPS   EVENTS   PRESS   BLOG   CONTACT   SUBSCRIBE

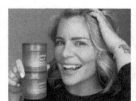

FEBRUARY 16, 2019

MY FAVORITE SKINCARE PRODUCTS

Let's be honest. I am 37, and there isn't a product on this earth I haven't tried.

My skincare regimen focuses on products that: fight acne, soothe, exfoliate, nourish, hydrate, and fight aging.

There is no such thing as a 1-2-3 step routine that never changes. Well, I take that back, There is no such thing as a 1-2-3 step routine that never changes, UNLESS you're a man,

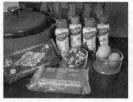

FEBRUARY 1, 2019

GETTING PROPER NUTRITION AS A BUSY ADULT

In this face paced world few of us young and older adults have the time or desire to cook every meal at home. And that's the reality. So, in my recent years of practice as a Nurse Practitioner, I've discovered that it's best to give recommendations that are not only realistic, but also adaptable for both young and older adults and all of their ever changing and busy agendas.

READ MORE →

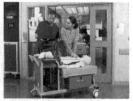

JANUARY 30, 2019

RQI AND HIGH-QUALITY CPR: THE NEW STANDARD OF RESUSCITATION, WITH A FOCUS ON QUALITY IMPROVEMENT

Knowing CPR and performing high-quality CPR are two different things.

2-year CPR training has long been the traditional practice, but is it optimal?

READ MORE →

Source: Reproduced with permission from Katie Duke. Retrieved from https://www.katiedukeonline.com/blog

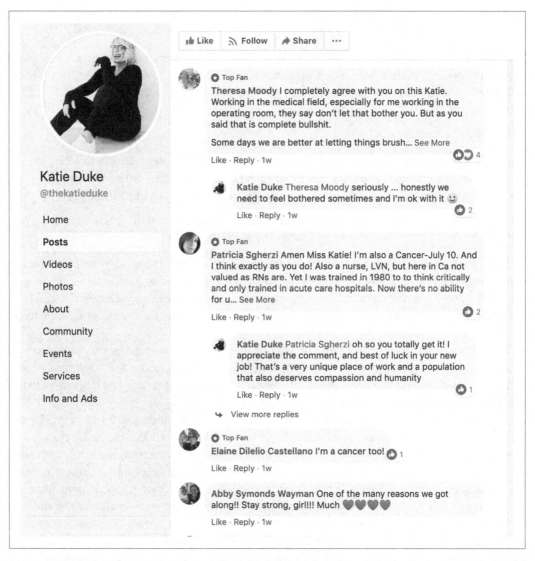

Source: Reproduced, with permission, from Katie Duke. Retrieved from https://www.facebook.com/pg/thekatieduke/posts/?ref=page_internal

---

 CALL TO ACTION

Identify three industry influencers whom you admire. How do they engage with their audience? How do they leverage their network to support their message?

PUTTING YOUR PERSONAL BRAND TO WORK ON ONLINE

After you lay the foundation for your own personal brand, start thinking about ways in which you might leverage your newfound digital supporters to benefit your organization. You can look at this through two lenses: information gathering and information sharing.

Information Gathering

One of the great things about the Internet is the sheer volume of information available; use this to your advantage. Spend time on a variety of social media channels, online forums, and other digital communities—not with the intent to engage, but with the intent to listen.

> *"When you talk, you're only repeating what you already know. If you listen, you may learn something new."* —Dalai Lama

Just as you are working to create a digital presence, so are many of your colleagues or employees. Schedule time each day or week to search for your organization's name, look at popular hashtags relevant to your line of work, scan your employees' or colleagues' social feeds and read through the comments of individuals who reply to your organization's or competitors' posts.

Use this information to keep a pulse on the overall perception of your organization. Do your employees generally post positive or happy messages? What do customers or community members say in relation to your organization or industry? Do you notice any red flags or potential issues lurking beneath the surface?

You should also pay close attention to your company's branded platforms (e.g., Twitter, Facebook page, LinkedIn page, press releases, website). A lot of thought and strategy goes into determining which content your organization shares publicly. More often than not, communications teams spend months planning campaigns and creating corresponding content to share online. And in the times when it is necessary to release an immediate public statement, know that the teams who write the announcements agonize over every word to ensure the audience interprets the message as intended.

Watch closely and you'll begin to understand the overarching themes that your organization speaks about, the tone and voice that your company's brand embodies, the values that they try to demonstrate in the content that they share. Take note of these characteristics and consider how you can embrace or support them within your own brand.

Information Sharing

Once you understand the campaigns and messages that your organization values, you can use this information to guide how you interact with, and support, your organization digitally. For example, you can help amplify important messages by sharing them with your network, leverage your status as a leader to comment on positive news in the community, act as a connector between other leaders in your company and influencers within your network, and congratulate individuals on recent accomplishments.

When sharing information about your organization, keep in mind Joe Pulizzi's 4-1-1 rule mentioned earlier. You should spend more time engaging and sharing other relevant content than you do sharing your own organization's messaging. Be intentional about helping to amplify other influencers' or organizations' content, when appropriate. Not only does this lend credibility to your name, but it also encourages a reciprocal response from supporters.

Regardless of the type of content that you share, always keep in mind how it reflects on you, both as an individual and as a leader in your company. For example, don't just share content based on a headline, make sure you read the article to understand the position of the author—and then add a thoughtful comment that explains why you chose to share the piece. If you choose to post photos or share other visual content, take the time to select a high-quality, professional visual. Most of all, add a personal touch or your own commentary as often as possible. You want your digital brand to feel authentic and transparent—not just a highlight of recent news.

REAL-WORLD EXAMPLE: CARRIE BASHAM YOUNG

Carrie Basham Young is the CEO of Talk Social To Me, a consulting firm that focuses on helping organizations launch, build, and accelerate employee engagement efforts and corresponding internal communications platforms. As an advocate for internal communications, human resources, and information technology (IT) leaders who support employee engagement, much of the content that Young shares ties back to her industry. However, she includes a healthy mix of content from her own organization, content from others in the industry, and content that offers a glimpse into her own life. By lifting up others, as well as publicly acknowledging kind gestures, Young projects herself not just as a strong leader, but also as a thoughtful, caring person. As such, she continues to grow her audience and keep her followers engaged.

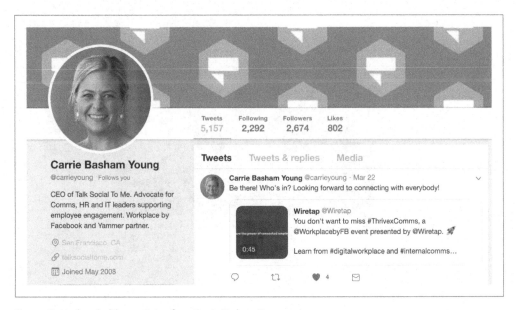

Source: Reproduced with permission from Carrie Basham Young.

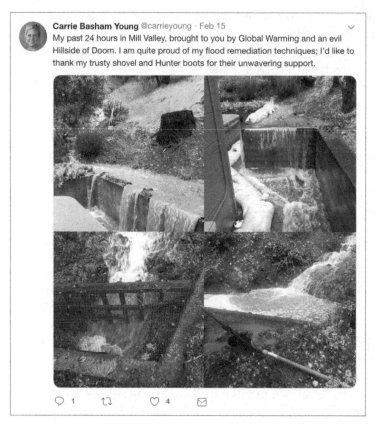

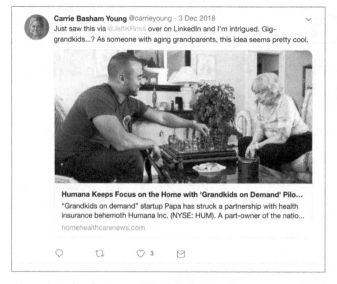

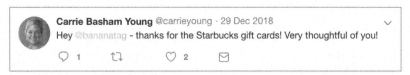

Source: Reproduced with permission from Carrie Basham Young. Retrieved from https:// twitter.com/carrieyoung/status/1079089382852780032

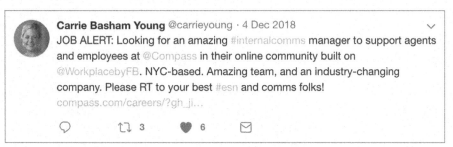

Source: Reproduced with permission from Carrie Basham Young. Retrieved from https://twitter.com/ carrieyoung/status/1070148881638318080

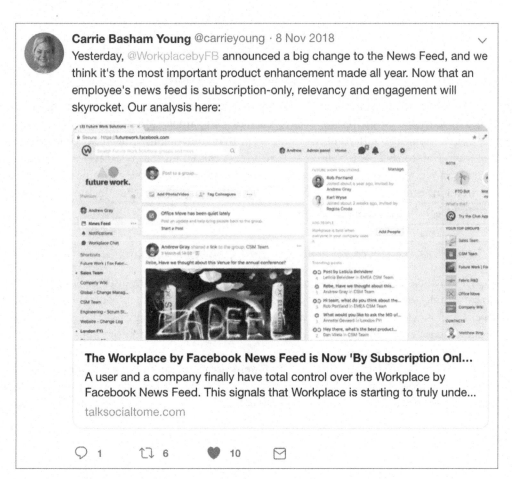

Source: Reproduced with permission from Carrie Basham Young. Retrieved from https://twitter.com/carrieyoung/ status/1060595269245448192

CALL TO ACTION

Try offering your audience a glimpse of your personal life. For example, share a photo, talk about an activity you're looking forward to, or share and comment on a piece of content that is unrelated to your profession. How does your audience react? Do they engage differently than when you share strictly professional content?

LEVEL UP BY COORDINATING WITH MARKETING EFFORTS

Your organization likely has a robust marketing and communications team that focuses on a variety of issues, from brand affinity and awareness to key industry initiatives to celebrating employees and company culture. There are a few ways that you can support your company's marketing efforts:

1. Self-identify important initiatives to amplify them.
2. Coordinate directly with marketing and communications.
3. Offer yourself as a thought leader.

Self-Identify Important Initiatives to Amplify Them

This strategy takes the least amount of up-front legwork on your end. Simply pay attention to internal announcements, upcoming events, current campaigns, and community activities related to your organization. If you hear of an event that someone in your network might enjoy, send an invitation to this person directly. If you see a campaign that resonates with you, comment on it, share it with your network broadly, or even post it to industry forums for discussion. If you attend an event, take a few photos of guests enjoying themselves. Include any relevant event branding or hashtags in your post and tag the host or notable guests.

Coordinate Directly With Marketing and Communications

Your organization's marketing and communications team spends months or longer creating robust campaigns with detailed communications plans to support them. Social media is likely just one tactic out of many that this team uses to achieve campaign goals. The synergy among all mediums (e.g., experiential, video, email, web, broadcast television or radio, social media, PR) drives the success of a given campaign.

Set up time with your marketing and communications team and ask members to identify and provide key messaging that they wish to promote. Chances are, they will jump at the opportunity to have an additional set of hands to help achieve their goals. You can offer to share messaging broadly on social media, as well as directly with relevant contacts in your networks. The team might also have suggestions regarding conversations on forums or upcoming articles that they want you to engage in or share.

Allow your marketing and communications team to draft suggested copy to use in your outbound messages, and then tweak the copy slightly to match your own personal brand voice—this is key to sounding authentic. Confirm any links, images, hashtags, or other assets that you should use in your posts. When engaging in conversations or commenting on articles, keep in mind the goals of the campaign and let those goals guide you in your responses. When in doubt, reach out to a marketing or communications leader for their input.

Offer Yourself as a Thought Leader

To establish credibility as a leading organization in the industry, your communications and media relations teams spend a lot of time trying to secure articles or quotes for its leaders in key industry and business publications. These come in a variety of forms: staying top-of-mind with journalists so that they reach out for quotes to include in articles they write or for broadcast segments; working with company leaders to write contributed, or *byline*, articles for trade publications; and pitching ideas or topics to encourage journalists to tell a story specifically around your organization.

You can support these efforts by offering to act as a thought leader on behalf of your organization. When you meet with your communications and media relations teams to discuss this, come prepared with a list of topics and areas of expertise that you feel comfortable speaking about. One of the easiest ways to get started in this area is to identify a topic that you want to write about and create an outline. Talk to the team about where this content might live. For example, is it an article that you wish to contribute to a trade publication—or an opinion piece that might live on a blog? Be sure to let the team know about any areas where you might need additional coaching (e.g., live media interviews, writing a scholarly article).

REAL-LIFE EXAMPLE: JASON MORGAN, PHD

Jason Morgan holds his doctorate in political methodology from The Ohio State University and is currently the Vice President of Behavioral Intelligence at Wiretap, a technology start-up focused on governance and compliance for enterprise collaboration. He leverages his academic background and leadership position to help establish Wiretap as a cutting-edge firm with best-in-class collaboration technology. Morgan often writes byline articles for trade publications, speaks on podcasts or at events on behalf of Wiretap, and contributes to the Wiretap blog. He works closely with the marketing and communications team to ensure he stays on message and aligns with the organization's goals.

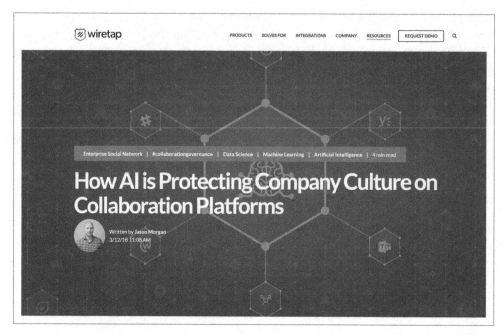

Source: Reproduced with permission from Aware. Retrieved from https://www.wiretap.com/blog/how-ai-is-protecting-company-culture-on-collaboration-platforms

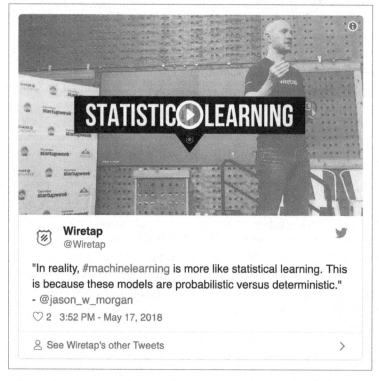

Source: Reproduced with permission from Aware. Retrieved from https://twitter.com/Wiretap/status/997203205628022786

Leadership and Followership—Social Media As a Strategic Choice in My Leadership

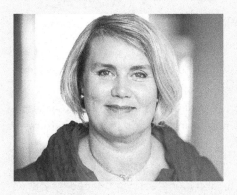

Vibeke Westh is the regional chairman for the Danish Nurses Organization in the Capital Region of Denmark.

The use of social media is one of the most important strategic management choices that can be made today. It is no longer an option whether or not to a senior executive is on social media, but he or she does need to determine how to communicate there. This is where you communicate efficiently, build your image, and this is where you ensure that your organization or cause gets more recognition. You can significantly improve your leadership through use of a conscious strategy. My assertion is that you can create a following, which ensures completely new support from your organization and partners, in addition to what you could have gotten previously.

I have no doubt that it is necessary to be authentic in your communication, so I have chosen to be the creator of my content. My philosophy is that it is the personal and direct contact that changes people and attitudes. As an elected leader, one must constantly contribute to shaping the history of the organization and the cause consistently and faithfully. But the way that you are present, how much and where, must be balanced. If you have a well-thought-out strategy for your leadership in social media, you can create a following.

Present Across Three Social Media Platforms

Most people have profiles on several social media platforms. Users of these platforms utilize some of them a lot, others almost never, and others several times every day.

I use social media professionally to influence the policy-making process, to build alliances, and to promote nurses' causes and community. I employ three platforms that I use very differently. These three platforms contribute in a variety of ways to achieve my goals, build alliances, and create a following. I am active on all three platforms, and I am online most of the time.

Twitter

- I focus exclusively on the strictly professional aspect of my leadership. I am different with regard to Facebook.

- On Twitter, there is a focus on attitudes and short uncensored messages. The messaging is direct and relatively impersonal or what we would call *professional* in a more classic sense.

(continued)

(continued)

LinkedIn

- On LinkedIn, it is possible to connect to people who I do not know personally, but who I want to follow professionally and may want to influence now or in the future.
- LinkedIn is very useful to ensure direct access to other managers.

Facebook

- On Facebook, I use a mix of personal and professional information to enhance my professional impact.
- Facebook can be a difficult media platform to use professionally because most people use Facebook privately, but it also offers many opportunities for a manager with management tasks like mine.

Don't Lose Sight of Your Purpose

It is easy to get caught up in the world of social media influencers; stay grounded by following your North Star. Refer often to the guidelines and values you defined at the onset of your journey, and periodically audit your behavior to ensure alignment.

One thing that you might easily overlook is how you engage with employees internally on a day-to-day basis. Your organization needs social influence inside the walls, just as much as it needs it externally. Make sure to take the time to participate in internal communication communities, share positive feedback with others *and* their managers, publicly acknowledge the hard work of other teams, and offer a hand up to employees at more junior levels. One of the most valuable things you can do for another person is offer your time and expertise to help him or her learn and grow.

The best leaders have a high consideration factor. They really care about their people."
—Brian Tracy

FROM THE FIELD: BRINGING IT ALL TOGETHER TO MAKE MAGIC HAPPEN

Throughout your personal branding journey, you will experience plenty of hits and misses—you'll learn which strategies work well to influence others, and which strategies flop. Occasionally, the stars will all align and, subsequently, you knock it out of the park. Think about your goals; what does knocking it out of the park look like in your mind?

Technology start-up Wiretap points to a single event to demonstrate how influencers working hand in hand with the marketing team generated unimaginable success. The company knew of an upcoming, exclusive event that key buyers from potential clients would attend. Traditional approaches to event presence (e.g., sponsorships, speaking positions) were unavailable, so Wiretap needed to find a way to leverage influence and buzz to reach the audience.

The marketing and communications team devised an experience after careful research regarding the location of the event. The team hired a large tour bus to park in front of the venue and wrapped the bus with graphics promoting the Wiretap message. They also identified key leaders who would likely attend the event, created a database with links to the leaders' social profiles, and packaged an exclusive gift for each leader. Leading up to the event, the marketing and communications team worked closely with other Wiretap employees to educate them on the campaign messaging and to provide specific action items for employees who wanted to support the efforts.

On the evening before the event, the communication plan went in to action. With the bus parked in front of the venue, key leaders from Wiretap infiltrated the lobby wearing branded shirts. They leveraged social media to share their location and invite guests to join the team for happy hour or dinner. The communication plan continued into the next day, with employee influencers engaging on social media to direct guests to find the Wiretap leaders on-site, tagging the previously identified key leaders to let them know a gift awaited, and helping to create buzz around the energy of the event.

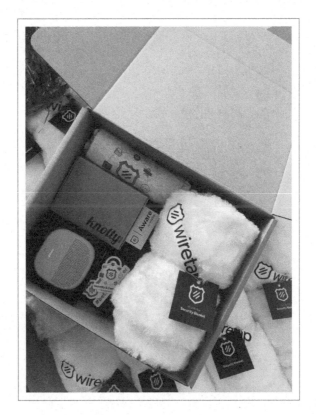

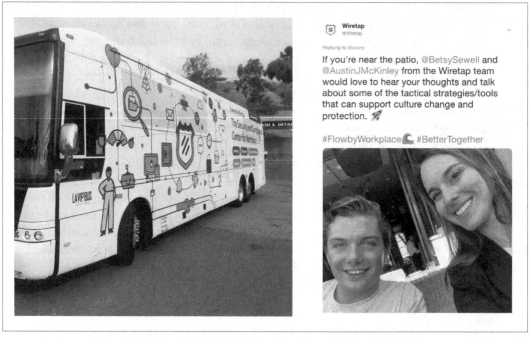

Source: Reproduced with permission from Aware. Retrieved from https://twitter.com/Wiretap/status/1049760747205611520

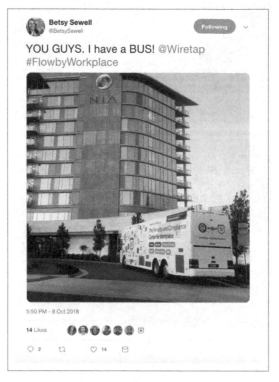

Source: Courtesy of Betsy Sewell. Retrieved from https://twitter
.com/BetsySewell/status/1049416658815602690

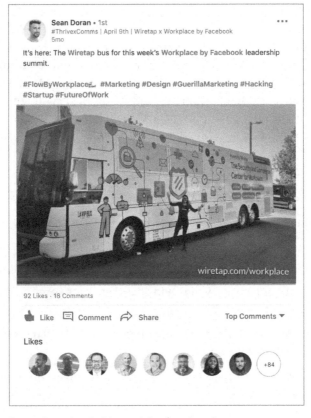

Source: Reproduced with permission from Sean Doran.

The carefully crafted guerilla marketing tactics, combined with organization leaders leveraging social media influence, created an incredible impact for Wiretap. As a result of these efforts, Wiretap gained:

- Three strategic, enterprise-level clients
- 35,000+ event-related social media impressions over 2 days
- Two "drive-by" meetings with industry analysts, resulting in mentions in two articles
- Two off-site interviews with journalists, resulting in inclusion in one story
- Strengthened partner relationship with Workplace by Facebook and key leaders

"Alone we can do so little; together we can do so much." —Helen Keller

FOR THE ENTREPRENEURS

Many, if not all, of the strategies and tactics presented in this chapter also apply to creating a brand for your business. First, you need to develop a foundation and plan for your brand. For example, clearly define your brand's tone and voice, so that messaging sounds consistent no matter who posts to the account. You'll also want to develop a content strategy and distribution plan, along with goals and KPIs, just as you would for your personal brand.

One thing to keep in mind as an entrepreneur launching a new brand: Digital and social media missteps are much harder to overcome as an organization than for a personal brand. As such, put the time and effort into thoughtful planning of all brand activities to minimize mistakes. However, when a mistake happens—and it will happen at some point—act swiftly, acknowledge the misstep and, most important, articulate how your brand will learn and change from the experience. Your audience will appreciate the authenticity and, we hope, will quickly forgive and forget.

KEY TAKEAWAY POINTS

- Creating a personal brand is critical to both personal success and the success of your organization.

- Leaders need to identify and define guidelines to drive their personal brand.

- Leaders need to create a plan for "when" and "how" they use social media or other platforms depending on their goals.

- Leveraging a personal brand for business influence requires coordination and communication to align with organization-wide efforts.

- Successful use of a digital personal brand requires engagement, nurturing, time, effort, and energy to do it right.

CALL TO ACTION

Using Social Media to Influence Policy

As the leader of a professional nursing organization, you are tasked with creating social media content that targets an upcoming state bill that seeks to expand the practice scope of nurse practitioners. You follow various state representatives and senators, and some also follow you as well. The bill is coming up for a vote in its first committee and is predicted to make it to the floor for a vote in the next week.

1. How do you leverage your social media accounts and followers to promote this legislation?

2. How would you craft your messaging? For those who support the legislation and for those who do not?

3. Who would you target for your messaging? How would you tailor your messaging for different groups?

REFERENCES

Pew Research Center. (2018a). Internet/broadband fact sheet. Retrieved from www.pewinternet .org/fact-sheet/internet-broadband

Pew Research Center. (2018b). Social media fact sheet. Retrieved from www.pewinternet.org/ fact-sheet/social-media

Index